Disturbances in Lipid and Lipoprotein Metabolism

Disturbances in Lipid and Lipoprotein Metabolism

EDITED BY **John M. Dietschy**

Department of Internal Medicine
University of Texas Southwestern Medical School
Dallas, Texas

Antonio M. Gotto, Jr.

Department of Medicine
Baylor College of Medicine
Houston, Texas

Joseph A. Ontko

Laboratory of Lipid and Lipoprotein Studies
Oklahoma Medical Research Foundation
Oklahoma City, Oklahoma

AMERICAN PHYSIOLOGICAL SOCIETY
Bethesda, Maryland, 1978

Library of Congress Catalog Card Number 77-93528

International Standard Book Number 0683-02557-0

Printed in the United States of America by
Waverly Press, Inc., Baltimore, Maryland 21202

Distributed for the American Physiological Society by
The Williams & Wilkins Company, Baltimore, Maryland 21202

Preface

There has been considerable progress during the past few years in gaining a better understanding of many aspects of lipid metabolism. The mechanisms of lipid solubilization and transport in body fluids are now fairly well elucidated through a number of fundamental studies on the characteristics of lipid interactions with carriers such as bile acid micelles, albumin, and a variety of lipoproteins. The general principles governing the monomolecular movement of lipids across cell membranes have been developed and the importance of the cellular uptake of lipoproteins by endocytotic processes has been recognized. Other studies have delineated the mechanisms of regulation of many intracellular enzymatic pathways involved in both the oxidation of lipids as a major source of cellular energy and in the synthesis of more complex lipids and their assembly into various classes of lipoproteins. The information in this book is based on material presented at a Symposium on Lipoprotein and Lipid Metabolism sponsored by the American Physiological Society, and the chapters are divided into four groups:

- The first chapter discusses the general principles involved in determining the rates of movement of lipids, simple or complex, across biological membranes.
- The second group of chapters deals with the problem of lipid absorption in the intestine and describes the process of fatty acid and sterol esterification and chylomicron synthesis in the intestinal mucosa and the events that occur as the chylomicron is metabolized in the peripheral circulation.
- The third set of chapters covers the complex process of the synthesis of very-low-density, low-density, and high-density lipoproteins in the liver and describes the important regulatory roles for certain of these lipoproteins in peripheral tissues; abnormalities in the physiology of certain lipoprotein classes encountered in clinical disorders of lipid metabolism in man are also discussed.
- The final chapters deal with the release, binding, and metabolism of fatty acids both in the liver and in muscle tissue.

This book is intended to serve as a source of basic information in the field of lipid metabolism both for the investigator working in this area and for the clinician who must deal with disordered lipid physiology in patients.

The Editors

Contents

Fatty Acid Transport and Metabolism

1

General Principles Governing Movement of Lipids Across Biological Membranes

JOHN M. DIETSCHY

*Department of Internal Medicine, University of Texas
Health Science Center, Dallas, Texas*

Two General Types of Transport Involved in Movement of Lipids Across Biological
    Membranes
Monomolecular Diffusion of Lipid Molecules Through an Infinite Number of Sites on
    the Cell Membrane
    Effect of solute interactions with other molecules in the cytosolic compartment and
        in the bulk phase on monomolecular diffusion rates
    Effect of membrane polarity on rates of monomolecular diffusion
    Dependency of maximal rates of monomolecular diffusion on polarity of the cell
        membrane
    Anomalous behavior of monomer diffusion of polar, small-molecular-weight solutes
        across biological membranes
Effect of Diffusion Barriers on Rates of Movement of Lipids Across Biological
    Membranes
    General principles of molecular movements across diffusion barriers in biological
        systems
    Relative importance of membrane and diffusion-barrier resistances in determining
        rates of lipid movement across biological membranes
    Effect of diffusion barriers on measurements of activation energies
    Effect of diffusion barriers on kinetics of lipid transport by a finite number of
        membrane sites
    Role of carrier molecules in overcoming diffusion-barrier resistance

THIS BOOK DEALS WITH MANY ASPECTS of lipid metabolism including the mechanisms of dietary triglycerides and cholesterol absorption, the formation and function of lipoproteins, and the metabolism of fatty acids. In all these processes one of the critical steps is the movement of some species of lipid across one or more cell membranes. Over the past 10 years there has been considerable progress in our understanding of the determinants of the rates at which nonelectrolytes penetrate biological membranes. Much of this information, however, has been published in journals principally dealing with membrane transport and has not generally been applied to the specific problems of how lipids enter and exit from cells. In this initial chapter certain general principles are outlined that dictate the rates of transmembrane movement of solute molecules and the relevancy of these principles to specific problems of lipid transport is discussed.

TWO GENERAL TYPES OF TRANSPORT INVOLVED IN MOVEMENT OF
LIPIDS ACROSS BIOLOGICAL MEMBRANES

Many complex types of transport systems have been described but only two probably are important in explaining the movement of lipids into and out of most types of tissues. The first is usually designated as "simple passive diffusion" and involves the movement of individual solute molecules across the lipid-protein matrix of the cell membrane. Since such movement occurs across an "infinite" number of sites in the membrane and is driven by the chemical activity of the molecule in the pericellular perfusate, the rate of such movement is usually a linear function of the concentration[1] of the solute molecule to which a given cell is exposed. As shown in *panel I* of Figure 1, the rate of movement (J) of the solute molecule from the outside of the cell into the cytosolic compartment is equal to the product of the concentration of the molecule in the bulk solution (C_2) and the passive permeability coefficient (P) for the particular solute crossing that particular membrane.

$$J = (P)(C_2) \tag{1}$$

The passive permeability coefficient describes the amount of solute that crosses 1 cm² of the cell membrane per unit time per unit concentration of

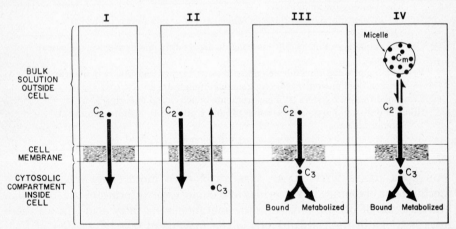

FIG. 1. Diagrammatic representation of several experimental situations encountered during monomolecular movement of a solute molecule across a biological membrane. C_2 represents the concentration of the solute molecule in solution perfusing the outside of the cell membrane; C_3 represents the concentration of the molecule in the aqueous phase in the cytosolic compartment inside the cell membrane. C_m in *panel IV* represents the concentration of the solute molecule within the micellar phase and K is a conventional partitioning coefficient dictating the relationship between C_m and C_2 such that $K = C_m/C_2$.

---

[1] As with all transport phenomena the velocities of the various processes depend on the chemical activities of the solutes in solution and not, strictly speaking, on their chemical concentrations. For convenience, however, in this chapter the terms "concentration" or "monomolecular concentration" mean chemical activity in the specific sense.

the solute to which the membrane is exposed and so has units such as nanomoles per square centimeter per second/(nanomoles per cubic centimeter), which reduces to the conventional units used for P of centimeters per second. When this value is multiplied by the concentration term, J describes a flux rate with the units of mass of solute moving across 1 cm² of membrane per unit time, e.g., nanomoles per square centimeter per second. However, in nearly all experimental systems utilized to study lipid transport the membrane surface area is unknown and the rate of movement is normalized to some other parameter of cell mass such as milligrams of protein (e.g., tissue culture cells), grams wet weight (e.g., perfused liver or epididymal fat-pad), or 10^6 cells (e.g., isolated liver cells). Under these conditions the experimentally determined flux rates and passive permeability coefficients are designated J_d and P_d, respectively, and have units such as nanomoles per gram tissue per second (J_d) and nanomoles per gram tissue per second/ (nanomoles per cubic centimeter) (P_d). In such measurements it is tacitly assumed that the surface area of the cell membranes across which transport is occurring has a constant relationship to the parameter of tissue mass utilized and, further, that this relationship does not change under different experimental conditions. This relationship can be designated as S_m so that J_d/S_m equals J and P_d/S_m equals P. Thus, for example, if a flux rate of 10 nmol/g tissue per s has been experimentally determined (J_d) and if S_m is known to equal 100 cm²/g tissue, then a flux rate of 0.1 nmol/cm² per s can be calculated. However, since values for S_m are seldom known for many experimental preparations, most transport rates necessarily must be expressed as J_d and the corresponding passive permeability coefficients also must be normalized to the same parameter of tissue mass (P_d) and so will not have the conventional units of centimeters per second. Finally, it should be emphasized that P or P_d describes the ability of a particular solute to penetrate a particular biological membrane and has meaning independent of knowledge of C_2: in contrast, the magnitude of J or J_d has meaning only when one also knows the solute concentration at which the measurement was obtained.

The second type of transport important in the transmembrane movement of lipids involves the binding of specific lipoproteins to a finite number of sites on the cell membrane followed by cellular uptake of the entire particle by an endocytotic process (2, 3). The uptake of the chylomicron remnant by the liver (18) and of low-density lipoproteins (LDL) by the human fibroblast by such a process is discussed in detail elsewhere in this book. Since this process involves the interaction of solute molecules, in this case a lipoprotein, with a finite number of transport sites on the cell membrane the kinetics of uptake may be described by the following relationship

$$J = \frac{(J^m)(C_2)}{K_m + C_2} \qquad (2)$$

where J^m is the maximal velocity of transport the system can achieve and K_m defines the concentration of the solute molecule at the aqueous-membrane interface (C_2) at which half the value of J^m is achieved. Again, ideally both J and J^m should be expressed as the amount of solute transported per unit time per square centimeter of surface area; however, as discussed above this is usually not possible in most systems of importance to the study of lipid transport so that these two velocity terms again must be normalized to some other parameter of tissue mass and the terms J_d and $J_d{}^m$ must be substituted for J and J^m, respectively, in *equation 2*.

A third type of transport commonly encountered in cell membranes involves the cellular uptake of very polar molecules (and hence molecules having very low passive permeability coefficients) like monosaccharides and amino acids by a finite number of transport sites linked to an intracellular source of energy and manifesting kinetics identical to those described by *equation 2*. Currently, however, there is no convincing evidence that such "active transport" or other carrier-mediated systems are involved in the movement of individual lipid molecules across cell membranes. Hence, such transport mechanisms are not discussed further in this chapter.

MONOMOLECULAR DIFFUSION OF LIPID MOLECULES THROUGH AN INFINITE NUMBER OF SITES ON THE CELL MEMBRANE

Effect of Solute Interactions with Other Molecules in the Cytosolic Compartment and in the Bulk Phase on Monomolecular Diffusion Rates

As is evident from *equation 1* the rate of molecular diffusion is determined essentially by only two factors: the concentration of the solute molecule in the perfusate bathing the cell membrane and the passive permeability coefficient for the molecule. Since lipid molecules commonly undergo interactions with other molecules in the bulk perfusate and/or cytosolic compartment that markedly alter the monomolecular concentrations of the lipid in solution, these interactions have profound effects on the rate of transmembrane movement. As shown in *panel I* of Figure 1, the rate of movement of the solute from the bulk solution into the cell equals the product $(C_2)(P_d)$. However, as the molecule diffuses into the cell the concentration of the solute in the cell water begins to increase so that there is movement of the molecule out of the cell at a rate equal to $(C_3)(P_d)$, as shown in *panel II*.[2] Thus, at any point in time the net flux of the solute into the cell is given by the following expression:

$$J_d^{net} = (C_2 - C_3)(P_d) \qquad (3)$$

If the solute is neither bound within the cytosol nor metabolized then C_3

_____

[2] In this formulation the cell membrane is assumed to behave symmetrically with respect to passive permeability so that the same value of P can be utilized regardless of the direction of molecular diffusion. Most experimental data suggest that this assumption is correct.

must eventually equal C_2 and J_d^{net} must equal 0. Using a radiolabeled molecule one can still demonstrate the two unidirectional fluxes under this circumstance even though net movement has ceased. If, however, the solute is rapidly bound to a receptor molecule in the cytosol or is rapidly metabolized to some other species then C_3 is maintained lower than C_2 and there is a continuous net movement of the molecule to the cell at a rate described by *equation 3*. Finally, the direction of net movement can be reversed if the solute molecule is also being generated within the cell. For example, in the fed state the concentration of fatty acid outside the adipocyte is higher than that inside so that there is net entry of lipid into the cell. With stimulation of the hormone-sensitive lipase within the cell, however, C_3 greatly exceeds C_2 and there is net movement of fatty acid out of the cell.

Interactions of the solute with molecules in the bulk perfusate also can markedly influence the rate of both unidirectional and net solute movement. For example, in vivo steroid hormones usually are bound to carrier proteins in plasma and fatty acids are largely bound to albumin, whereas in experiments in vitro steroids and fatty acids commonly are added to the perfusate with various proteins, solvents, or detergents to increase their "solubility." In such cases, however, the term "solubility" is misleading: although the total amount of the solute dispersed in the aqueous phase may be high, the actual amount of the solute in true solution and available for reaction with the membrane (C_2) may still be exceedingly low. Furthermore, the interactions between the solute and the carrier molecule are often complex and if not taken into consideration may interject marked artifacts into the interpretation of the kinetics of the uptake process. An example of this is shown in *panel IV*, where it is assumed that a solute molecule is "solubilized" in the bulk perfusate by use of a detergent that forms micelles and that the ratio of the concentration of the solute in the micelle (C_m) and in the aqueous phase (C_2) can be defined in terms of a conventional partitioning coefficient (K). Under these conditions the following relationship would be true:

$$KC_2 = C_m \qquad (4)$$

This equation can be rewritten to yield

$$K\left(\frac{M_w}{V_w}\right) = \left(\frac{M_m}{V_m}\right) \qquad (5)$$

where M_w and M_m are the masses of the solute molecule in the water and micellar phases, respectively, and V_w and V_m represent the volumes of the aqueous and micellar phases, respectively.[3] Since M_m equals the total mass of solute in the system (M_t) minus that in the water phase (M_w), the expression $M_t - M_w$ can be substituted for M_m in *equation 5*, and after

---

[3] The volume of the micellar phase can be calculated from the concentration of detergent in the perfusate and its appropriate partial specific volume.

rearranging terms the following expression is obtained:

$$\frac{M_w}{V_w} = \frac{M_t}{KV_m + V_w}$$

(6)

From this expression the rate of uptake of the solute can be calculated since J_d^{net} is proportional to the term M_w/V_w, i.e., to C_2 (assuming for the purposes of this illustration that C_3 is 0). The curves shown in Figure 2 have been derived with this equation and illustrate the effect of altering the relative concentration of the detergent and solute on rates of uptake of the solute molecule. In *panel I* the concentration of the detergent is kept constant while that of the solute is increased. As is evident, under this circumstance J_d^{net} increases in a linear relationship to the total concentration of the solute in the perfusate but the magnitude of the uptake rate is markedly dependent on K. When the total concentration of the solute is kept constant while the concentration of the detergent is increased, the rate of uptake declines in a curvilinear fashion and, again, the absolute value of J_d^{net} is influenced markedly by K. Of particular importance is the set of curves shown in *panel III*, where the concentrations of both the solute and the detergent have been increased in parallel so that the ratio between the two is constant. In this circumstance the relationship between J_d^{net} and the total concentration of solute superficially resembles a "saturable" kinetic curve. Thus, the point to

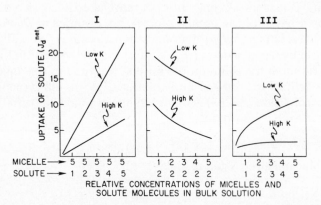

FIG. 2. Theoretical relationship between the rate of uptake of a solute molecule and the concentration of that molecule in the perfusate under circumstances where the solute is partially solubilized in a detergent micelle. *Panel I* illustrates the situation where the micellar concentration is kept constant while the solute concentration is progressively increased. *Panel II* shows the opposite situation, where the solute concentration is kept constant while the micellar concentration is increased. *Panel III* illustrates the situation in which the concentration of both the micelles and solute is increased in parallel so that the molar ratio between these two components of the solution remains constant. In each case results are shown for 2 experimental situations where the partitioning coefficient for the solute molecule into the micellar phase is either high or low. In this diagram the units of solute uptake and concentration are arbitrary relative values. These illustrations, however, are based on specific calculations (given in ref. 22).

be emphasized is that when uptake rates of lipids are measured from a solution containing other molecules with which the solute can interact, the observed values of J_d may be determined as much by events within the bulk solution as by the kinetic characteristics of the transport system in the biological membrane under study. Under such circumstances it is nearly impossible to interpret the meaning of relative rates of uptake of different lipids or of the kinetic characteristics of the uptake process unless appropriate mathematical or experimental corrections can be made to distinguish the true concentration of the lipid in solution (C_2) from the total concentration of the molecule (C_t) in the perfusate (22).

Effect of Membrane Polarity on Rates of Monomolecular Diffusion

The second major factor influencing the rate of molecular diffusion of lipids across cell membranes is the passive permeability coefficient for the solute (*equation 1*). The value of P is unique for a given solute passing through a given membrane and is determined by the polar characteristics of both the solute and the membrane: thus, for a particular solute molecule P can be described by the expression (8, 10, 28):

$$P = K_m\left(\frac{D_m}{d_m}\right) \tag{7}$$

where K_m, D_m, and d_m represent, respectively, the partitioning coefficient for the solute molecule between the lipid phase of the cell membrane and the aqueous phase of the perfusate, the diffusion coefficient for the solute in the membrane, and the effective thickness of the membrane (8). The partitioning coefficient is the overwhelmingly important term in determining P since d_m is relatively constant for most biological membranes, and for most solutes D_m varies over a narrow range but the values of K_m may vary over a range as great as 10^{10} (8, 28). Thus, the values of P vary directly with the value of K_m for a particular cell membrane. Recognition of this relationship has provided a useful way of assessing and comparing the "functional" polarity of membranes from different biological systems. For example, as illustrated diagrammatically in Figure 3, the logarithms of the passive permeability coefficients for a series of fatty acids in a particular cell membrane have been plotted against the logarithms of the partitioning coefficients of these same fatty acids into three different bulk organic solvents. As illustrated by *line A*, the addition of each —CH₂— group to the solute has the same relative effect on increasing the movement of the molecule across the membrane or in increasing its partitioning into the bulk solvent: hence, the "effective" polarity of the solvent and cell membrane must be approximately the same. In contrast, *lines B* and *C*, respectively, show the results obtained with two solvents that are either less or more polar than the cell membrane. For example, in *B*, the addition of each —CH₂— group to the fatty acid chain has a twofold greater effect on increasing $\ln K$ than in increasing $\ln P$: since

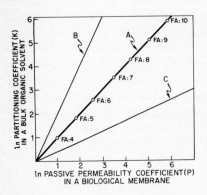

FIG. 3. Comparison of passive permeability coefficients (P) for a series of fatty acids with the partitioning coefficients of these same molecules between bulk buffer solution and bulk organic solvent. Logarithm of K is plotted in arbitrary units on the vertical axis; logarithm of P is shown on the horizontal axis. *Line A* represents the situation in which the polarity of the bulk solvent and membrane lipids is identical, *line B* represents the situation where the organic solvent is less polar, and *line C* represents the situation where the solvent is more polar than the membrane. Designation beside each data point represents a fatty acid containing the number of carbon atoms noted.

the —CH₂— group principally undergoes hydrophobic interactions with components of the solvent and the cell membrane, it follows that in this case the membrane behaves as a more polar structure than the bulk solvent. Comparisons of this type have been made between a number of different solvents and a variety of different cell membranes and, in general, the membranes of most mammalian cells have been found to be relatively polar structures. Thus, in a number of instances the membranes behave in a manner similar to a bulk solvent like isobutanol rather than a very nonpolar solvent such as diethyl ether, benzene, or triglyceride (4, 8, 9, 19).

While useful, such comparisons are cumbersome to undertake and require that a number of different measurements of K and P be made with various homologous series of solute molecules. More recently, a second method has been commonly employed to describe the effective polarity of biological membranes; it involves determination of the manner in which the addition of a particular substituent group to any solute molecule alters the rate of movement of that solute across a biological membrane or alters the partitioning of the solute into a bulk organic solvent (8, 9, 17, 19, 28). In both instances the following equation describes the relationship between the partitioning of a solute between a cell membrane (K_m) or a bulk solvent (K) and the aqueous phase of the perfusate and several thermodynamic parameters (8, 28):

$$K_m \text{ or } K = e^{-\Delta F_{w \to 1} /RT} \tag{8}$$

where $\Delta F_{w \to 1}$ is the free-energy change associated with the movement of 1 mol of solute from the perfusate to the membrane (or solvent), R is the gas constant, and T is the absolute temperature. Although it is difficult to obtain absolute values of $\Delta F_{w \to 1}$ for a solute, the manner in which this thermodynamic parameter is changed by the addition of a substituent group to the solute can be experimentally measured: thus, the change in $\Delta F_{w \to 1}$, i.e., the incremental free-energy change ($\delta \Delta F_{w \to 1}$), brought about by the addition of the substituent group s to the solute is given by the following two expressions:

$$\delta\Delta F^s_{w\to 1} = -RT \ln \frac{P^s}{P^0} \tag{9}$$

$$\delta\Delta F^s_{w\to 1} = -RT \ln \frac{K^s}{K^0} \tag{10}$$

Equation 9 yields the incremental free-energy change associated with the addition of group s to a solute based on the measurement of the passive permeability coefficients for the solute with (P^s) and without (P^0) the substituent group. *Equation 10* gives the same value for substituent group s based on measurements of the effect of this group on partitioning of the solute into a bulk solvent.

In practice, $\delta\Delta F_{w\to 1}$ can be measured for nearly any substituent group such as —CH_2—, —OH, —NH_2, and —COOH. The addition of a polar group such as a hydroxyl function capable of hydrogen bonding with water molecules in the bulk perfusate generally reduces the passive permeability coefficient or the partitioning coefficient obtained with a given solute and so yields a positive value for $\delta\Delta F_{w\to 1}$. In contrast, the addition of a nonpolar substituent group such as the methylene group that is forced out of the aqueous phase by entropy effects and undergoes hydrophobic interactions within the membrane or bulk solvent generally increases the value of P and K and gives a negative value for the incremental free-energy change.[4] Since at 37°C the value of RT is approximately 616 cal/mol, a nonpolar substituent group that increases P or K by a factor of 5-, 25-, or 125-fold is associated with a $\delta\Delta F_{w\to 1}$ value of approximately -1000, -2000, and -3000 cal/mol, respectively. Conversely, a polar group that reduces P or K by a factor of 0.20, 0.04, or 0.008 would yield $\delta\Delta F_{w\to 1}$ values of $+1000$, $+2000$, and $+3000$ cal/mol, respectively.

From this discussion it is apparent that measurement of $\delta\Delta F_{w\to 1}$ values for various substituent groups provides a sensitive method for characterizing the effective polarity of a particular cell membrane and for comparing it to the membranes of other cell types and to various bulk solvents. Such data are now available for a number of different tissues and solvents and representative values for the hydroxyl and methylene groups are summarized in Figure 4. The addition of the hydroxyl function decreased the permeability coefficient for solute movement across the membranes of the muscle cell, adipocyte, gallbladder, and intestine by a factor that varied from 0.14 to 0.61: these values correspond to $\delta\Delta F^{OH}_{w\to 1}$ values of approximately $+300$ to $+1200$ cal/mol. In contrast, this substituent group reduced partitioning of the solute into very nonpolar solvents like triglyceride, ether, and olive oil by factors ranging from 0.035 to 0.011, yielding $\delta\Delta F^{OH}_{w\to 1}$ values varying from

---

[4] A detailed consideration of the intermolecular forces that provide the thermodynamic explanation for the effect of various substituent groups on permeability and partitioning coefficients is beyond the scope of this chapter. For a complete discussion of these aspects see references 8 and 28.

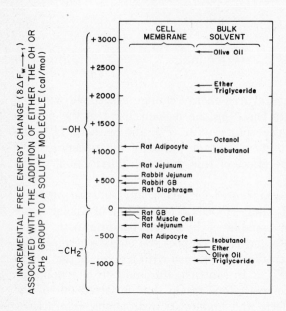

FIG. 4. Incremental free-energy changes ($\delta\Delta F_{w\rightarrow 1}$) associated with addition of either —OH or —CH_2— groups to a solute molecule. Addition of the hydroxyl function decreases the rate of membrane permeation and is associated with positive values; addition of the methylene group enhances the rate of membrane permeation and is associated with negative values. Effect of addition of these 2 substituent groups on permeation of various probe molecules across cell membranes of a variety of tissues is shown in the 1st column; effect of addition of these same groups on partitioning of various probe molecules into bulk organic solvents is shown in the 2nd column. Data are based on observations from a number of different laboratories (summarized in ref. 17).

+2070 to +2800 cal/mol. These data indicate that the membranes of at least this group of cells behave as relatively polar structures (perhaps because they are relatively hydrated) and not as very hydrophobic "lipid" membranes. This view is supported by the results obtained with the methylene group and also shown in Figure 4. Again, the addition of this substituent group has much less of an effect in increasing the passive permeability coefficients ($\delta\Delta F_{w\rightarrow 1}^{CH_2}$ are all less than −550 cal/mol) than one would expect if the cell membranes behaved as a very nonpolar structure analogous to the nonpolar solvents. Thus, data obtained in a number of different laboratories for many different cell membranes suggest that these membranes behave as relatively polar structures at least with respect to the manner in which they affect the rate of transmembrane, monomolecular solute diffusion (7, 11, 14, 15, 17, 19, 21).

Dependency of Maximal Rates of Monomolecular Diffusion on Polarity of the Cell Membrane

The recognition that many biological membranes behave as relatively polar structures has profound implications in many experimental settings where the metabolic effects of various lipids or sterols are studied with different types of cell preparations under in vitro conditions. These implications can best be understood by examining a specific set of data taken from the literature (21) and shown diagrammatically in Figure 5. In this example the passive permeability coefficients for the transmembrane movement of a homologous series of saturated fatty acids have been determined experimentally and it was found that P increased by a factor of 1.58 for each —CH_2—

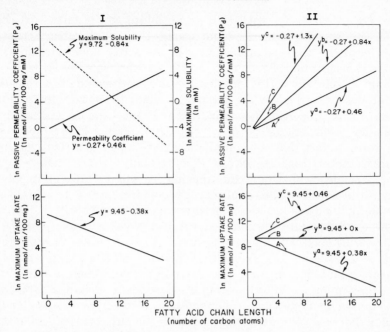

FIG. 5. Effect of relative polarity of a solute molecule on its maximum rate of transmembrane movement. Panels in *column I* represent actual experimental data obtained on uptake of fatty acids of various chain lengths into the intestinal mucosal cell (22). Upper panel shows the logarithm of passive permeability coefficients and maximum aqueous solubilities of the homologous series of saturated fatty acids; lower panel shows the logarithm of the maximum uptake rate, which equals the passive permeability coefficient times the maximum solubility for each individual fatty acid. Panels in *column II* illustrate the effect of altering polarity of the biological membrane. *Curves A, B,* and *C* show theoretical results obtained where the membrane is made progressively less polar so that the addition of each —CH₂— group to the fatty acid chain increases the passive permeability coefficient by a factor of 1.58 (*A*), 2.32 (*B*), and 3.67 (*C*). These values correspond to $\delta\Delta F_{w\rightarrow 1}$ values of −283, −517, and −801 cal/mol for the —CH₂— group in these 3 respective situations. Results are based on experimental data in which the permeability coefficients and uptake rates were normalized to 100 mg dry wt of intestinal tissues (22).

group added to the fatty acid chain. Thus, as shown by the solid line in *panel I,* the logarithm of P plotted against the fatty acid chain length has a slope of +0.46. In this same study the maximum solubility of each fatty acid was determined in the perfusate and, as shown by the dashed line, maximum solubility decreased by a factor of 0.43 (slope of the semilogarithmic plot of −0.84) for each —CH₂— group added to the fatty acid. Since the rate of uptake of any of these fatty acids is equal to the product of the concentration of the fatty acid in the perfusate and its appropriate passive permeability coefficient (*equation 1*), it follows that the maximum rate of uptake must equal the product of the maximum solubility of each fatty acid in the perfusate times its passive permeability coefficient. When such values are calculated for each fatty acid, as seen in the lower solid line of *panel I,* the maximum rate of uptake decreases by a factor of 0.68 (slope of the semilogarithmic plot of -0.38) for each CH_2 group added to the fatty acid chain. Thus, for this homologous series of fatty acids the highest rates of transport are seen with the more polar members of the series under circumstances where the concentration of each fatty acid in the perfusate has been elevated to its limit of solubility. This relationship derives from the fact that as — CH_2— groups are added to the fatty acid chain the maximum solubility decreases out of proportion (slope of -0.84) to the increase in the passive permeability coefficient (slope of $+0.46$). This latter relationship in turn results from the fact that the cell membrane behaves as a relatively polar structure so that in this instance $\delta\Delta F_{w \to 1}^{CH_2}$ equals only -283 cal/mol.

The dependency of the maximal monomeric uptake rates on membrane polarity is illustrated by the set of curves shown in Figure 5, *panel II*, where the membrane is made progressively less polar so that $\delta\Delta F_{w \to 1}^{CH_2}$ is increased from the experimentally determined value of -283 cal/mol (*curve A*) to -517 (*curve B*) and -801 (*curve C*) cal/mol. In *curve B* the membrane has been made less polar to the extent that the addition of a CH_2 group results in an exactly equal incremental increase in P and decrement in solubility so that the maximum uptake rate becomes independent of chain length (*curve B, lower panel II*). Only when the membrane is made even less polar than this are higher rates of uptake observed with the fatty acids of longer chain length (*curve C*).

These observations are particularly relevant to the study of the uptake, metabolism, or metabolic effects of different lipids or steroids that are added to the perfusate of a cell preparation in amounts likely to exceed their true solubility in the buffer. Such a situation, for example, might occur when various steroids are dissolved in a solvent and then added to the fluid perfusing a tissue-culture or isolated-cell preparation. Under these circumstances it will be very difficult to make valid judgments about the relative rates of metabolism or the relative effects of different members of a homologous series of lipids in altering a particular cellular pathway since the rates of entry of the various lipids into the cells will vary markedly. In general, in this situation it is anticipated that the more polar members of a series of solutes will have the highest rates of cellular uptake and therefore will be metabolized and/or exert greater metabolic effects within the cells under study than would the less polar members of the series.

Anomalous Behavior of Monomer Diffusion of Polar, Small-Molecular-Weight Solutes Across Biological Membranes

In Figures 3 and 5, it has been assumed that the permeability coefficients for a homologous series of fatty acids follow a regular and predictable pattern based on the number of methylene groups in the fatty acid chain. In these instances, the addition of each —CH_2— group increases P by a constant amount so that ln P is a linear function of the number of carbon atoms in the fatty acid. A similar relationship can be seen for steroids, where, for example, ln P varies as a linear function of the number of hydroxyl groups added to the sterol nucleus. Although such behavior has been described for the penetration of many different classes of solutes across biological membranes, it also has been consistently reported that for any homologous series of molecules the more polar members of the series, with smaller molecular weights, have anomalously high permeability coefficients. For example, data such as those shown in Figure 6 have been found in membranes of the intestine, gallbladder, adipocyte, and muscle cell (14, 17, 21). For the fatty acids with more than six carbon atoms in the chain there is a linear relationship between ln P and chain length. This relationship is not true, however, for the fatty acids with shorter chain lengths that typically manifest much higher passive permeability coefficients than would be extrapolated from the behavior of the series members of higher molecular weights. Such "anomalously" high rates of monomolecular diffusion have been reported in nearly all biological membranes that have been studied for many types of small-molecular-weight molecules, including short-chain-length alcohols and fatty acids, urea, methyl urea, foramide, and acetamide (4, 8, 9, 11, 14, 17, 19, 21, 29). Although such behavior has been attributed in the past to carrier-mediated diffusion or to aqueous "pores" within the cell membrane, current data suggest that these high permeability coefficients are due to an inherent property of biologic membranes that allows small molecules to pass relatively more rapidly between the structural components of the membranes than solutes of larger molecular weight (28). Although this phenomenon is not particularly important in studies dealing with medium- and long-chain-length fatty acids and with steroids, it may become relevant in studies involving the movement of the small-molecular-weight metabolic products of lipids across cell membranes.

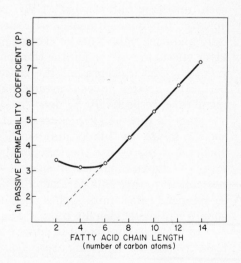

FIG. 6. Relationship of the passive permeability coefficient to the chain length of various saturated fatty acids. This diagram illustrates that the shorter chain length, more polar members of this homologous series have higher passive permeability coefficients than would be expected from the linear extrapolation of the results obtained with fatty acids containing 6 or more carbon atoms.

EFFECTS OF DIFFUSION BARRIERS ON RATES OF MOVEMENT OF LIPIDS
ACROSS BIOLOGICAL MEMBRANES

*General Principles of Molecular Movement Across Diffusion
Barriers in Biological Systems*

Nearly all of the discussion thus far has been based on *equation 1*,
which states that the rate of diffusion of a lipid across a membrane is
determined by the concentration of the solute in the perfusate and its
passive permeability coefficient. This simple situation is probably never
encountered in biologic systems under either in vitro or in vivo conditions
since the concentration of the solute molecule measurable in the bulk
solution perfusing a particular tissue or cell preparation is usually not the
same as the concentration of the solute molecule "seen" by the cell membrane. This is true because there is usually a diffusion barrier, be it simple
or complex, interposed between the cell surface and the bulk perfusion
medium. Because of the physicochemical characteristics of lipid molecules
with their limited solubility and high passive permeability coefficients, such
diffusion barriers markedly influence the rate at which these solutes enter
and exit from cells and have led to the evolution of a whole series of carrier
substances, the major function of which is to overcome the resistance
encountered by lipid movement through these barriers.

The simplest situation is shown diagrammatically in *panel I* of Figure 7
and involves the movement of a solute molecule from the bulk phase of the
perfusate across a single cell membrane into the cytosolic compartment.
However, interposed between the bulk perfusate and the membrane surface
are layers of water that are not subject to the same gross mixing that takes
place in the bulk perfusate and through which diffusion is the sole means for
molecular movement (5). Obviously, there is no sharp demarcation between
such "unstirred water layers" (UWL) and the bulk solution of the perfusate:
however, functional dimensions for these layers can be measured experimentally and such values are of critical importance in dealing with unstirred-
layer effects in any membrane transport system (6, 21, 23). Thus, in Figure
7 C_1, C_2, and C_3 represent the concentrations of the solute in the bulk
perfusate, at the aqueous-membrane interface, and just inside the cell
membrane, respectively; S_w denotes the functional surface area of the UWL,
d equals its functional thickness, and D is the diffusion coefficient for the
specific solute. In this formulation S_w is similar to the S_m term described
earlier but represents the functional surface area of the unstirred water
layer overlying a particular amount of tissue or cells; this term must be
normalized to the same parameter of tissue mass utilized in the J_d term and
so commonly has units such as square centimeters per gram of tissue or
square centimeters per 10^6 cells.

In the situation shown in *panel I* the net movement of solute from C_1 to
C_3 is given by the following expression:

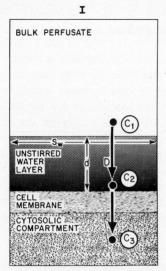
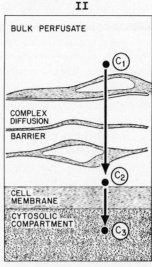

FIG. 7. Diagrammatic representation of the major parameters of diffusion barriers in biological systems. *Panel I* represents the simplified situation in which a solute molecule is moving from a bulk perfusate into the cystolic compartment of a cell. In so doing it must cross 2 diffusion barriers, the UWL outside the cell and the cell membrane itself. C_1, C_2, and C_3 represent the concentration of the solute molecule in the bulk perfusate, at the aqueous-membrane interface, and in the cystosolic compartment, respectively. S_W and d represent the effective surface area and effective thickness, respectively, of the UWL; D is the diffusion coefficient for the solute molecule. *Panel II* represents the more complex situation where the solute molecule must move from the bulk perfusate (e.g., serum within a capillary) to a target cell (e.g., an adipocyte) through a complex diffusion barrier made up of many different tissue spaces and cell membranes. In this situation S_w and d will be profoundly affected by the actual anatomical pathway that the solute molecule must follow through the diffusion barrier.

$$J_d^{net} = (C_1 - C_2)\left(\frac{S_w D}{d}\right) = (C_2 - C_3)P_d \qquad (11)$$

The first term describes the net rate of movement of the solute across the unstirred water layer; the second term gives the net flux of the molecule across the cell membrane. In the steady state these two flux rates must be equal and C_2 may assume any value between the limits of C_1 and 0. This value can be calculated from the following expression:

$$C_2 = C_1 - \left(\frac{dJ_d^{net}}{S_w D}\right) \qquad (12)$$

The term $dJ_d^{net}/S_w D$ essentially represents the resistance encountered by the solute in crossing the UWL: the higher this resistance, the lower the value of C_2. This resistance term is complex, however, and is determined by the physical dimensions of the UWL (d/S_w), by the diffusivity of the solute molecule in the aqueous phase (D), and by the net velocity of solute transport across the system (J_d^{net}).

In many physiological situations, both in vivo and in vitro, the diffusion barrier overlying a particular tissue essentially consists entirely of such unstirred water layers. This is probably the case, for example, in epithelial membranes such as intestine, gallbladder, choroid plexus, and bladder and when isolated cells are studied under in vitro conditions. Under both in vivo and in vitro conditions the unstirred water layers overlying the surface of such epithelial membranes commonly vary in thickness from approximately 100 to 800 μm, depending on the rate of mixing of the bulk phase, and it is seldom possible to reduce this thickness to less than 75 μm even with the most vigorous mixing that can reasonably be employed under in vitro conditions (6, 12–14, 19, 21, 25, 30). On the other hand, the thickness of the UWL surrounding individual cells suspended in an incubation medium is probably considerably less than 10–20 μm (16, 17).

In many other tissues, the diffusion barriers are much more complex (*panel II*). For example, any solute that must move from capillary blood to a target tissue such as an adipocyte or muscle cell must necessarily pass through a complex series of cell membranes and aqueous spaces. The total resistance encountered during this diffusion process equals the sum of the resistances encountered in diffusing through each membrane in series, i.e., $(1/P_d)^1 + (1/P_d)^2 + (1/P_d)^3 + \cdots$, plus the sum of the resistances encountered in diffusing through each aqueous space, i.e., $(d/S_wD)^1 + (d/S_wD)^2 + (d/S_wD)^3 + \cdots$. Furthermore, if the solute has limited solubility in the blood then the rate at which it can be delivered to the capillaries of the tissue also may be limited and this limitation can be taken as yet another resistance to uptake of the solute by the target cells. This latter resistance term is a function of the reciprocal of the product of the volume of blood flow per unit of time to the target tissue (V) and the concentration of the solute in the bulk phase of the blood, i.e., $1/VC_1$ (27).[5] Thus, in many anatomically intact tissues the rate of cellular uptake is profoundly influenced by the magnitude of the total resistance to molecular movement imposed by such complex diffusion barriers, and this total resistance is made up of such factors as the rate of blood flow to a particular organ, the solubility of the solute in blood, and the rate of diffusion of the molecule across a series of unstirred water layers and cell membranes.

Relative Importance of Membrane and Diffusion-Barrier Resistances in Determining Rates of Lipid Movement Across Biological Membranes

It is apparent from *equations 11* and *12* that two extreme situations may be encountered in various membrane systems. First, the rate of movement of the solute molecule across the diffusion barrier may be very

---

[5] This term is actually more complex than stated here; for a more complete discussion of this expression see reference 27.

rapid relative to its rate of movement across the cell membrane: i.e., $S_w D/d$ may be very much larger than P_d. In this case unstirred-layer resistance is negligible and the rate of molecular penetration through the cell membrane becomes totally rate limiting to cellular uptake as described by the following equation:

$$J_d^{net} = (C_1 - C_3)P_d \qquad (13)$$

Second, the rate of movement of the solute molecule might be very much faster through the cell membrane than across the UWL: i.e., P_d is very much larger than $S_w D/d$. In this case the value of $dJ_d^{net}/S_w D$ in *equation 12* essentially equals the value of C_1 and therefore the value of C_2 approaches 0. In this case the rate of solute movement across the diffusion barrier becomes wholly rate limiting to cellular uptake and is described by the following equation:

$$J_d^{net} = (C_1 - C_3)\left(\frac{S_w D}{d}\right) \qquad (14)$$

These two extreme situations as well as the intermediate condition where both the UWL and membrane resistances influence uptake rates are shown graphically in Figure 8, where the logarithm of the value of J_d^{net}/D has been plotted as a function of the fatty acid chain length at several different values for unstirred-layer resistance. In these examples the concentration gradient between C_1 and C_3 is assumed to be the same for each fatty acid. *Curve A* represents the extreme case (*equation 13*) where S_w/d is infinitely great and unstirred-layer resistance is therefore negligible. In this situation J_d^{net} is determined by the passive permeability coefficient for each fatty acid so that the term $\ln J_d^{net}/D$ increases as an essentially linear function of the fatty acid chain length. However, there is significant deviation from this behavior as the diffusion barrier begins to exert a finite resistance. In the first example (*curve B*) fatty acids with 2–8 carbon atoms have such low passive permeability coefficients that membrane permeation is still totally rate limiting and the value of $\ln J_d^{net}/D$ still falls on the linear portion of the curve (the segment of *line B* to the left of *point x*). In contrast, the passive permeability coefficients for fatty acids with 18, 20, and 22 carbon atoms are so high that uptake becomes totally diffusion limited as described by *equation 14*. In this case J_d^{net}/D reaches a constant and limiting value dictated by S_w/d (the portion of *curve B* to the right of *point y*). The portion of *curve B* between *points x* and *y* delineates those fatty acids where the UWL and cell membrane both contribute in determining the rate of cellular fatty acid uptake. When a UWL of even greater resistance is introduced in front of the membrane then, as shown by *curve C*, the diffusion barrier becomes totally rate limiting to cellular uptake for all fatty acids greater than 10 carbon atoms.

The important principle illustrated by Figure 8 is that the higher the

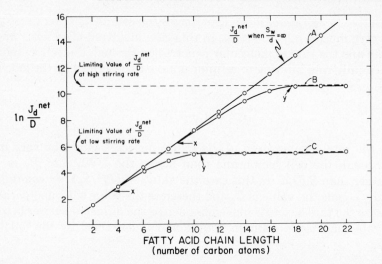

FIG. 8. Diagrammatic representation of the effect of diffusion barriers of varying resistance on the cellular uptake of fatty acids of different chain length. In this example the concentration gradient across the cell membrane is assumed to be the same for each fatty acid. Under these conditions the rate of net uptake (J_d^{net}) will equal the product of the passive permeability coefficient of each fatty acid times its concentration gradient. If no diffusion barrier is present outside the cell membrane then the uptake rate will be essentially a linear function of the fatty acid chain length (*curve A*). *Curve C* represents the theoretical findings anticipated when the bulk solution is stirred at a very low rate so that the diffusion barrier is relatively thick; *curve B* represents the results anticipated at a higher rate of stirring. For the latter 2 curves *point x* illustrates the point at which the diffusion barrier begins to exert significant resistance and uptake rates begin to deviate from the linear relationship illustrated by *curve A*. At *point y* diffusion of fatty acids across the UWL becomes totally rate limiting to cellular uptake so that J_d^{net} is proportional to D and the quantity J_d^{net}/D becomes constant. These theoretical curves are based on actual experimental data derived in several types of epithelial tissues (19, 21, 26).

passive permeability coefficient for a particular solute molecule the more likely that diffusion barriers, rather than the cell membrane, will be rate limiting to monomolecular uptake. Characteristically the passive permeability coefficients are very high for most lipids including the long-chain fatty acids, various sterols, and steroid hormones. It therefore follows that under in vivo conditions the rate-limiting step to the cellular uptake of these compounds is likely to be diffusion across the various complex diffusion barriers between the sites of lipid production and the target cells where they are taken up and utilized.

Effect of Diffusion Barriers on Measurement of Activation Energies

This recognition that either the cell membrane or the diffusion barrier outside of the cell may limit the rate of lipid uptake in a particular tissue has important implications with respect to the interpretation of temperature effects on the transmembrane movement of solutes. In general, in the past the passive monomolecular diffusion of a solute across a biological membrane has been said to have low Q_{10} values and correspondingly low activation energies. Furthermore, in some instances an abrupt change in apparent activation energy has been found when the temperature was lowered and this effect has been attributed to a temperature-related phase change in the lipid molecules making up the structure of the cell membrane. Such behavior is illustrated by the "experimental curve" in *panel II* of Figure 9. At higher temperatures the slope of the line is shallow, corresponding to a change in the rate of solute uptake of approximately 1.2 for each 10°C change in temperature (an activation energy of only about 2800 cal/mol); as the temperature is lowered, however, a "transition" point apparently is reached below which the line acquires a steeper slope that may correspond to a Q_{10} value varying from 2.0 to 4.0 and to activation energies varying from approximately 10,700 to 21,000 cal/mol. However, when such data are corrected for unstirred-layer effects (*curve B*), the transition point disappears and a single linear regression curve is produced that has a steep slope corresponding to a high activation energy for the passive penetration of this solute across the cell membrane (1, 28). Such data suggest that in many instances both the low activation energies and the apparent transition points reported for passive solute uptake across biological membranes are

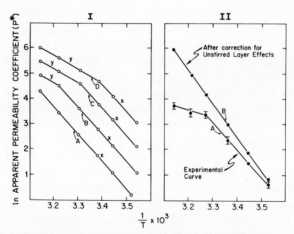

FIG. 9. Diagrammatic representation of the effect of diffusion barriers on apparent "transition temperatures" and on activation energies for solute molecules with various permeability coefficients. Logarithm of the apparent permeability coefficient (P^*) has been plotted against the reciprocal of the absolute temperature. *Panel I* shows results that might be obtained with 4 different solute molecules that penetrate a biological membrane at different rates. *Curve A* represents a molecule having the lowest passive permeability coefficient; *curve D* represents a molecule with a much higher P value. In this diagram the segment of each curve labeled x has a relatively steep slope and therefore yields a high value for the activation energy; the segments labeled y have lower slopes and correspondingly lower values for activation energies. In *panel II, curve A* illustrates results obtained when experimental data on uptake are plotted and *curve B* shows results obtained after correction of the experimental data for unstirred-layer effects. These theoretical relationships are based on actual experimental data (e.g., 1).

artifacts due to failure to recognize that the uptake of the solute is diffusion limited at physiological temperatures. Thus, at higher temperatures the low Q_{10} value simply reflects the low activation energy for the diffusion of the solute through the aqueous environment of the UWL. As the temperature is decreased, a point is reached at which penetration through the cell membrane, rather than through the diffusion barrier, becomes rate limiting and the apparent activation energy abruptly increases. Thus the transition point shown in *panel II* (Fig. 9) actually corresponds to the point where the major resistance to molecular uptake of the solute shifts from the UWL to the cell membrane (1).

Since the resistance encountered by a solute in crossing the diffusion barrier also is a function of the passive permeability coefficient of that molecule (and hence the J_d^{net} term in *equation 12*) it follows that the apparent transition temperature seen in a given membrane should vary inversely with the P value for a series of solute molecules. This situation is illustrated by the series of curves shown in *panel I* of Figure 9. *Curve A* represents the situation encountered with a compound having such a low passive permeability coefficient that the cell membrane is rate limiting to uptake at all temperatures. As solutes with progressively higher P values are tested, an apparent transition point is seen (the change in slope between the line segments labeled x and y). This apparent transition temperature is not constant, however, but occurs at a progressively lower temperature for each more permeant solute tested. In each case, correction for UWL resistance would eliminate this transition point and yield curves reflecting the true activation energies for the passive penetration of these solutes through this particular biological membrane (1).

These data illustrate two important generalizations concerning the effect of diffusion barriers on the determination of activation energies. First, it now seems likely that the passive penetration of biological membranes by various lipid molecules is very dependent on temperature and manifests high activation energies. It has been reported, for example, that the activation energy for such uptake increases by 2500–3600 cal/mol for each —CH_2— group added to a solute molecule (1). Low activation energies previously reported for such processes probably reflect failure to make appropriate corrections for unstirred-layer effects. Second, some previous reports suggesting that temperature-dependent changes in the activation energy for passive uptake reflect phase transitions in the lipid structure of the cell membrane also are likely to be in error and result from failure to make these corrections.

Effect of Diffusion Barriers on Kinetics of Lipid Transport
by a Finite Number of Membrane Sites

Thus far in this section the influence of diffusion barriers on the passive monomolecular uptake of lipids into cells has been examined. However, such barriers also have profound effects on the kinetic characteristics of the second type of lipid transport, which depends on the interaction of a specific lipoprotein fraction with a finite number of receptor sites on the cell membrane. In the simplest case, the kinetics of such a transport system are described by *equation 2* so that the rate of uptake (J_d) bears a hyperbolic relationship to the concentration of the solute molecule present at the aqueous-membrane interface (C_2), and the kinetics of a particular transport system are described in terms of the maximal transport rate that can be achieved $(J_d{}^m)$ and the concentration of the solute molecule necessary to reach half of this limiting rate (K_m). This equation, it should be emphasized, is written in terms of C_2, the concentration of the solute molecule "seen" by the membrane. In the presence of a diffusion barrier, however, this equation must be rewritten in terms of C_1: i.e, the concentration of the molecule present in the bulk perfusate. Since $C_2 = C_1 - (dJ_d/S_wD)$, this expression can be substituted for C_2 in *equation 2* to give:

$$J_d = \frac{J^m\left(C_1 - \dfrac{dJ_d}{S_wD}\right)}{K_m + \left(C_1 - \dfrac{dJ_d}{S_wD}\right)} \tag{15}$$

When solved for J_d this equation yields the quadratic expression (20):

$$J_d = (0.5)(D)\left(\frac{S_w}{d}\right)\left[C_1 + K_m + \frac{dJ_d{}^m}{S_wD}\right.$$
$$\left. - \sqrt{\left(C_1 + K_m + \frac{dJ_d{}^m}{S_wD}\right)^2 - 4C_1\left(\frac{dJ_d^m}{S_wD}\right)}\,\right] \tag{16}$$

Thus, under most physiological circumstances where the membrane transport sites are separated from the bulk perfusate by a diffusion barrier, it is this equation that describes the relationship between the rate of uptake and the concentration of the solute (or lipoprotein) in the bulk perfusing medium. It should be emphasized, therefore, that the value of J_d is influenced by the resistance of the diffusion barrier, given by the expression $dJ_d{}^m/S_wD$, as well as by the values of the K_m and $J_d{}^m$ terms.

This formulation has four important consequences. First, in the presence of a significant diffusion-barrier resistance J_d becomes essentially a linear function of C_1 and the "saturable" appearance of the kinetic curve is lost. This effect is illustrated by the series of curves derived from *equation 16* shown in *panel I* of Figure 10. When the resistance term (i.e., $dJ_d{}^m/S_wD$) is low, as in *curve A*, the rate of uptake exhibits saturation kinetics with respect to C_1. However, when the resistance term is increased 500-fold, as in *curve D*, J_d increases in essentially a linear fashion with respect to the concentration of the solute molecule in the bulk solution. Thus, in the presence of a major diffusion barrier such linear kinetics are to be anticipated and should not be construed as evidence against the possibility that the uptake process involves translocation by a finite number of transport sites.

Second, the presence of a significant diffusion barrier leads to gross overestimation of the true K_m value for the transport process. This effect also is shown in *panel I* of Figure 10, where the true K_m value for the system is assumed to equal 1.0 concentration units: as the resistance of the diffusion barrier is increased over a 500-fold range, the apparent K_m value $(K_m{}^*)$ increases from 1.0 to 26.2 concentration units. In fact, as shown in *panel II*, under these circumstances the apparent K_m value increases linearly with the resistance of the overlying diffusion barrier as given by the following equation (20, 24):

$$K_m{}^* = K_m + 0.5 \left(\frac{dJ_d{}^m}{S_w D}\right) \qquad (17)$$

Stated in a different way, if no diffusion barrier were present then this transport system would achieve 80% of the maximal transport rate $(J_d{}^m)$ at a solute concentration of 4 units. In the presence of the high-resistance barrier *(curve D)*, the solute would have to be raised to 45 concentration units in the bulk perfusate to attain the same rate of transport.

Third, in the presence of a significant diffusion resistance the apparent K_m becomes a dependent variable of $J_d{}^m$. This effect is illustrated by the series of curves shown in *panel I* of Figure 11, where the true K_m value is again set equal to 1 concentration unit. As seen in *panel I*, under circumstances where the diffusion-barrier resistance is low increasing the value of $J_d{}^m$ 10-fold has only a minimal effect in increasing the apparent K_m value to 1.2 concentration units. However, a similar increase in $J_d{}^m$ under circumstances where the diffusion-barrier resistance is increased 50-fold *(panel II)*

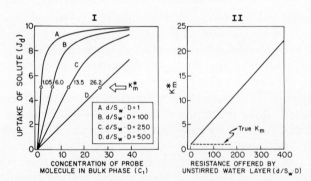

FIG. 10. Effect of diffusion barriers of various resistances on the kinetics of transport through a finite number of sites on a biological membrane. In *panel I* the rate of solute uptake is plotted in arbitrary units on the vertical axis and the concentration of the solute molecule in the bulk perfusate (C_1) is plotted in arbitrary units on the horizontal axis. It is assumed that the true K_m value for the transport process equals 1.00 and this illustration shows the effect of increasing the resistance of unstirred water layers overlying the transport sites 500-fold on apparent K_m values $(K_m{}^*)$. In *panel II* the $K_m{}^*$ values are plotted against the resistance of the UWL as given by $d/S_w D$. These theoretical curves are based on values for the various parameters of transport likely to be encountered in biologic systems (given in detail in ref. 20).

FIG. 11. Effect of maximal transport rates $(J_d{}^m)$ on apparent K_m values in the presence of a diffusion barrier of low and high resistance. As in Fig. 10, the true K_m value for the transport system is assumed to equal 1.00. In *panel I,* under circumstances where the diffusion barrier over the transport sites exerts only a very low resistance, increasing the maximal transport rate 10-fold has only a minimal effect in increasing $K_m{}^*$ from 1.0 to 1.2. However, as shown in *panel II,* if the resistance of the diffusion barrier overlying the transport sites is increased by 50-fold then $K_m{}^*$ increases over 9-fold under circumstances where $J_d{}^m$ is increased 10-fold. Thus, in the presence of a significant diffusion barrier the apparent K_m for the transport system has become a dependent variable of $J_d{}^m$.

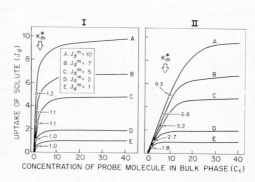

results in an increase in $K_m{}^*$ to 9.3 concentration units. Thus, since the $J_d{}^m$ term enters into the total resistance term in *equations 16* and *17, K_m* varies directly with $J_d{}^m$.

Fourth, the presence of a diffusion barrier will lead to overestimation of maximal transport rates $(J_d{}^m)$ if these values are estimated from double-reciprocal plots. As shown in Figure 12, in the absence of a diffusion barrier the relationship between J_d and C_1 is described by *equation 2* and takes the form of *curve A* in *panel I.* When replotted in the double-reciprocal form (*panel II*) such a curve becomes linear and has an intercept on the vertical axis that equals $1/J_d{}^m$. However, when a diffusion barrier is present over the transport sites then *equation 16* describes the relationship between J_d and C_1 and yields, for example, a curve such as B in *panel I.* Since *equation 16* does not take the form of a rectangular hyperbola, plotting these data in the double-reciprocal form does not transform *curve B* into a straight line: rather, as seen in *panel II* the curve turns sharply upward as it approaches the vertical axis to intercept at $1/J_d{}^m$. However, if, as is commonly done, the experimental points are used to construct a linear regression curve and this curve is extrapolated to the vertical axis (dashed line) then an artifactually high value for $J_d{}^m$ will be obtained. Thus, if it is experimentally difficult to measure directly the maximal transport rate for a particular transport system (because, for example, of limited solubility of the solute) then estimation of this value from double-reciprocal plots will lead to an artifactually high value for $J_d{}^m$ if a diffusion barrier is interposed between the bulk solution and the transport sites (23, 24).

Finally, it should be emphasized that *equation 16* and the various examples of curves derived from this equation are based on the assumption that the diffusion barrier has a homogenous structure in which reasonable values D, d, and S_w apply, e.g., when the barrier is simply an unstirred

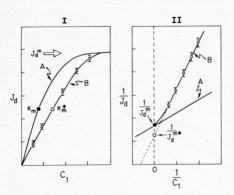

FIG. 12. Effect of diffusion barriers on determination of maximum transport velocities ($J_d{}^m$) by use of double-reciprocal plots. *Panel I* shows 2 kinetic curves for uptake of a solute molecule in the absence (*A*) and presence (*B*) of a significant diffusion barrier. In the presence of the diffusion barrier K_m is shifted to the right but both curves achieve the same value of $J_d{}^m$. These same 2 curves are replotted in *panel II* as the reciprocal of these two variables. Linear extrapolation of the data points in *curve B* gives a value for $J_d{}^m$ much higher than the true maximal transport rate, i.e., $1/J_d{}^{m*}$ is artifactually lower than $1/J_d{}^m$.

water layer. If, however, movement of the solute through the barrier cannot be described in terms of this simple diffusion equation, e.g., if the barrier exerts a sieving effect or has some type of carrier-facilitated transport, then the mathematical treatment is still more complex than that given in *equation 16* although the same general principles still apply.

Role of Carrier Molecules in Overcoming Diffusion-Barrier Resistance

From these considerations it is likely that the uptake of most lipids is limited by their diffusion across various barriers overlying the target cells regardless of whether the actual mechanism of cellular uptake is by mono-molecular diffusion or by a transport process involving a finite number of receptor sites. In order to overcome these resistances to cellular uptake a number of different carrier structures have evolved that greatly facilitate the uptake rates for a variety of different lipids. Several are shown diagrammatically in Figure 13. *Panel I* shows the simplest example that might be encountered, where a detergent micelle is utilized as a carrier to facilitate the uptake of a particular lipid molecule across a simple UWL interposed between the bulk perfusate and the membrane of the target cell. This type of system exists in the intestine, where bile acid micelles are utilized to facilitate fatty acid and sterol absorption. As an example of the magnitude of the effect of having the micelle present, one can calculate the rate of fatty acid absorption that takes place in the absence and in the presence of the detergent. The maximal rate of stearic acid uptake that can be achieved without bile acid can be calculated from *equation 14* to equal 1.35 nmol/min per 100 mg tissue (assuming that the maximum solubility of the fatty acid in solution equals 4.37 μM, that S_w equals 11.7 cm²/100 mg tissue, and that d is 137 μm (22). In the presence of a bile acid micelle a much higher total concentration of fatty acid can be achieved in the bulk solution and a large mass of this solute, solubilized in the micelle, diffuses up to the aqueous-membrane interface. If this results in an aqueous concentration of the fatty

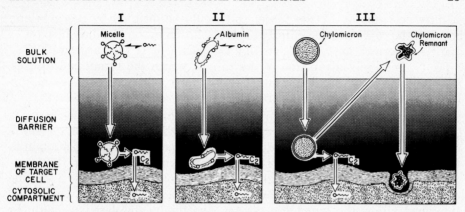

FIG. 13. Diagrammatic representation of how 3 different macromolecular structures act to overcome the resistance encountered by solute molecules in crossing several different diffusion barriers. *Panel I* is based on the situation in the gastrointestinal tract where the bile acid micelle acts as a carrier to bring a large mass of cholesterol, free fatty acids, and β-monoglyceride across the UWL adjacent to the microvillus border to the aqueous-membrane interface. *Panel II* illustrates a similar situation where albumin carries a large mass of free fatty acids from some source (e.g., the adipocyte) to a target tissue (e.g., a muscle cell): in this situation the diffusion barrier represents the entire vascular space between the site of origin and the site of disposition of the fatty acids. *Panel III* represents the more complex situation where the chylomicron delivers fatty acids to one site (e.g., the adipocyte or muscle cell) and dietary cholesterol to a second site (e.g., the liver).

acid in equilibrium with the micelle (C_2) of 4.37 μM, then the rate of uptake in this instance can be calculated from *equation 1* to equal 12.8 nmol/min per 100 mg tissue (utilizing a P value for stearic acid of 2930 nmol/min per 100 mg tissue per mM). Thus, the presence of the bile acid has facilitated uptake of the fatty acid by a factor of 9.5. Since the magnitude of the diffusion-barrier resistance varies directly with the passive permeability coefficient for a particular solute (*equation 12*) it follows that the relative effect of a bile acid micelle in facilitating lipid absorption in the gut should increase with increasing hydrophobicity of the particular lipid. Such an effect has been demonstrated since, for example, the presence of the detergent enhances intestinal uptake of the fatty acids with 8, 12, 16, and 20 carbon atoms by factors of 1.05, 1.48, 3.53, and 25.8, respectively, and of the still more hydrophobic cholesterol molecule by a factor of approximately 145.

Panel II of Figure 13 shows a similar model that might be encountered under in vitro conditions where albumin, rather than a bile acid micelle, is utilized to deliver a lipid molecule to the target tissue. Such a system also is important in vivo where albumin acts as a major carrier for overcoming the resistance to net fatty acid movement between the sites of production, e.g., the adipocyte, and the sites of utilization, e.g., muscle cell. Obviously, in this case the albumin-fatty acid complex would maintain a relatively higher monomer concentration of fatty acid in the aqueous environment of the capillary blood than would be present if albumin were absent. The net rate of fatty acid uptake by the target cell would be dictated by the gradient between the concentration of fatty acid in solution in the capillary blood (C_2) and its concentration in the cytosolic compartment of the target cell (C_3). Since C_3 is largely a function of the rate at which the target cell utilizes fatty acid, the magnitude of the net flux of fatty acid across this system is largely determined by the rate of cellular metabolism of the compound.

A third example is shown in *panel III* of Figure 13, where the carrier is a lipoprotein and, in this case, specifically the chylomicron. This system is complex since the same carrier delivers two components of the lipoprotein to two different anatomical sites. The particle is synthesized within the intestine and transports dietary triglyceride and cholesterol across the various diffusion barriers represented by the tissue spaces within the core of the intestinal villus, the lymphatic system, and finally the vascular space. In the capillaries of tissues like muscle and adipose tissues an enzyme, lipoprotein lipase, hydrolyzes the triglycerides and generates a locally high concentration of fatty acids (C_2 in the diagram). Since these same tissues either store the fatty acids as triglyceride or rapidly oxidize them as a source of energy the concentration of fatty acids in the cytosolic compartment of the target cell probably is maintained at a very low level so that there is rapid net uptake of fatty acids across the capillary wall. Obviously during this process fatty acids must cross several cell membranes and tissue spaces rather than a single membrane as shown diagrammatically in *panel III*, but molecules such as long-chain fatty acids have such high passive permeability coefficients that diffusion through even a series of biological membranes probably constitutes little impediment to the net movement of these molecules. With hydrolysis of a portion of the triglyceride content of the chylomicron and significant alterations in its peptide composition the chylomicron remnant is formed and is carried to the sinusoidal membrane of the hepatocyte, where apparently it is taken up intact by an endocytotic process (18). Thus, this particular lipoprotein acts as a carrier that markedly facilitates the net rate of movement of triglyceride and cholesterol from the intestinal epithelial cell to the peripheral sites of utilization.

One final point concerning the movement of lipoproteins from the serum across diffusion barriers to a target cell deserves emphasis. As the chylomicron remnant moves from the capillary blood to the surface of the hepatocyte relatively little diffusion resistance is encountered since the diffusion distance across the space of Disse cannot be more than 1–2 μm. Hence, the apparent K_m value for the uptake process is very close to the true K_m value. Thus, as illustrated by *curve A* in Figure 14, if K_m for the transport process is 10 mg/dl then the maximal rate of uptake is achieved with elevation of the serum level of the lipoprotein to only about 40 mg/dl. On the other hand, if a significant barrier were interposed between the capillary blood and the target cell then serum levels in excess of 160 mg/dl would have to be achieved in order to reach the same uptake rate even though the true K_m value for the transport process on the target cell is the same. This again

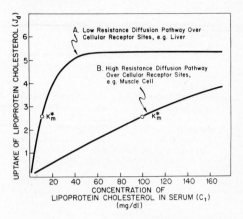

FIG. 14. Effect of diffusion barriers of different resistances on uptake of cholesterol carried in lipoproteins. In this example the transport mechanism responsible for lipoprotein uptake is assumed to have a true K_m value of approximately 10 mg/dl. Rate of uptake is given in arbitrary units; concentration values are given in mg/dl.

emphasizes that the functional kinetics for such a transport system are influenced as much by the diffusion barriers overlying the target tissue as by the characteristics of the transport sites on the cell membrane.

These studies were supported by Public Health Service research grants HL 09610, AM 16386, and AM 19329.

REFERENCES

1. BINDSLEV, N., AND E. M. WRIGHT. Effect of temperature on nonelectrolyte permeation across the toad urinary bladder. *J. Membrane Biol.* 29: 265–288, 1976.
2. BROWN, M. S., S. E. DANA, AND J. L. GOLDSTEIN. Regulation of 3-hydroxy-3-methylglutaryl coenzyme A reductase activity in human fibroblasts by lipoproteins. *Proc. Natl. Acad. Sci. US* 70: 2162–2166, 1973.
3. BROWN, M. S., AND J. L. GOLDSTEIN. Familial hypercholesterolemia: defective binding of lipoproteins to cultured fibroblasts associated with impaired regulation of 3-hydroxy-3-methylglutaryl coenzyme A reductase activity. *Proc. Natl. Acad. Sci. US* 71: 788–792, 1974.
4. COLLANDER, R., AND H. BARLUND. Permeabilitatsstudien an chara ceratophylla. *Acta Botan. Fennica* 11: 5, 1932.
5. DAINTY, J. Water relations of plant cells. *Advan. Botan. Res.* 1: 279–326, 1963.
6. DIAMOND, J. M. A rapid method for determining voltage-concentration relations across membranes. *J. Physiol., London* 183: 83–100, 1966.
7. DIAMOND, J. M., AND Y. KATZ. Interpretation of nonelectrolyte partition coefficients between dimyristoyl lecithin and water. *J. Membrane Biol.* 17: 121, 1974.
8. DIAMOND, J. M., AND E. M. WRIGHT. Biological membranes: the physical basis of ion and nonelectrolyte selectivity. *Ann. Rev. Physiol.* 31: 581–646, 1969.
9. DIAMOND, J. M., AND E. M. WRIGHT. Molecular forces governing non-electrolyte permeation through cell membranes. *Proc. Roy. Soc., London Ser. B* 172: 273–316, 1969.
10. LIEB, W. R., AND W. D. STEIN. The molecular basis of simple diffusion within biological membranes. *Current Topics Membranes Transport* 2: 1–39, 1971.
11. NACCACHE, P., AND R. I. SHA'AFI. Patterns of nonelectrolyte permeability in human red blood cell membrane. *J. Gen. Physiol.* 62: 714–736, 1973.
12. READ, N. W., C. D. HOLDSWORTH, AND R. J. LEVIN. The role of jejunal unstirred layer thickness in interpretation of changes in electrogenic glucose absorption in coeliac disease. *European J. Clin. Invest.* 4: 311, 1976.
13. READ, N. W., R. J. LEVIN, AND C. D. HOLDSWORTH. Measurement of the functional unstirred layer thickness in the human jejunum in vivo. *Brit. Soc. Gastroenterol.* 17: 387, 1976.
14. SALLEE, V. L., AND J. M. DIETSCHY. Determinants of intestinal mucosal uptake of short- and medium-chain fatty acids and alcohols. *J. Lipid Res.* 14: 475–484, 1973.
15. SAVITZ, D., AND A. K. SOLOMON. Tracer determinations of human red cell membrane permeability to small nonelectrolytes. *J. Gen. Physiol.* 58: 259, 1971.
16. SHA'AFI, R. I., G. T. RICH, V. W. SIDEL, W. BOSSERT, AND A. K. SOLOMON. The effect of the unstirred layer on human red cell water permeability. *J. Gen. Physiol.* 50: 1377–1399, 1967.
17. SHERRILL, B. C., AND J. M. DIETSCHY. Permeability characteristics of the adipocyte cell membrane and partitioning characteristics of the adipocyte triglyceride core. *J. Membrane Biol.* 23: 367–383, 1975.
18. SHERRILL, B. C., AND J. M. DIETSCHY. Uptake of lipoproteins of intestinal origin in the isolated perfused liver. *Circulation* 54, Suppl. II: 91, 1976.
19. SMULDERS, A. P., AND E. M. WRIGHT. The magnitude of nonelectrolyte selectivity in the gallbladder epithelium. *J. Membrane Biol.* 5: 297–318, 1971.
20. THOMSON, A. B. R., AND J. M. DIETSCHY. Derivation of the equations that describe the effects of unstirred

water layers on the kinetic parameters of active transport processes in the intestine. *J. Theoret. Biol.* 64: 277–294, 1977.

21. WESTERGAARD, H., AND J. M. DIETSCHY. Delineation of the dimensions and permeability characteristics of the two major diffusion barriers to passive mucosal uptake in the rabbit intestine. *J. Clin. Invest.* 54: 718–732, 1974.

22. WESTERGAARD, H., AND J. M. DIETSCHY. The mechanism whereby bile acid micelles increase the rate of fatty acid and cholesterol uptake into the intestinal mucosal cell. *J. Clin. Invest.* 58: 97–108, 1976.

23. WILSON, F. A., AND J. M. DIETSCHY. The intestinal unstirred layer: its surface area and effect on active transport kinetics. *Biochim. Biophys. Acta* 363: 112–126, 1974.

24. WINNE, D. Unstirred layer, source of biased Michaelis constant in membrane transport. *Biochim. Biophys. Acta* 298: 27–31, 1973.

25. WINNE, D. Unstirred layer thickness in perfused rat jejunum in vivo. *Experientia* 32: 1278–1279, 1976.

26. WINNE, D. The influence of unstirred layers on intestinal absorption. In: *Intestinal Permeation.* Amsterdam: Excerpta Med., 1977, p. 58–64.

27. WINNE, D., AND H. OCHSENFAHRT. Die formale kinetik der resorption unter Berucksichtingung der Darmdurchblutung. *J. Theoret. Biol.* 14: 293, 1967.

28. WRIGHT, E. M., AND N. BINDSLEV. Thermodynamic analysis of nonelectolyte permeation across the toad urinary bladder. *J. Membrane Biol.* 29: 289–312, 1976.

29. WRIGHT, E. M., AND J. M. DIAMOND. Patterns of non-electrolyte permeability. *Proc. Roy. Soc., London, Ser. B* 172: 227–271, 1969.

30. WRIGHT, E. M., AND J. W. PRATHER. The permeability of the frog choroid plexus to nonelectrolytes. *J. Membrane Biol.* 2: 127–149, 1970.

2

Intestinal Absorption of Lipids: Influence of the Unstirred Water Layer and Bile Acid Micelle

A. B. R. THOMSON

Department of Medicine, University of Alberta, Edmonton, Alberta, Canada

DIETARY LIPIDS REPRESENT a major portion of the total daily caloric intake of man and animals and play an important role in the nutritional and physiological processes of the body. Over the last decade significant advances in the understanding of the normal mechanisms of fat absorption have led to a clearer perception of the pathophysiology of malabsorption. In this chapter, the major steps of triglyceride and cholesterol absorption are considered first and then a more detailed analysis is made of the influence of the unstirred water layer and the bile acid micelle.

NUTRITIONAL ASPECTS

The normal dietary intake of fat in the adult in the Western hemisphere varies from 60 to 100 g/day. Most is in the form of triglycerides, with the remainder comprised of phospholipids and cholesterol esters. The majority of the triglycerides contain saturated or unsaturated fatty acids (FAs) with chain lengths greater than 14 carbon atoms, linked through ester bonds to glycerol in the 1, 2, and 3 position. The 0.5–1.0 g of cholesterol esters ingested each day is mixed with similar amounts of endogenous cholesterol from saliva, gastric secretions, bile, and sloughed intestinal epithelial cells. After mixing in the intestinal lumen, there is no apparent physiological distinction between the exogenous and endogenous cholesterol.

The absorption of dietary triglycerides is extremely efficient, with a coefficient of absorption of more than 95%. On the other hand, cholesterol absorption is much less efficient, only 20–50% being absorbed. A logical approach to the normal mechanism of lipid absorption would be to consider first the role of pancreatic and biliary secretions in the biochemical events that occur in the intestinal lumen and to consider second the role of the unstirred water layer and the bile salt micelle in the physiological process of mucosal uptake (Fig. 1). A subsequent section deals with the role of the intestinal mucosal cell in reesterification of fatty acids and monoglyceride to triglyceride and of cholesterol to cholesterol esters; then, the synthesis and release of the chylomicrons are discussed.

ROLE OF PANCREATIC AND BILIARY SECRETIONS

Emulsification and Lipolysis

Emulsification of dietary lipid begins in the stomach by mechanical means and continues in the upper bowel, where the coarse emulsion is mixed with pancreatic juice and bile. Bile salts are poor emulsifying agents (24), but the addition of lecithin and monoglycerides results in a lowering of interfacial tension and continued emulsification. An emulsion contains particles, diameter 2000–50,000 Å, that can be seen under the microscope, scatter light, and therefore are visible to the naked eye. As emulsification

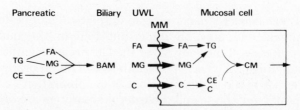

FIG. 1. Diagrammatic representation of the normal mechanism of lipid absorption. The major events occur in the intestinal lumen, or adjacent to or within the intestinal mucosal cell. Abbreviations: TG, triglyceride; CE, cholesterol ester; FA, fatty acid; MG, monoglyceride; C, unesterified cholesterol; BAM, mixed bile acid micelle; UWL, unstirred water layer; MM, microvillus membrane; CM, chylomicron. *1) Pancreatic*: emulsification and hydrolysis of TG and CE by pancreatic esterases. *2) Biliary*: solubilization of FA, MG, and C in BAM. *3) UWL*: diffusion of BAM across UWL up to MM. *4) MM*: diffusion of FA, MG, and C across the MM. *5) Mucosal cell*: reesterification, synthesis, and release of chylomicron.

proceeds, so also does lipolysis take place, thus providing more polar lipid for further emulsification and eventual micellar solubilization.

The major pancreatic enzymes involved in lipolysis include triglyceride lipase, cholesterol esterase, and phospholipase. The hormone coordinating the secretion of these pancreatic enzymes with the passage of food into the upper intestine is cholecystokinin-pancreozymin (CCK-PZ). Cholecystokinin is thought to be present in duodenal mucosal cells, and the hormone is released by the entry of fat and other food substances into the upper small bowel, resulting in the contraction of the gallbladder and release of pancreatic enzymes. The major properties and the physiological importance of pancreatic lipase have been reviewed (3, 13), and only a brief outline is given here.

Because of its substrate stereospecificity, pancreatic lipase (PL) hydrolyzes only the 1 and 3 ester bonds of the triglyceride (TG) molecule, thereby producing free fatty acid (FFA) and 2-monoglyceride (MG); subsequent hydrolysis of the MG probably occurs only after isomerization of the fatty acid to the 1 position (Fig. 2). Pancreatic lipase acts at the oil-water interface of the emulsion droplets; the rate of hydrolysis is proportional to the interfacial area, with activity depending on the surface concentration of adsorbed enzyme and the surface concentration of sterically accessible triglyceride (1). Pancreatic lipase has little specificity for any particular TG, but the reaction rate is greater when the substrate is medium-chain TG (30). The effect of bile salts on PL remains controversial. They may inhibit PL by preventing the lipophilic bonding of PL to TG at the oil-water interface; this inhibition of PL by bile salts may be prevented by a heat-stable acidic polypeptide cofactor, colipase (mol wt 13,000) (4). On the other hand, bile salts may enhance the activity of PL by preventing the hydrophobic interactions between protein and lipid that might lead to denaturation and therefore

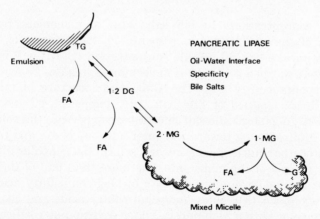

FIG. 2. Pancreatic lipase in the hydrolysis of triglycerides in the intestinal lumen. Hydrolysis of the 1 and 3 ester bonds begins at the oil-water interface of the emulsion droplets, and the end products of this reaction, in the presence of bile acids, form a mixed micelle. Abbreviations: TG, triglyceride; DG, diglyceride; MG, monoglyceride; FA, fatty acid; and G, glycerol.

inactivation of PL (5). Despite this dispute over in vitro findings, bile salts do not seem to be important for the in vivo activity of PL, since lipolysis proceeds rapidly in the absence of bile (42, 50), and lipolysis does not limit the rate of transport (27).

Dietary cholesterol is largely in the form of esters, and hydrolysis by pancreatic esterase proceeds optimally when the pH in the intestinal lumen is 6.6–8. Once the dietary and endogenous cholesterol has been absorbed into the mucosal cell, reesterification occurs. This proceeds at an optimal rate when the pH is 5–6.2. Most of the available information suggests that pancreatic and mucosal esterase are similar enzymes; note that pH conditions in the intestinal lumen favor hydrolysis of cholesterol esters, whereas in the mucosal cell the reaction proceeds in the opposite direction (31). There is evidence that bile salts can enhance both hydrolysis and esterification (66), possibly by a molecular interaction between bile salts and cholesterol esterase, leading to polymerization of the enzyme monomer to its active form (39). There is no substrate specificity for hydrolysis, but esterification occurs most readily when the unsaturated fatty acids oleic, linoleic, and linolenic are available as substrates, compared with the saturated fatty acids palmitic and stearic, and little esterification occurs in the presence of acids of shorter chain length (70).

As a result of the attack of the major pancreatic enzymes, monoglyceride, glycerol, cholesterol, lysolecithin, and fatty acids are released into the aqueous environment in the intestinal lumen (40). However, the water solubility of these end products of hydrolysis is very low, and only small amounts would be dissolved in the aqueous phase if bile acids were not present to bring about micellar solubilization.

Micellar Solubilization

At low concentrations the bile salts exist as monomers, but after the contraction of the gallbladder in response to the presence of food in the upper intestine the critical micelle concentration (CMC) will be exceeded, and negatively charged 30- to 100-Å molecular aggregates known as micelles will form spontaneously (71). The CMC and structure of micelles vary according to the species of bile salt, pH, temperature, and counterion concentration. In general bile salt micelles are spherical, the polar hydroxyl and amino groups facing toward the outer aqueous phase and the nonpolar steroid hydrocarbon nuclei facing inward to form the nonpolar interior of the micelle. At the pH of the upper intestine more than half of the fatty acids are in their ionized form since the pK_a of long-chain fatty acids in a bile micelle is about 6.5 (33). Since long-chain fatty acids and cholesterol are relatively unpolar with a high micelle:water partitioning coefficient, most of the end products of hydrolysis will be present in the bile acid micelle rather than in solution in the aqueous phase (34).

Bile acids are C_{24} carboxylic acids and are the end products of cholesterol metabolism. The chemical structures of the individual bile acids differ from each other in the number of α-hydroxyl groups linked to the nonpolar steroid nucleus at positions 3, 7, and 12 (Fig. 3). The trihydroxyl bile acid cholic acid has hydroxyl groups at positions 3, 7, and 12; chenodeoxycholic and deoxycholic acid have hydroxyl groups at 3 and 7 and at 3 and 12, respectively; lithocholic acid has a hydroxyl at the 3 position. In man the "primary" bile acids are those synthesized in the liver, and these include conjugates of cholic (40%) and chenodeoxycholic acid (40%). The "secondary" bile acids, deoxycholic and lithocholic acid, are produced in the intestinal lumen from bacterial 7α-dehydroxylation of the primary bile acids. Each of these bile acid species is present in human bile as peptide conjugates of the amino acids glycine and taurine. In the adult the glycine conjugates predominate (3:1), whereas the taurine conjugates predominate in the child. Conjugation results in a reduction of the value of the dissociation constants (pK_a) from pH 6.0 for the bile acids to pK_a 4 for the glycine and pK_a 2 for taurine conjugates. This renders them more soluble at the pH of the upper small intestine.

The bile salt molecules themselves are in rapid equilibrium between the micellar aggregate and the surrounding aqueous environment (6, 7); the small amount of fatty acid and sterol not dissolved in the micelle remains in the water phase and is in dynamic equilibrium with the lipids in the micelle. Thus the first important role of the bile acid micelle is to solubilize lipids.

Enterohepatic Circulation of Bile Salts

Since bile acid metabolism is central to the issue of lipid absorption, it is mandatory to consider the enterohepatic circulation of bile salts. Each day

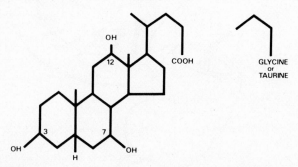

FIG. 3. Structure of primary (1°) and secondary (2°) bile acids. Hydroxyl groups are at the α-3, 7, or 12 position on the cholesterol molecule, and the different bile acid species are present in human bile as peptide conjugates of the amino acids glycine and taurine.

Hydroxyl Group	Name	
3–7–12	Cholic	} 1°
3–7	Chenodeoxycholic	
3–12	Deoxycholic	} 2°
3	Lithocholic	

approximately 0.5 g of the two primary bile acids, cholic acid and chenodeoxycholic acid, are synthesized by the liver from cholesterol (Fig. 4). After being conjugated with glycine or taurine, they are secreted from the hepatocyte into the canalicular bile. In the intestinal lumen some of the primary bile acids are acted on by bacterial enzyme systems, resulting in the secondary bile acids. The total bile acid pool in man is about 3 g, and this is stored in the gallbladder and delivered into the intestinal lumen when the gallbladder contracts during ingestion of a meal. As previously described, mixed micelles are formed, their contents are absorbed, and most of the bile salts are themselves subsequently absorbed in the terminal ileum by an active transport mechanism, but smaller amounts are taken up by both ionic and nonionic diffusion across the intestinal and colonic epithelium (57). The pool of bile acids circulates in this manner about 6 times daily, so that the liver secretes about 18 g of bile each day, even though the size of the bile salt pool is smaller and the amount of primary bile acids newly secreted

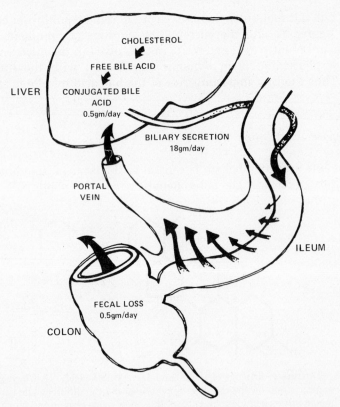

FIG. 4. Quantitative aspects of the enterohepatic circulation of bile salts in man. Each day about 3 g of primary and secondary bile acids are secreted by the hepatocyte and circulate 6–8 times, resulting in a total hepatic secretion of 12–18 g of bile acid into the proximal small intestine. This enterohepatic circulation is maintained by reabsorption of bile acids by an active transport mechanism in the terminal ileum and by both ionic and nonionic diffusion in the small and large intestine. Fecal loss of bile acids is usually matched by de novo synthesis of bile acids in the liver from cholesterol.

each day is even smaller still (2). Although there is an extremely efficient enterohepatic circulation, reabsorption is incomplete and about 5% of the circulating bile salts pass into the large intestine where they are degraded by the normal resident flora to the secondary bile salts (18, 63). Some of these bile salts are lost in the stools, and the daily 0.5-g fecal loss of bile salts is normally replaced by hepatic de novo synthesis of bile acids from cholesterol.

MUCOSAL UPTAKE OF LIPID

The general features of bile acid and fatty acid absorption have been known for some time (44) and it is generally appreciated that the bile acid uptake can occur against a chemical gradient in the ileum but not in the jejunum; that fatty acid uptake occurs at all levels of the small intestine; and that bile acid either facilitates lipid absorption, as is the case with long-chain fatty acids, or is absolutely required for intestinal uptake, as in the case of steroids such as cholesterol (23, 58). It remains debatable whether the mixed micelle crosses the intestinal brush border intact or whether the lipids of the micelle are absorbed independent of the bile acid constituents (28, 60, 79). Indeed, the mechanism of membrane translocation of lipids remains poorly understood, with such widely varying hypotheses as simple passive diffusion and a more complex process that involves binding to specific cell membrane receptor sites (48, 55, 58). Further consideration of the mechanism of lipid absorption must center around the role of the unstirred water layer and the bile acid micelle.

Intestinal Unstirred Water Layers

Only recently has it been appreciated that adjacent to all biological membranes there is a layer of relatively unstirred water through which movement of solute molecules is determined only by diffusional forces (8, 10). Such an unstirred water layer (UWL) exerts a major portion of the total resistance encountered by a probe molecule during its passage from the bulk extracellular water phase in the intestinal lumen into the cell interior (16, 86). This resistance is determined by three parameters: the effective thickness of the UWL, its effective surface area, and the free diffusion coefficient of the probe molecule in the UWL (73, 82). The effective thickness of this layer varies from 100 to 400 μm in various epithelial surfaces in vitro (32, 41), including gallbladder (14–16, 72), choroid plexus (85), cornea (29), frog skin (11), and intestine (19, 20, 73, 82). Preliminary results indicate that the UWL resistance is even greater in the in vivo perfused rat (84) and human jejunum (51).

The second dimension of the UWL is its effective surface area. For an anatomically simple, flat membrane, the surface of the UWL is equal to that of the underlying membrane. Because of the presence of villi and microvilli, however, the situation is somewhat more complex for the intestinal mucosa.

Here, the UWL lies both over and between the intestinal villi. The ratio of the effective surface area of the unstirred layer to that of the underlying mucosal cell is at least 1:500 (73, 82). Since solute molecules must first pass through the relatively small area of the UWL before reaching the much greater surface area of the villi and microvilli, the unstirred layer becomes an effective barrier to intestinal absorption. The importance of this barrier must be considered in relation to active and passive transport processes (Fig. 5). Failure to correct for the effect of the resistance of the UWL will lead to serious errors in the estimation of the true Michaelis constant (K_m) of active transport processes (25, 46, 47, 51, 52, 82, 83). These recent theoretical and experimental considerations have confirmed that the characteristics of the uptake of an actively transported molecule are a complex function of the resistance of both the UWL and the mucosal cell membrane. Indeed, there appear to be serious limitations in the interpretation of much of the previously published data dealing with active transport processes in the intestine, since these studies failed to account for the effect of the UWL.

It is now abundantly clear that the UWL also plays a major role in passive transport processes. Several recent studies (19, 25, 46, 47, 51, 52, 73, 80, 82–84) have clearly demonstrated that a UWL with the dimensions described above may offer sufficient resistance to constitute the major rate-limiting step for intestinal uptake of a number of passively transported probe molecules. For example, this unstirred diffusion barrier is of major importance in determining the rate of absorption of such physiologically

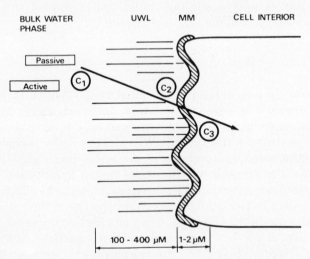

FIG. 5. Diagrammatic representation of pathway for absorption of a molecule from the bulk water phase in the intestinal lumen into the cell interior across the unstirred water layer (UWL) and through the microvillus membrane (MM) of the mucosal cell. Concentrations of a given probe molecule in the bulk water phase, adjacent to the aqueous-lipid membrane interface, and just beyond the microvillus membrane in the cell interior are given by C_1, C_2, and C_3, respectively. Approximate thickness of the UWL is between 100 and 400 μm (11, 14, 15, 19, 20, 29, 32, 41, 51, 72, 76, 81, 84, 85), compared with the relatively small thickness of the MM, 1–2 μm.

important molecules as long-chain fatty acids, saturated alcohols, bile acids, and cholesterol (22, 47, 73, 75). Let us consider the basis for this critically important observation.

As a molecule moves from the bulk water phase of the intestinal contents into the cell interior it must penetrate at least two membranes, a UWL adjacent to the aqueous-lipid interface and the lipid cell membrane itself. The UWL consists of a series of water lamellae extending outward from the cell membrane, each progressively more stirred, until they blend imperceptibly with the bulk water phase of the intestinal contents. Although the boundary between the well-mixed bulk water phase and UWL is not distinct, it can be assigned a finite functional thickness; this operational value is the equivalent thickness of a single layer in which transport occurs only by diffusion. The cell membrane itself usually is considered a bimolecular leaflet of lipid molecules associated in some manner with structural protein units (9). With passive transport, molecules must cross this membrane by passive diffusion through polar channels within the cell membrane or between adjacent cells, or by passive diffusion through the lipid sheet itself. In both types of passive transport net solute movement takes place only in the direction of the prevailing electrochemical gradient and is usually linear with respect to concentration of solute molecules in the bulk water phase. There is no competition between structurally related compounds and there is no inhibition of uptake by metabolic inhibitors, anoxia, or absence of electrolytes (35, 38, 54, 56, 59, 74, 75).

Since the two "membranes" (the UWL and the brush border) are in series, the rates and characteristics of absorption of such solutes as fatty acids are determined by the interaction of these two resistances. In a particular situation either the UWL or the lipid cell membrane may become primarily rate limiting to uptake. Movement across the UWL is a simple diffusion process in which the rate of movement is determined by the functional thickness of the UWL (d), the aqueous diffusion constant of the molecule (D) in the UWL, which is assumed to equal the free diffusion coefficient, and the concentration gradient between the bulk water phase and the lipid cell membrane. If C_1 and C_2 represent the concentrations of the molecule in the bulk water phase and at the aqueous-membane interface, respectively (Fig. 5), the flux of a probe molecule across the UWL (J) will be given by the formula:

$$J = (C_1 - C_2)\frac{D}{d} \qquad (1)$$

In the presence of significant UWL resistance the concentration of the probe molecule at the aqueous-membrane interface is reduced below the concentration of the molecule in the bulk phase; the magnitude of this reduction can be calculated by rearranging *equation 1* to give:

$$C_2 = C_1 - J\frac{(d)}{D} \qquad (2)$$

Once the molecule reaches the aqueous-membrane interface, the velocity of passive unidirectional flux across the cell surface is determined by the permeability coefficient for the molecule (P) and the concentration gradient across the lipid membrane. A lipid molecule has more free energy in an aqueous than in a lipid environment and so there is a tendency to pass from water to lipid. If C_2 and C_3 represent the concentrations of the molecule just outside and inside the membrane, respectively, then the flux of a probe molecule across the membrane will be given by the formula:

$$J = (C_2 - C_3)\, P \qquad\qquad (3)$$

Now, it is apparent that in a steady state the rate of movement of a molecule across these two membranes will be equal, and thus *equation 1* equals *equation 3*:

$$J = (C_1 - C_2)\frac{D}{d} = (C_2 - C_3)\, P \qquad\qquad (4)$$

In this equation the flux term J has the units of mass crossing unit area per unit time. Often the area of the diffusion membrane is unknown, and the experimentally determined flux rate Jd across an unstirred water layer or membrane of unknown surface area is related to some parameter of tissue mass that is assumed to bear a constant relationship to the surface area of the water layer or membrane. Commonly, Jd is normalized to wet or dry weight of tissue, unit length, or protein content. We have chosen the term Sm to represent the functional surface area of a given membrane relative to some other parameter such as tissue mass. The units of this term must correspond to the appropriate units of Jd. Similarly, we have chosen the term Sw to represent the functional surface area of the UWL, and it too must have units corresponding to those of Jd. Thus the term:

$$J = Jd/Sm \qquad\qquad (5)$$

corrects the experimentally measured flux to membrane surface area, and the term:

$$J = Jd/Sw \qquad\qquad (6)$$

corrects the experimentally measured flux to the surface area of the UWL overlying a particular membrane. Substituting *equations 5* and *6* into *equation 4*,

$$Jd = (C_1 - C_2)\frac{D}{d}\cdot Sw = (C_2 - C_3)\, P\cdot Sm \qquad\qquad (7)$$

The term D/d can be viewed as the "permeability coefficient" of the UWL, whereas P is the permeability coefficient for the "lipid" membrane.

For the movement of a molecule from the bulk intestinal contents into the interior of the mucosal cell, two extreme conditions may prevail: D/d may be very much larger than P, in which case the rate of movement across the cell membrane is rate limiting to absorption; alternatively, P may be very much larger than D/d, in which case the rate of diffusion across the UWL is rate limiting to cellular uptake.

UNSTIRRED LAYERS AS THE RATE-LIMITING "MEMBRANE" FOR MUCOSAL CELL UPTAKE OF CERTAIN HIGHLY PERMEANT MOLECULES

Let us consider the special circumstance where $P \gg D/d$ and the UWL becomes rate limiting to the overall uptake rate. In this case C_1 is much larger than C_2, $C_1 - C_2$ approaches C_1, and the rate of absorption into the cell is given by the formula:

$$Jd = \frac{C_1 \cdot D \cdot Sw}{d} \qquad (8)$$

This equation predicts that when diffusion is limited by the UWL: $a)$ Jd will be proportional to D for any given value of C_1, d, and Sw; and $b)$ the value Jd/D will vary directly with Sw and indirectly with d for any given value of C_1. These predictions have been borne out experimentally (82). As shown in Figure 6, the quantity Jd/D approaches a constant value when uptake of the longer chain-length members of the series was measured. Thus, in the unstirred situation the aqueous diffusion barrier is rate limiting for the absorption of the 8:0, 10:0, and 12:0 alcohols. In the stirred condition, only the uptake of the 10:0 and 12:0 alcohols was diffusion limited. Second, the mean value of Jd/D in the diffusion-limited situation is increased at least 10-fold by vigorous stirring, a change that would be anticipated if stirring reduced the effective value of d and increased that of Sw.

DETERMINATION OF PASSIVE PERMEABILITY COEFFICIENTS IN THE PRESENCE OF UNSTIRRED LAYERS

Previous work has suggested that fatty acid and steroid absorption in the intestine occurs by passive mechanisms, with a linear relationship between concentration and uptake, up to the limit of solubility in the micelle, no evidence of competition for uptake, a low Q_{10}, and failure of either metabolic inhibitors or glucose to affect uptake (35, 38, 54, 56, 59, 73, 75). Although most workers believe that the mucosal uptake of lipids occurs by a process of diffusion, for completeness it must be mentioned that there is some controversial evidence that this may be an energy-dependent process. Mishkin et al. (48) have shown that the initial uptake of micellar fatty acid may involve reversible binding to superficial sites such as the glycocalyx or microvillus membrane. Smith and co-workers (64, 65) have presented evidence that uptake into the mucosa of everted rat sacs occurs against a

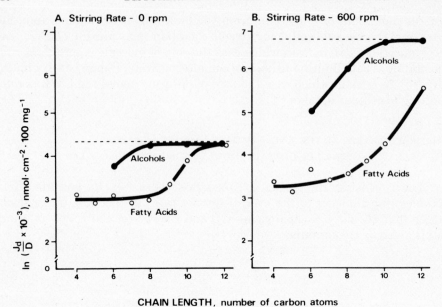

CHAIN LENGTH, number of carbon atoms

FIG. 6. Relationship between the rates of uptake of a homologous series of fatty acids and alcohols and the number of carbon atoms in each compound. In these 2 panels ln of the quantity $Jd/D \times 10^{-3}$ determined for a series of fatty acids and alcohols is plotted as a function of the chain length of each compound. A and B show such data in the unstirred and stirred (600 rpm) situation, respectively. In addition, the 2 limiting values have been calculated that denote the maximum rates of passive uptake at the 2 stirring rates that any compound can achieve: at these rates the UWL becomes absolutely rate limiting to absorption. [From Westergaard and Dietschy (73).]

concentration gradient, and Sylven (67) has shown that there is preferential uptake of cholesterol versus β-sitosterol in vivo and that this selectivity can be abolished by rendering the intestinal loop ischemic, by poisoning with cyanide, or by hypothermia. It is indeed possible, however, that these findings can best be explained by postulating that membrane permeability is dependent on energy supply. Nonetheless, the consensus of opinion suggests that the absorption of lipids takes place by a passive process (56).

Now let us consider the second extreme, where $D/d \gg P$, and the microvillus membrane becomes rate limiting to the overall uptake rate. In this case *equations 3* and *5* prevail and:

$$Jd = (C_2 - C_3) P \cdot Sm \qquad (9)$$

Since the lipid molecule is quickly metabolized within the cell or transported from it (40, 70), it is likely that $C_2 \gg C_3$, $C_2 - C_3$ approaches C_2, and:

$$Jd = C_2 \cdot P \cdot Sm \qquad (10)$$

The value of C_2 can be expressed in terms of C_1 by rearranging *equations 2* and *6*; thus:

$$Jd = (C_1 - C_2)\frac{D}{d} \cdot Sw \qquad (11)$$

and:

$$C_2 = C_1 - \frac{Jd \cdot d}{D \cdot Sw} \qquad (12)$$

Equation 12 is then substituted into *equation 10*, and:

$$Jd = C_1 - \frac{Jd \cdot d}{D \cdot Sw} \cdot P \cdot Sm \qquad (13)$$

It is essential to emphasize that the transport characteristics of a membrane are described in terms of the passive permeability coefficient (P). In the absence of an unstirred layer:

$$P = \frac{J}{C_1} \qquad (14)$$

and with the use of experimental values:

$$P = \frac{Jd/Sm}{C_1} \qquad (15)$$

However, in the presence of a UWL:

$$P = \frac{Jd/Sm}{C_2} \qquad (16)$$

The value of C_2 can be expressed in terms of C_1 with *equation 12*, and:

$$P = \frac{Jd/Sm}{C_1 - \dfrac{Jd \cdot d}{D \cdot Sw}} \qquad (17)$$

The magnitude of the experimentally determined membrane permeability coefficient (P^*) is determined from the relationship:

$$P^* = Jd/C_1 \qquad (18)$$

From consideration of *equations 17* and *18*, it is apparent that for any given membrane with fixed magnitude of Sm, and in the presence of an unstirred layer, the true membrane permeability P will be underestimated from the experimentally determined passive permeability coefficient by the magnitude of $Jd \cdot d/D \cdot Sw$. Thus, on the basis of these considerations, the magnitude of the error introduced into calculations of passive permeability coefficients, if unstirred layer resistance is ignored, is proportional to Jd and d and inversely proportional to Sw and D. These predictions are borne out by experimental data derived from studies in the intestine (73), where passive permeability coefficients were determined from a homologous series of saturated alcohols with chain lengths varying from 6 to 12 carbons.

The marked variation in rates of uptake of bile acid monomers, fatty acids, and fatty alcohols (73) brought about by relatively minor changes in chemical structure (Fig. 6) may be understood in terms of the factors that control the movement of molecules from the aqueous phase of the UWL to the lipid phase of the cell membrane. Diamond and Wright (16) have shown that permeability coefficients are proportional to the partitioning coefficient K for the molecule between these two phases; K is itself proportional to $e^{-\Delta Fw \rightarrow 1/RT}$, where $Fw \rightarrow 1$ is the free-energy change involved in transferring 1 mol of solute from the aqueous to the lipid phase, R is the gas constant, and T is the absolute temperature. It is impossible to determine absolute values for $\Delta Fw \rightarrow 1$, but it is possible to determine the incremental free energy of solution, i.e., the increment by which addition of a —CH_2— or —OH group changes the value of $\Delta Fw \rightarrow 1$. Thus, $\ln P$ is proportional to $\Delta Fw \rightarrow 1$ and, as shown in Figure 6, the value of P increases by approximately 1.52 for each carbon atom that is added to the hydrocarbon chain (73). From this relationship one can extrapolate and obtain permeability coefficients for the relatively insoluble long-chain fatty acids. Now, although the P values obtained by extrapolation are very high, such rates of uptake are never achieved, since diffusion of fatty acids across the UWL is slower than the potential rates of permeation across the lipid cell membrane, so that the UWL becomes rate limiting to absorption; this is demonstrated in Figure 6, in which the rate of uptake of the probe molecule reaches a limiting value for fatty acids of chain length 12 or greater.

Since unstirred layers clearly constitute a significant barrier to diffusion of solute molecules up to the microvillus border of the intestine, measurement of passive permeability coefficients in this organ therefore requires correction for UWL resistance in order to obtain reliable values denoting the passive permeability characteristics of the microvillus membrane. Therefore, the rate of flux of the probe molecule across the microvillus membrane appears to take place by a passive process in which the rate of flux of the compound across the microvillus membrane must be determined by its concentration at the aqueous-membrane interface times its appropriate permeability coefficient (73). However, the concentration of a hydrophobic molecule in the aqueous milieu of the intestinal lumen will itself be limited by its maximum solubility in water. With a homologous series of fatty acids, the addition of each —CH₂— group is associated with an increase in jejunal permeability by a factor of 1.52 (73), but solubility falls by a factor of approximately 2.32 (9). It follows that the product of passive permeability times maximum solubility declines, and the relative rate of mucosal absorption will fall with decreasing polarity and solubility (Fig. 7). If there were no UWL in the intestine, the maximum uptake that could be achieved for any lipid would equal the product of its passive permeability coefficient times the maximum aqueous solubility of that lipid. Since, in the case of the fatty acid series, maximum solubility decreases by a factor of 2.32 for each —CH₂— group added to the hydrocarbon chain, while the passive permeability coefficient increases by a factor of only 1.52, it follows that the value of the maximum uptake decreases for each carbon atom added to the fatty acid chain (Fig. 7). In the intestine, however, there is a UWL of significant dimensions, and the maximum uptake is reduced to the extent that this diffusion barrier exerts an additional resistance to the moelcular uptake. Thus, under conditions of constant thickness and surface area of the UWL, uptake will vary as a function of the passive permeability and free diffusion coefficients for a particular probe molecule. Consequently the maximum uptake observed in the presence of a UWL is considerably less for the more hydrophobic molecules than would be predicted if no UWL were present in the intestine (Fig. 7). Thus, in the presence of a UWL, the maximum rate of absorption will be described by a line below the theoretical line, and the deviation between these two lines represents a manifestation of UWL resistance. Note that this UWL effect is quantitatively unimportant for the polar members of

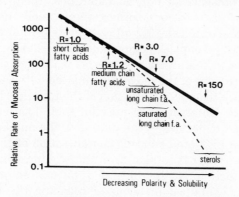

FIG. 7. Relative rates of mucosal absorption of lipid molecules of different polarity in the presence and absence of bile acid micelles. Solid line shows relative rate of intestinal mucosal cell uptake for compounds of differing polarity and solubility in the presence of bile acid micelles; dashed line shows the rates expected in the absence of bile acid. For each group of lipids the ratio R defines the degree to which the presence of bile acid micelles facilitates absorption. This ratio is close to 1 for short- and medium-chain-length fatty acids: i.e., bile acid micelles do not significantly enhance mucosal uptake of these compounds. The ratio progressively increases, however, with fatty acids of longer chain length and sterols so that the presence of bile acid micelles significantly enhances the uptake of these particular compounds into the intestinal mucosal cell. [From Westergaard and Dietschy (74, 75).]

the series but quantitatively very important for the less polar members of the series, such as long-chain fatty acids and cholesterol.

ROLE OF BILE ACID MICELLE IN LIPID ABSORPTION

Having established that fatty acid absorption occurs by passive mechanisms and that under physiological conditions it is the UWL and not the lipid cell membrane that is rate limiting to uptake of long-chain fatty acids and cholesterol, the next feature of fat absorption that requires clarification is the manner in which the addition of bile acid micelles to the bulk water phase enhances fat uptake into the intestinal absorptive cell. Lipids have low solubility in the bulk solution and because of very low free-energy changes associated with movement of these solutes from the aqueous to the membrane phase, they usually can passively penetrate cell membranes at very high rates. Indeed for such compounds the resistance encountered in crossing the unstirred layers may exceed that encountered in crossing the cell membrane itself, so that this diffusion barrier becomes absolutely rate limiting to cell uptake (54, 73). In various studies carried out in animals as well as in man it has been demonstrated that bile acids play an important role in facilitating the absorption of various dietary fats by the gastrointestinal tract. The micelle can solubilize very large amounts of fatty acid, monoglyceride, and sterol. There are quantitative differences, however, in the dependency of various lipids on the presence of micelles. Fatty acids of medium chain length, for example, are absorbed nearly as well in the absence as in the presence of bile acid micelles. As the chain length is increased the fatty acids become progressively more dependent on the presence of the bile acid micelle for efficient uptake into the mucosal cell, and in the case of very nonpolar compounds such as cholesterol essentially no absorption occurs in the absence of bile acids (23, 38, 40, 58, 62, 70, 78). Because of the greater size of the micelle, compared with the monomolecular species, the resistance to aqueous diffusion of the micelle will be higher than that of the monomer. However, with micellar solubilization the ratio of the number of solubilized molecules in the micelle to the number in monomolecular solution will be high, the aqueous concentration of the monomers will be high, and the net effect is to maintain a maximum monomer concentration. Thus, the function of the bile acid micelle in augmenting lipid absorption must be explained in terms of reducing the resistance of the UWL (Figs. 6 and 7). Furthermore such a formulation must explain the quantitative differences that exist in the dependency of different lipids on the presence of bile acids in the intestinal lumen for efficient absorption (Fig. 7).

In the presence of adequate amounts of pancreatic enzymes, long-chain fatty acids and free cholesterol are generated from dietary lipids and partitioned into bile acid micelles. These mixed micelles then diffuse toward the microvillus membrane at a rate determined by the unstirred layer resistance, $d/D \cdot Sw$. Since the lipolytic products exist in two phases at the membrane interface, i.e., dissolved as monomers in the aqueous phase and carried in the structure of the bile acid micelle, at least three different mechanisms may explain events that might occur during the uptake step.

Micellar Phase

The first possibility is that the micelle might be taken up into the cell intact. This seems unlikely since the various constituent molecules in the mixed micelle are absorbed at essentially independent rates, and the ratio for uptake of any two lipid solutes does not necessarily agree with the ratio in the micelle (12, 35, 36, 59, 61, 69, 77, 80), and therefore there is no evidence that the uptake step occurs through a process akin to pinocytosis.

Lipid-Protein Phase

The second possibility is that the bile acid micelle interacts with or binds to the microvillus membrane during a direct "collision" between the micelle and the cell membrane. The micelle and membrane presumably would interact in such a way that water is excluded from the interface between the two structures, after which the solubilized lipids would move directly into the cell but the bile acid component of the mixed micelle would return to the intestinal lumen. If this model correctly describes events during lipid absorption into the intestinal mucosal cell, then the rate of absorption would be proportional to the concentration or mass of fatty acid, monoglyceride, and cholesterol in the micellar phase. This model does not fit the data derived experimentally (75).

Aqueous Phase

Finally, the absorption of lipids solubilized in the micelle might occur from the monomer phase of these molecules, which are in rapid equilibrium with the aggregated molecules in the micelle, with no direct interaction between the micelle and the microvillus membrane. Thus, as lipid molecules are absorbed, they would be replaced by movement of other molecules from the bile acid micelle into the aqueous phase, with partitioning of lipid molecules from the micelle into the aqueous phase occurring more rapidly than uptake of the solutes into the mucosal cell. If this model is correct, then uptake is proportional to the mass of the lipid probe molecule in the aqueous phase. This formulation is predicted on the assumption that the various probe molecules exist in aqueous solution in the monomer form, for which there is abundant evidence (38, 53). Thus, the micelle would merely act as a solubilizer to convey the water-insoluble lipid molecule up to the cell surface, where the maximum monomer concentration would be maintained. Theoretical and experimental evidence suggests that this latter model is indeed correct (75):

1) Mw, and therefore the rate of unidirectional flux, increases linearly when the concentration of the probe molecule is increased while the concentration of the bile acid is kept constant (Fig. 8*A*); *2)* when the concentration of the bile acid is increased but that of the probe molecule is kept constant, there should be a reciprocal decrease in the mass of the lipid in the aqueous phase (Fig. 8*B*); *3)* when the concentration of both the bile acid and the probe molecule is increased in parallel, the mass of the lipid in the aqueous phase, *Mw*, should show only a slight initial rise and then remain essentially constant (Fig. 8*C*); *4)* greatly increasing the total concentration of FA 12:0 in solution by adding bile acid is associated with an increase in uptake that is no greater than would be predicted if the only function of the micelle was to overcome the resistance of the UWL and to maintain a maximum monomer concentration at the aqueous-membrane interface (9); *5)* finally, the close relationship between the experimentally measured maximum uptake rates and those predicted theoretically from the product of the passive permeability coefficient and the maximum aqueous solubility for a particular fatty acid

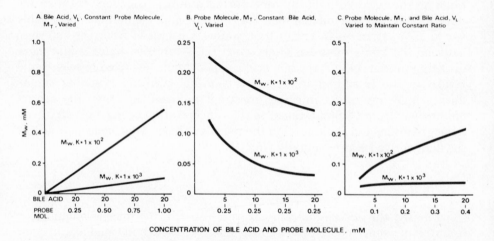

FIG. 8. Theoretical curves illustrating the manner in which the mass of a probe molecule in the water phase (*Mw*) varies under different experimental circumstances. Mass of the probe molecule in the water phase (*Mw*), as well as in the lipid phase (*M_L*), and therefore *Jd*, should increase linearly when the concentration of the lipid probe molecule is increased while the concentration of the micellar solvent is kept constant; this was the case for the probes FA 12:0, FA 16:0, and FA 18:0 (*A*). When the concentration of the bile acid is increased but that of the lipid probe molecule is kept constant, there should be a reciprocal decrease in *Mw*, as was observed experimentally for FA 16:0 (*B*); if the second model were correct (lipid-protein phase), then there should be a curvilinear increase in *M_L*, which did not occur. This decrease in *Jd* with increasing concentration of bile acids may be explained by the decreased monomolecular concentration in equilibrium with the micelles, since the excess of micellar solution renders the micelle relatively unsaturated with lipid. For FA 18:0, *Mw* showed only a slight initial rise and then remained essentially constant (*C*), as predicted for uptake from an obligatory aqueous rather than lipid phase. Accurate partition coefficients, *K*, for the long-chain fatty acids are unknown, and these curves were generated (9) with 2 arbitrary values of *K*. [The derivation of these curves is given by Westergaard and Dietschy (75).]

(75) strongly argues that uptake of long-chain fatty acids occurs from the aqueous phase.

If the function of the bile acid micelle is to overcome the resistance of the UWL and to maintain the maximum possible monomer concentration at the aqueous-membrane interface, then the relative effect of the bile acid micelle in facilitating uptake of a particular lipid is directly related to the magnitude of the resistance encountered by that molecule in crossing the UWL. The magnitude of this effect has been determined (75) by taking the rates of uptake in the presence and in the absence of bile acid. Thus, the presence of bile acid has little effect on the uptake of FAs 4:0–10:0, has a moderate effect on FAs of medium chain length, and has a more marked effect on long-chain FAs and cholesterol. Thus, in the absence of the micelle, short- and medium-chain-length FAs are absorbed at essentially normal rates, there is a moderate degree of malabsorption of long-chain-length FAs, and there is essentially no absorption of very polar compounds like cholesterol. These findings correlate well with the theoretical predictions indicated in Figures 7 and 8 and with observations made in intact animals and in man (26, 38, 50, 62, 70).

INTESTINAL TRANSPORT OF BILE ACIDS

Since the intestinal transport of bile acids is itself a key to the maintenance of a normal enterohepatic circulation (Fig. 4), it is necessary to consider the characteristics of the active and passive transport mechanisms for bile acids.

Active Transport of Bile Acids Across the Ileum

Bile acid absorption across the ileum appears to be by a carrier-mediated, energy-linked transport system that by current criteria must be considered an active process (21, 37, 43–45, 49). The demonstration of competitive inhibition of the active transport of one bile acid by another structurally related bile acid strongly suggests that ileal absorption of different bile acids occurs via a single transport system. Schiff, Small, and Dietschy (57), however, have shown in an in vitro preparation of rat intestine that the kinetic parameters of this system are quite different for the various bile acids: a) the V_{max} is greatly influenced by the number of hydroxyl groups on the steroid nucleus, with the trihydroxyl bile acids having the highest maximal transport rate and the monohydroxyl bile acids having the lowest rate; b) the magnitude of the apparent affinity constant $K_m{}^*$ of each bile acid is lower for the conjugated than for the unconjugated bile acids and is lower for those bile acids with the lower V_{max}. The influence of V_{max} on the magnitude of $K_m{}^*$ is likely related in part to the effect of the UWL (68), but the possibility cannot be excluded that there may be more than one transport system for bile acids in the ileum.

We have considered the profound effect of other UWLs on passive transport processes. What effect does the UWL have on active transport? For active transport processes, failure to correct for the effect of the resistance of the UWL will lead to serious errors in the estimation of both the true Michaelis constant (K_m) and the maximal transport rate (J_m). Under the circumstances of active absorption, the experimentally determined unidirectional flux across the cell membrane is given by expressions describing two components: the first component gives the magnitude of the active flux and the second component gives the magnitude of the passive flux (80). The active component must be derived by subtracting the passive flux from the experimentally determined values. This in turn requires accurate values for the appropriate permeability coefficients. As previously considered, the UWL results in an underestimation of passive permeation, and thus the correction for the contribution of the passive component to the total experimentally determined absorption process is too low. This in turn leads to an overestimation of the maximal transport rate (J_m) of the membrane carrier. Since the estimation of the apparent Michaelis constant (K_m^*) of an active transport process requires careful delineation of J_m, errors in J_m resulting from inappropriate correction of the passive component will in themselves lead to errors in the estimation of K_m.

In addition, it is likely that the UWL has a profound effect on the kinetic parameters of active transport processes themselves. An equation has been derived that predicts the effect of several variables on the observed velocity of active transport in a given experimental circumstance (68). Three of these variables $(d$, effective thickness of the UWL; Sw, effective area of the UWL; and D, free-diffusion coefficient of the probe molecule) are the direct consequence of the presence of the UWL, while the remaining three variables $(K_m$, true Michaelis constant; J_m, observed maximal transport rate, contributed by each of n segments of the villus) are derived from properties of the membrane. By substituting physiologically appropriate values for each of these variables into this equation, it has been possible to predict the manner in which variation in each parameter influences the kinetic curves for active transport. For example (Fig. 9), variations in the magnitude of the resistance of UWL, produced by varying the dimensions of the effective thickness or surface area of the UWL, has a profound effect on the magnitude of the estimate of K_m^* but not J_m. Early experimental work has fully substantiated these theoretical considerations and has confirmed that the true affinity constant of the membrane carrier for D-glucose is much less than predicted from the K_m^* values obtained at different stirring rates (Fig. 9). Thus failure to correct for the effect of the UWL clearly is likely to result in a major quantitative as well as qualitative error in the estimation of kinetic parameters of intestinal transport processes. This is particularly important since in almost all previous work dealing with transport in the gastrointestinal tract it has been assumed that the kinetic parameters describing the active uptake of a particular solute reflect the properties of the membrane transport carrier itself. However, it is now apparent that the characteristics of uptake of a molecule are a complex function of the

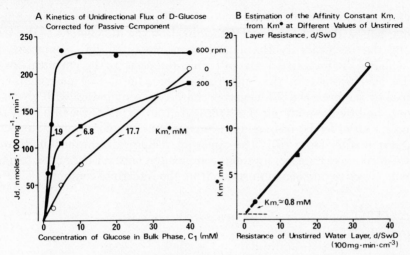

FIG. 9. Estimation of the true Michaelis constant for active transport of D-glucose. A: three theoretical curves obtained when $d/Sw \cdot D$ was varied from 1 to 500 100 mg/min per cm³. In these calculations $J_d{}^m$ was 100 nmol/100 mg per min and K_m was 1 mM. B: values of $K_m{}^*$, shown in A, were then plotted as a function of the effective resistance offered by the unstirred layer $(d/Sw \cdot D)$. It is evident from this plot that when $d/Sw \cdot D$ equals zero, $K_m{}^*$ equals K_m. Thus, by experimentally determining $K_m{}^*$ at various values of $d/Sw \cdot D$, it becomes possible to extrapolate to zero resistance and thereby obtain an estimate of the true Michaelis constant of the transport process. [From Thomson and Dietschy (68).]

resistances offered by at least two membranes in series, the unstirred water layer and the microvillus membrane. Therefore, the experimentally determined transport kinetics describe the characteristics of a membrane carrier only under the special circumstances where the resistance of the UWL approaches zero. It must be stressed that all currently available evidence indicates that this special circumstance is never achieved in any type of preparation that has been utilized for the study of transport in the gastrointestinal tract. Indeed, in vivo the dimensions of the UWL are probably so large that transport reflects the magnitude of the resistance of the UWL and not the characteristics of the membrane transport process. Furthermore, even in highly stirred in vitro preparations, UWL resistance is still very significant, and therefore this barrier will markedly influence the observed kinetic characteristics of active transport processes. Thus there are serious limitations in the interpretation of much of the previously published data dealing with active transport processes in the intestine, including that related to bile salts, since these studies failed to account for the effect of the UWL. Since the kinetic parameters are significantly distorted by the presence of the UWL, then many of the conclusions drawn on the basis of these data must be reevaluated.

Passive Transport of Bile Acids Across Small Bowel and Colon

Bile acids are passively absorbed in the jejunum and colon (17, 21, 44), and in addition there is a passive transport component superimposed on the active transport system in the colon (37, 57). The kinetic relationships of passive bile acid absorption are determined by the dimensions of the UWL and by the permeability characteristics of the lipid cell membrane; the permeability characteristics are in turn influenced by the chemical species of bile acid present in the bulk phase. In general (57) permeability is reduced by the presence of a negative charge, by conjugation with glycine or taurine, and by the addition of a hydroxyl group. Thus those bile acids that are poorly absorbed by passive diffusion are more readily absorbed by active transport in the ileum (57). The apparent reciprocal relationship between active and passive transport systems complement one another and so together promote effective bile acid absorption from the intestinal contents.

Effect of UWL on Uptake of Bile Acids from
Solutions Containing Micelles

The UWL has a profound effect on the unidirectional flux of fatty acid and cholesterol in the intestine (Figs. 6 and 7). There are several lines of evidence that the UWL may also be rate limiting for the uptake of bile acids from micellar solutions (19). First, the rate of uptake of a bile acid ceases to increase in a linear relationship to the concentration of bile acid in the bulk water phase once the critical micelle concentration is achieved. Second, stirring the bulk phase enhances bile acid uptake from micellar solutions to a much greater degree than from monomer solutions. Third, expanding the size of the bile acid micelle with another amphipath depresses bile acid uptake, but stirring again greatly increases uptake from any particular solution of mixed micelles. Together these findings suggest that the UWL exerts a major resistance to the passive uptake of bile acids from solutions containing bile acid micelles. Thus the UWL is a major determinant of uptake of bile acids from micellar solutions; the UWL exerts a modest influence on uptake from monomer solutions of nonpolar bile acids with very high permeability coefficients, and the UWL has essentially no effect on absorption from monomer solutions of very polar bile acids.

REESTERIFICATION, CHYLOMICRON SYNTHESIS, AND RELEASE

Once the contents of the mixed micelle have been discharged and absorbed, the long-chain fatty acids are activated to their CoA derivative by the enzyme fatty acid:CoA lipase. The activated long-chain FA thioesters are then esterified to triglycerides either by the monoglyceride or the L-α-glycerophosphate pathway (40). Cholesterol is similarly reesterified in the soluble fraction of the mucosal cell by acylation with long-chain fatty acids in the presence of cholesterol esterase. The resynthesized triglycerides, phospholipids, and cholesterol esters are combined with free cholesterol, and a small amount of a specific protein synthesized in the microsomes, to form the final products of fat absorption, chylomicrons and very-low-density lipoproteins (VLDL). The mechanism by which chylomicrons and VLDL are transported out of the mucosal cells is still poorly understood. However, once outside the cells they diffuse to central lacteals and then are transported to the peripheral circulation by way of the thoracic duct, to be utilized or stored in the body.

CLINICAL APPLICATION OF PHYSIOLOGICAL PRINCIPLES
OF FAT ABSORPTION

Fat malabsorption may be caused by a host of different diseases that produce a defect in any one of several physiological steps (Fig. 1). Any disease that causes significant reduction of pancreatic exocrine tissue such as chronic pancreatitis, cancer of the pancreas, or mucoviscidosis may result in insufficient secretion of pancreatic lipase, as well as other pancreatic enzymes, so that during a meal defective lipolysis ensues. Since undigested triglycerides are poorly solubilized in the bile acid micelles, severe steatorrhea results.

Since bile acids form micelles that enhance the rate of fat absorption, an insufficient intraluminal bile acid concentration during a meal may result in mild steatorrhea. Extrahepatic or intrahepatic biliary obstruction, intestinal stasis, or ileal resection or disease commonly lead to insufficient micellar solubilization, with steatorrhea. The reasons for steatorrhea developing in patients with biliary obstruction is self-evident. The intestinal stasis syndrome may arise from a variety of causes, each of which is associated with massive overgrowth of anaerobic bacteria, which are capable of deconjugation and dehydroxylation of bile acids. Since unconjugated bile acids either precipitate or are rapidly absorbed from the proximal small intestine or colon, there is a marked decrease in the effective concentration of bile acids in the intestinal lumen, below the critical micellar concentration, and micelles are not formed.

The UWL is a physiological event in search of a pathological entity. It is possible, though unproved, that in diseases such as scleroderma and diabetes mellitus, where there is hypomotility of the small intestine, there may be an increased UWL resistance and hence steatorrhea. The degree to which changes in UWL resistance may be instrumental in the production of steatorrhea in these and other diseases is currently unknown. It is of interest to speculate that the reduction in the apparent magnitude of the UWL resistance in patients with celiac disease (51) represents a compensatory mechanism to partially counter the deleterious effects of loss of mucosal surface area of the small bowel, as well as possible loss of the biochemical integrity of the mucosal cells.

Defective chylomicron formation occurs in the rare congenital disease abetalipoproteinemia. As a result of the inability of the mucosal cell to synthesize the protein moiety associated with chylomicrons, triglycerides accumulate in the mucosal cells. A defect in chylomicron transport from the mucosal cell into the lymphatics occurs in diseases that block these channels.

On this basis, moderate steatorrhea occurs in intestinal lymphangiectasia, in retroperitoneal fibrosis or lymphoma, and in Crohn's disease. Thus, fat absorption is a complex process, but knowledge of the basic physiology of this process will allow the clinician to follow a more rational approach to the investigation and diagnosis of patients with steatorrhea.

SUMMARY

It is proposed that lipid absorption occurs according to the following model (Fig. 10): in the intestinal lumen, fatty acids and free cholesterol are released as a result of the activity of pancreatic enzymes acting at the surface of lipid emulsions. These lipolytic products partition into the bile acid micelles, forming mixed micelles that diffuse down their concentration gradient, across the UWL, and up the aqueous-membrane interface of the microvillus membrane. In the presence of the micelle the monomer concentration at this interface is maintained at a maximum concentration, which is that of a saturated monomolecular solution. The lipids are passively absorbed from their monomer phase; the rate of uptake is thus determined by the aqueous concentration of the molecule present at the microvillus surface, as well as by the membrane passive permeability coefficient appropriate for each lipid. A large concentration gradient across the membrane is provided both by the constant partitioning of fatty acid and cholesterol out

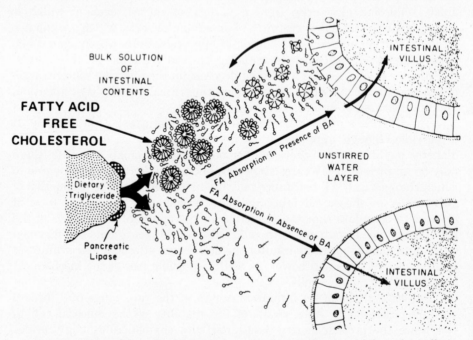

FIG. 10. Model of the role of intestinal unstirred water layer and bile acid micelle in absorption of lipid. [Modified from Westergaard and Dietschy (74).]

of the mixed micelle and by the rapid esterification of the lipid once inside the mucosal cell. Bile acid monomers will also be in equilibrium with the mixed micelles; since the rate of mucosal uptake of these bile acids is low in the proximal intestine, these molecules will diffuse back into the bulk phase in the intestinal lumen, where they will be utilized for the creation of new mixed micelles as additional amounts of free cholesterol and fatty acids are generated from hydrolysis of dietary lipids. Thus, the principal role of the bile acid micelle in facilitating lipid absorption is to solubilize large amounts of lipids, to overcome the resistance of the UWL, and to provide a vehicle from which lipids are partitioned into a monomer phase prior to their passive absorption into the mucosal cell.

REFERENCES

1. BENZONANA, G. AND P. DESNUELLE. Etude cinetique de l'action de la lipase pancreatique sur les triglycerides en emulsion. Essai d'une enzymologue en milieu heterogene. *Biochim. Biophys. Acta* 105: 121–136, 1965.
2. BERGSTRÖM, S., AND H. DANIELSSON. Formation and metabolism of bile acids. In: *Handbook of Physiology. Alimentary Canal.* Washington, D.C.: Am. Physiol. Soc., 1968, sect. 6, vol. V, p. 2391–2407.
3. BORGSTROM, B. Influence of bile salt, pH, and time on the action of pancreatic lipase; physiological implications. *J. Lipid Res.* 5: 522–531, 1964.
4. BORGSTROM, B., AND C. ERLANSON. Pancreatic juice co-lipase. *Biochim. Biophys. Acta* 242: 509–513, 1971.
5. BROCKERHOFF, H. On the function of bile salts and proteins as cofactors of lipase. *J. Biol. Chem.* 246: 5828–5831, 1971.
6. CAREY, M. C., AND D. M. SMALL. The characteristics of mixed micellar solutions with particular reference to bile. *Am. J. Med.* 49: 590–608, 1970.
7. CAREY, M. C., AND D. M. SMALL. Micelle formation by bile salts. *Arch. Internal Med.* 130: 506–527, 1972.
8. COLLANDER, R. The permeability of nitella cells and non-electrolytes. *Physiol. Plant Pathol.* 7: 420–445, 1954.
9. CULLITON, B. J. Cell membranes: a new look at how they work. *Science* 175: 1348–1350, 1972.
10. DAINTY, J. Water relations of plant cells. *Advan. Botany Res.* 1: 279–326, 1963.
11. DAINTY, J., AND F. R. HOUSE. Unstirred layers in frog skin. *J. Physiol., London* 182: 66–78, 1966.
12. DAWSON, A. M., AND J. P. W. WEBB. Oleic acid absorption from micellar solutions and emulsions in the rat. *Proc. Soc. Exptl. Biol. Med.* 142: 906–908, 1973.
13. DESNUELLE, P., AND P. SAVARY. Specificities of lipases. *J. Lipid Res.* 4: 369–384, 1963.
14. DIAMOND, J. M. A rapid method for determining voltage-concentration relations across membranes. *J. Physiol., London* 183: 83–100, 1966.
15. DIAMOND, J. M., AND E. M. WRIGHT. Molecular forces governing non-electrolyte permeation through cell membranes. *Proc. Roy. Soc. London, Ser. B* 172: 273–316, 1969.
16. DIAMOND, J. M., AND E. M. WRIGHT. Biological membranes: the physical basis of ion and non-electrolyte selectivity. *Ann. Rev. Physiol.* 31: 581–646, 1969.
17. DIETSCHY, J. M. Mechanisms for the intestinal absorption of bile acids. *J. Lipid Res.* 9: 297–309, 1968.
18. DIETSCHY, J. M. The biology of bile acids. *Arch. Internal Med.* 130: 473, 1972.
19. DIETSCHY, J. M. Mechanisms of bile acid and fatty acid absorption across the unstirred water layer and brush border of the intestine. *Helv. Med. Acta* 37: 89–102, 1973.
20. DIETSCHY, J. M., V. L. SALLE, AND F. A. WILSON. Unstirred water layers and absorption across the intestinal mucosa. *Gastroenterology* 61: 932–934, 1971.
21. DIETSCHY, J. M., H. S. SALOMON, AND M. D. SIPERSTEIN. Bile acid metabolism. I. Studies on the mechanisms of intestinal transport. *J. Clin. Invest.* 45: 832–846, 1966.
22. DIETSCHY, J. M., AND H. WESTERGAARD. The effect of unstirred water layers on various transport processes in the intestine. In: *Intestinal Absorption and Malabsorption,* edited by T. Z. Csaky. New York: Raven, 1975, p. 197–207.
23. DIETSCHY, J. M., AND J. D. WILSON. Regulation of cholesterol metabolism. *New Engl. J. Med.* 282:1128–1138, 1241–1249, 1970.
24. DREHER, K. D., J. H. SCHULMAN, AND A. F. HOFMANN. Surface chemistry of the monoglyceride-bile salt system. *J. Colloid Interface Sci.* 25: 71–83, 1967.
25. DUGAS, M. C., K. RAMASWAMY, AND R. K. CRANE. An analysis of the d-glucose influx kinetics of *in vitro* hamster jejunum, based on considerations of the mass-transfer coefficient. *Biochim. Biophys. Acta* 383: 576–589, 1975.
26. FERNANDES, J., J. H. CAN DE KAMER, AND H. A. WEIJERS. Differences in absorption of the various fatty acids studied in children with steatorrhea. *J. Clin. Invest.* 41: 488–494, 1962.
27. GALLAGHER, N., J. WEBB AND A. M. DAWSON. The absorption of 14C-oleic acid and 14C-triolein in bile fistula rats. *Clin. Sci.* 29: 75–82, 1965.
28. GORDON, S. G., P. B. MINER, JR., AND F. KERN, JR. Characteristics of conjugated bile salt absorption by hamster jejunum. *Biochim. Biophys. Acta* 248: 333–342, 1971.
29. GREEN, K., AND T. OTOU. Direct measurements of membrane unstirred layers. *J. Physiol., London* 207: 93–102, 1970.
30. GREENBERGER, N. J., J. B. RODGERS, AND K. J. ISSELBACHER. Absorption of medium and long chain triglycerides. Factors influencing their hydrolysis and transport. *J. Clin. Invest.* 45: 217–227, 1966.
31. HERANDEX, H. H., AND I. L. CHAIKOFF. Purification and properties of pancreatic cholesterol esterase. *J. Biol. Chem.* 228: 447–457, 1975.

32. HINGSON, D. J., AND J. M. DIAMOND. Comparison of nonelectrolyte permeability patterns in several epithelia. *J. Membrane Biol.* 10: 93–135, 1972.

33. HOFMANN, A. F. Functions of bile in the alimentary canal. In: *Handbook of Physiology. Alimentary Canal.* Washington, D.C.: Am. Physiol. Soc., 1968, sect. 6, vol. V, p. 2507–2533.

34. HOFMANN, A. F. The function of bile salts in fat absorption. *Biochem. J.* 69: 57–68, 1963.

35. HOFFMAN, N. E. The relationship between uptake in vitro of oleic acid and micellar solubilization. *Biochim. Biophys. Acta* 196: 193–203, 1970.

36. HOFFMAN, N. E., AND V. J. YEOH. The relationship between concentration and uptake by rat small intestine in vitro for two micellar solutes. *Biochim. Biophys. Acta* 233: 49–52, 1971.

37. HOLT, P. R. Intestinal absorption of bile salts in the rat. *Am. J. Physiol.* 207: 1–7, 1964.

38. HOLT, P. R. Medium chain triglycerides. *Disease-a-Month* June: 3–30, 1971.

39. HYUN, J., N. STEINBERG, C. R. TREADWELL, AND G. V. VAHOUNY. Cholesterol esterase—a polymeric enzyme. *Biochim. Biophys. Res. Commun.* 44: 819–825, 1971.

40. JOHNSTON, J. M. Mechanism of fat absorption. In: *Handbook of Physiology. Alimentary Canal.* Washington, D.C.: Am. Physiol. Soc., 1968, sect. 6, vol. III, p. 1353–1375.

41. KIDDER, G. W. III. Unstirred layer in tissue respiration: application to studies of frog gastric mucosa. *Am. J. Physiol.* 219: 1789–1795, 1970.

42. KNOBEL, L. K., AND J. H. RYAN. Digestion and mucosal absorption of fat in normal and bile deficient dogs. *Am. J. Physiol.* 200: 313–317, 1963.

43. LACK, L. Some recent observations concerning ileal bile salt transport. In: *Bile Salt Metabolism,* edited by L. Schiff, J. B. Carey, Jr., and J. M. Dietschy. Springfield, Ill.: Thomas, 1969, p. 25.

44. LACK, L., AND I. M. WEINER. In vitro absorption of bile salts by small intestine of rats and guinea pigs. *Am. J. Physiol.* 200: 313–317, 1961.

45. LACK, L., AND I. M. WEINER. The intestinal action of benzmalecene: the relationship of its hypocholesterolemic effect to active transport of bile salts and other substances. *J. Pharmacol. Exptl. Therap.* 139: 248–258, 1963.

46. LEWIS, L. D., AND J. S. FORDTRAN. Effect of perfusion rate on absorption, surface area, unstirred water layer thickness, permeability and intraluminal pressure in rat ileum *in vivo. Gastroenterology* 68: 1509–1516, 1975.

47. LUKIE, B. E., H. WESTERGAARD, AND J. M. DIETSCHY. Validation of a chamber that allows measurement of both tissue uptake rates and unstirred layer thicknesses in the intestine under conditions of controlled stirring. *Gastroenterology* 67: 652–661, 1974.

48. MISHKIN, S., M. YALOVSKY, AND J. I. KESSLER. Stages of uptake and incorporation of micellar palmitic acid by hamster proximal intestinal mucosa. *J. Lipid Res.* 13: 155–168, 1972.

49. PLAYOUST, M. R., AND K. J. ISSELBACHER. Studies on the transport and metabolism of conjugated bile salts by intestinal mucosa. *J. Clin. Invest.* 43: 467–476, 1964.

50. PORTER, H. P., D. R. SAUNDERS, G. TYTGAT, O. BRUNSER, AND C. E. RUBIN. Fat absorption in the bile fistula man. A morphological and biochemical study. *Gastroenterology* 60: 1008–1019, 1971.

51. READ, N. W., R. J. LEVEN, AND C. D. HOLDSWORTH. Measurement of the functional unstirred layer thickness in the human jejunum in vivo. *Gut* 17: 387, 1976.

52. REY, F., F. DRILLET, J. SCHMITZ, AND J. REY. Influence of flow rate on the kinetics of the intestinal absorption of glucose and lysine in children. *Gastroenterology* 66: 79–85, 1974.

53. SALLEE, V. L. Apparent monomer activity of saturated fatty acids in micellar bile salt solutions measured by a polyethylene partitioning system. *J. Lipid Res.* 15: 56–64, 1974.

54. SALLEE, V. L., AND J. M. DIETSCHY. Determinants of intestinal mucosal uptake of short- and medium-chain fatty acids and alcohol. *J. Lipid Res.* 14: 475–484, 1973.

55. SALLEE, V. L., AND J. M. DIETSCHY. The role of bile acid micelles in absorption of fatty acids across the intestinal brush border. *J. Clin. Invest.* 50: 80a, 1972.

56. SALLEE, V. L., F. A. WILSON, AND J. M. DIETSCHY. Determination of unidirectional uptake rates for lipids across the intestinal brush border. *J. Lipid Res.* 13: 184–192, 1972.

57. SCHIFF, E. R., N. C. SMALL, AND J. M. DIETSCHY. Characterization of the kinetics of the passive and active transport mechanisms for bile acid absorption in the small intestine and colon. *J. Clin. Invest.* 51: 1351–1362, 1972.

58. SENIOR, J. R. Intestinal absorption of fats. *J. Lipid Res.* 5: 495–521, 1964.

59. SIMMONDS, W. J. The role of micellar solubilization in lipid absorption. *Australian J. Exptl. Biol. Med. Sci.* 50: 403–421, 1972.

60. SIMMONDS, W. J., A. F. HOFMANN, AND E. THEODOR. Absorption of cholesterol from a micellar solution: intestinal perfusion studies in man. *J. Clin. Invest.* 46: 874–890, 1967.

61. SIMMONDS, W. J., T. G. REDGRAVE, AND R. L. S. WILLIX. Absorption of oleic and oleic and palmitic acids from emulsions and micellar solutions. *J. Clin. Invest.* 47: 1015–1025, 1968.

62. SIPERSTEIN, M. D., I. L. CHAIKOFF, AND W. O. REINHARDT. C^{14}-cholesterol. V. Obligatory function of bile in intestinal absorption of cholesterol. *J. Biol. Chem.* 198: 111–114, 1952.

63. SMALL, D. M. The enterohepatic circulation of bile salts. *Arch. Internal Med.* 130: 552, 1972.

64. SMITH, A. L., R. HAUK, AND F. R. TREADWELL. Uptake of cholesterol and cholesterol esters by inverted sacs of rat intestine. *Am. J. Physiol.* 193: 34–40, 1958.

65. SMITH, A. L., AND C. R. TREADWELL. Effect of bile acids and other factors on cholesterol uptake by inverted intestinal sacs. *Am. J. Physiol.* 195: 773–778, 1958.

66. SWELL, A. L., H. FIELD, AND C. R. TREADWELL. Role of bile salts in activity of cholesterol esterase. *Proc. Soc. Exptl. Biol. Med.* 84: 417–420, 1953.

67. SYLVEN, C. Influence of blood supply on lipid uptake from micellar solutions by the rat small intestine. *Biochim. Biophys. Acta* 203: 365–375, 1970.

68. THOMSON, A. R. B., AND J. M. DIETSCHY. Derivation of the equations that describe the effects of unstirred water layers on the kinetic parameters of active transport processes in the intestine. *J. Theoret. Biol.* 64: 277–294, 1977.

69. THORNTON, A. G., G. U. VAHOUNY, AND C. R. TREADWELL. Absorption of lipids form mixed micellar bile salt solutions. *Proc. Soc. Exptl. Biol. Med.* 127: 629–000, 1968.

70. TREADWELL, C. R., AND G. V. VAHOUNY. Cholesterol absorption. In: *Handbook of Physiology. Alimentary Canal.* Washington, D.C.: Am. Physiol. Soc., 1968, sect. 6, vol. III, p. 1407–1438.

71. VAN DEEST, B. W., J. S. FORDTRAN, S. G. MORAWSKI, AND J. D. WILSON. Bile salt and micellar fat

concentration in proximal small bowel contents of ileectomy patients. *J. Clin. Invest.* 47: 1314, 1968.

72. WEDNER, H. J., AND J. M. DIAMOND. Contributions of unstirred layer effects to apparent electrokinetic phenomena in the gallbladder. *J. Membrane Biol.* 1: 92–108, 1969.

73. WESTERGAARD, H., AND J. M. DIETSCHY. Delineation of the dimensions and permeability characteristics of the two major diffusion barriers to passive mucosal uptake in the rabbit intestine. *J. Clin. Invest.* 54: 718–732, 1974.

74. WESTERGAARD, H, AND J. M. DIETSCHY. Normal mechanisms of fat absorption and derangements induced by various gastrointestinal diseases. *Med. Clin. North Am.* 58: 1413–1427, 1974.

75. WESTERGAARD, H., AND J. M. DIETSCHY. The mechanism whereby bile acid micelles increase the rate of fatty acid and cholesterol uptake into the intestinal mucosal cell. *J. Clin. Invest.* 58: 97–108, 1976.

76. WESTERGAARD, H., AND J. M. DIETSCHY. Structure of the unstirred water layer (UWL) in the intestine (abstr.). *Clin. Res.* 20: 736, 1972.

77. WILLIX, R. L. S. Solute fluxes in fat absorption. *J. Pharm. Sci.* 59: 1439–1444, 1970.

78. WILSON, F. A., AND J. M. DIETSCHY. Differential diagnostic approach to clinical problems of malabsorption. *Gastroenterology* 61: 911–931, 1971.

79. WILSON, F. A., AND J. M. DIETSCHY. The role of micelle uptake during bile acid and fat absorption by the intestinal mucosa. *Clin. Res.* 19: 406, 1971.

80. WILSON, F. A., AND J. M. DIETSCHY. Characterization of bile acid absorption across the unstirred water layer and brush border of the rat jejunum. *J. Clin. Invest.* 51: 3015–3025, 1972.

81. WILSON, F. A., AND J. M. DIETSCHY. The effect of unstirred layer on the kinetics of active transport in the rat intestine (abstr.). *Clin. Res.* 20: 783, 1972.

82. WILSON, F. A., AND J. M. DIETSCHY. The intestinal unstirred layer: its surface area and effect on active transport kinetics. *Biochim. Biophys. Acta* 363: 112–126, 1974.

83. WINNE, D. Unstirred layer, source of biased Michaelis constant in membrane transport. *Biochim. Biophys. Acta* 298: 27–31, 1973.

84. WINNE, D. Unstirred layer thickness in perfused rat jejunum in vivo. *Experientia* 32: 1278–1279, 1976.

85. WRIGHT, E. M. The permeability of the frog choroid plexus to non-electrolytes. *J. Membrane Biol.* 2: 127–149, 1970.

86. WRIGHT, E. M., AND J. N. DIAMOND. Patterns of non-electrolyte permeability. *Proc. Roy. Soc. London, Ser. B* 172: 227–271, 1969.

3

Esterification Reactions in the Intestinal Mucosa and Lipid Absorption

JOHN M. JOHNSTON

Department of Biochemistry and Obstetrics-Gynecology and the Cecil H. and Ida Green Center for Reproductive Biology Science, University of Texas Southwestern Medical School, Dallas, Texas

THE MOLECULAR BASIS for the understanding of lipid absorption has been developed in the last 20 years. The major emphasis here is placed on the esterification reactions as they relate to lipid absorption in the mucosa cell. The aim of this chapter is to update the present state of the art on esterification reactions as they pertain to the absorption of lipids. This topic has been the subject of several recent reviews [Borgström (2), Brindley (4), Ockner and Isselbacher (28), and Johnston (16)].

The previous chapter discussed the physicochemical mechanism by which the products of lipid digestion, namely, monoacylglycerols, fatty acids, cholesterol, and lysophosphatides, traverse the unstirred water layer to come in contact with the plasma membrane (chapt. 2). It has been recognized for a number of years that the uptake of lipids for the mucosal cell is a passive process (17). Until recently, little information has been available concerning the mechanism by which the products of digestion, present in the brush border of the enterocyte, are translocated to the endoplasmic reticulum (ER). Numerous investigations have established that this subcellular location is the site for the resynthesis of triacylglycerols, cholesterol esters, and glycerophospholipids. Recently, Ockner and associates (30) have suggested a mechanism to explain this process. They have isolated a fatty acid-binding protein (FABP) from the cytosolic fraction of the enterocyte and have suggested that the function of this protein is the transfer of fatty acids from the brush-border membrane to the smooth endoplasmic reticulum (SER). The presence of FABP in the mucosal cell, which is similar but not identical to a previously described protein designated Z (22), not only provides a mechanism for translocation of fatty acids from the brush border to the SER but also may function to prevent the accumulation of intracellular unbound fatty acids. Free fatty acids are known to have a deleterious effect on numerous cellular metabolic processes. The FABP may also be important in facilitation of the esterification process of long-chain fatty acids. This conclusion was based on the fact that a significant conversion of C10:0 and C12:0 fatty acids to their corresponding acyl-CoA forms occurs (5) when intestinal microsomes are used as the enzyme source, whereas in vivo experiments suggest that these fatty acids rapidly appear in the portal circulation without undergoing esterification (28). Since FABP preferentially binds long-chain fatty acids, it may facilitate their esterification. Consistent with the view that FABP functions in the translation process is the observation that FABP is present in higher concentrations in the proximal portion of the small intestine than in the distal portions of the small bowel. In addition, increasing quantities of FABP are present in the tip cells of the villus compared with the crypt cells (30). The amount of FABP can also be increased in the lower ileum by the administration of large quantities of triacylglycerols (29).

TRIACYLGLYCEROL BIOSYNTHESIS IN THE INTESTINAL MUCOSAL CELL

Prior to the utilization of fatty acid in esterification, the long-chain fatty acids must be activated to their CoA derivative. The enzyme catalyzing this reaction is long-chain fatty acid:CoA ligase (EC 6.2.1.3).

The enzyme has been demonstrated in the microsomal fraction of the small intestine in all species examined. The enzyme is more active when long-chain saturated fatty acids are employed as substrates (5). The intestinal mucosa also contains an enzyme that will activate medium-chain fatty acids (44). The fatty acid-AMP complex is thought to be an intermediate in the formation of fatty acid-CoA. However, some reports have suggested the involvement of an enzyme-CoA intermediate (1, 35).

There are at least three distinct mechanisms for the synthesis of triacylglycerols in the intestinal mucosa. These employ glycerol-3-PO_4, dihydroxyacetone-PO_4 (DHAP), and monoacylglycerol as the acyl acceptors. Phosphatidic acids are produced by both the glycerol-3-PO_4 and DHAP pathways. The contribution of the DHAP pathway to the synthesis of triacylglycerols has not been established in the enterocyte although the pathway has been demonstrated in this cell (36).

The reaction sequence for the synthesis of triacylglycerols via the glycerol-3-PO_4 pathway is illustrated in Figure 1. The phosphatidic acids formed in the intestinal mucosal cell remain strongly bound to the ER (19). The microsomal-bound phosphatidic acids are further hydrolyzed to the sn-1,2-diacylglycerols via the action of the cytosolic L-α-phosphatidate phosphohydrolase (EC 3.1.3.4) (20). Although phosphatidate phosphohydrolase activity is also found in the microsomal fractions, present evidence seems to suggest that the cytosolic enzyme is responsible for the major activity associated with triacylglycerol biosynthesis (20, 41). This enzyme is thought to be the

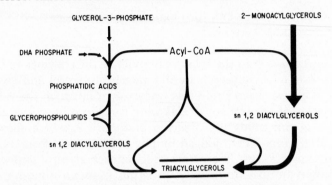

FIG. 1. Pathways of triacylglycerol biosynthesis in the intestinal mucosal cell. Heavy arrow denotes major pathway of triacylglycerol biosynthesis in the enterocyte.

major cytosolic stimulatory factor for triacylglycerol synthesis by the glycerol-3-PO_4 pathway (42).

The first direct evidence for the biosynthesis of triacylglycerols from monoacylglycerols in the intestinal mucosa (7) was suggested in 1960 (Fig. 1). It has been shown in a variety of species, including rat, hamster, chicken, pig, cat, guinea pig, sheep, and man, that the monoacylglycerol pathway is the major pathway for the synthesis of triacylglycerols in the intestinal mucosa. The sn-2-monoacylglycerol is the major isomer produced by the action of pancreatic lipase and absorbed into the enterocyte (25). The sn-2-monoacylglycerols are acylated in a stepwise manner to form triacylglycerols, with the intermediate formation of the sn-1,2-diacylglycerols (18) employing microsomes as the enzyme source. With intestinal everted sacs used as the enzyme source, it was recently found that the sn-1-position is preferentially acylated (31) although a significant formation of sn-2,3-diacylglycerol was also found.

Although the glycerol-3-PO_4 and monoacylglycerol pathways both utilize acyl-CoA as the acyl donor and diacylglycerols as intermediates for triacylglycerol biosynthesis, evidence has been presented suggesting that the two pathways operate quite independently in the mucosal cell (19). It also should be emphasized that the monoacylglycerol pathway is a much more efficient mechanism for the synthesis of triacylglycerols from an energetic standpoint since 4 high-energy phosphate bonds are required for the biosynthesis of a triacylglycerol molecule employing monoacylglycerol as the acyl acceptor compared with approximately 10 high-energy phosphate bonds for the synthesis of triacylglycerol via the glycerol-3-PO_4 pathway. The subcellular location of the enzymes responsible for triacylglycerol biosynthesis has been documented by a number of laboratories to be the endoplasmic reticulum. Several reports have appeared in the last few years suggesting that the brush border may be the location of triacylglycerol biosynthesis (8, 10, 37, 43). However, more recent electron-microscopic and biochemical studies strongly suggest that triacylglycerol biosynthesis occurs almost exclusively in the ER (38, 39).

INTERRELATIONSHIP BETWEEN GLYCEROL-3-PO$_4$ AND
MONOACYLGLYCEROL PATHWAYS

In order to ascertain the relative activity of the enzymes responsible for the synthesis of triacylglycerols by the monoacylglycerol and glycerol-3-PO$_4$ pathways, a comparative study was undertaken in which the relative rates of esterification of the two substrates were compared in several tissues (33). The results of this study are depicted in Figure 2, which shows that the acylation of glycerol-3-PO$_4$, judged by phosphatidic acid formation, is fairly constant in most tissues. In contrast the monoacylglycerol pathway shows a wide variation in specific activity, ranging from an almost undetectable level in the liver to activities far exceeding those of glycerol-3-PO$_4$ in the intestinal mucosa. The marked difference in the activities of the two pathways suggested to us that, although the pathways share certain intermediates in the biosynthesis of triacylglycerols such as acyl-CoA and diacylglycerols, they probably function quite independently. This conclusion also was supported by the following observations: *1*) no significant acylation of glycerol-3-PO$_4$ could be detected with the enzyme complex triacylglycerol synthetase, which acylated monoacylglycerols (34); *2*) the glycerol-3-PO$_4$ pathway could be utilized for both triacylglycerols and glycerophospholipids but the monoacylglycerol pathway produced almost exclusively triacylglycerols (19); and *3*) the *sn*-1,2-diacylglycerols synthesized by both pathways did not equilibrate (18).

The lack of equilibration by the two diacylglycerols produced by the different pathways may be explained by the fact that the microsomes employed in these studies were derived from cells that contained relatively different capacities to esterify glycerol-3-PO$_4$ and monoacylglycerols. Mansbach (23) has reported that microsomes obtained from villous tip and crypt cells have different specific activities for the synthesis of phosphatidylcholine by the two pathways. We therefore investigated the relative rates of esterification of glycerol-3-PO$_4$ and monoacylglycerol employing microsomes obtained mostly from either the tip or crypt cells of the intestinal villus. Marker enzymes were utilized to establish the relative enrichment of the tip and crypt cells used (15). The results of this study are illustrated in Figure 3. Although the specific activity of the monoacylglycerol transacylase was

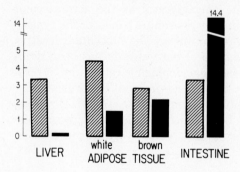

FIG. 2. Relative specific activities of glycerol-3-PO$_4$ (striped bars) and monoacylglycerol (solid bars) acylation by microsomal fraction obtained from various tissues. Data are expressed as picomoles of product formed per milligram of protein per minute.

increased in the microsomes derived from the tip cells compared with the crypt cells, increased activity of glycerol-3-PO_4 esterification was also found in the tip cells. Further experiments are necessary to clarify whether the differences in activity of the tip and crypt cells for the two biosynthetic pathways can account for the failure of equilibration of the two diacylglycerol pools (18). We also have examined the activity of monoacylglycerol hydrolase in microsomes obtained from the tip and crypt cells. The results of this study, illustrated in Figure 4, show that the hydrolase activity has an inverse relationship to the monoacylglycerol transacylase activity. We suggested several years ago (6) that the physiological function of the monoacylglycerol hydrolase in the intestinal mucosa was to hydrolyze any monoacylglycerols that were in excess of available fatty acids for triacylglycerol biosynthesis via the monoacylglycerol pathway. The fatty acids released from the monoacylglycerols could then be utilized for triacylglycerol biosynthesis via the glycerol-3-PO_4 pathway.

Several years ago we suggested that the kinetic parameters (34) of the enzymes responsible for the acylation of monoacylglycerols and glycerol-3-PO_4 may explain the preferential utilization of monoacylglycerol for triacyl-

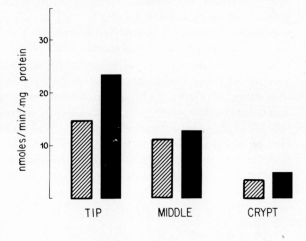

FIG. 3. Relative specific activities of glycerol-3-PO_4 (striped bars) and monoacylglycerol (solid bars) acylation employing the microsomal fraction obtained from various fractions of the intestinal villus.

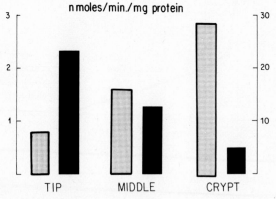

FIG. 4. Relative specific activities of monoacylglycerol hydrolase (stippled bars, left-hand scale) and monoacylglycerol transacylase (solid bars, right-hand scale) present in the microsomal fraction obtained from various fractions of the intestinal villus.

glycerol biosynthesis (21). Recent observations from our laboratory suggest an additional relationship between the two pathways (33). These results were obtained from investigations in which the monoacylglycerol and glycerol-3-PO$_4$ pathways were studied in the same incubation vessel. A decrease in acylation of glycerol-3-PO$_4$ was observed when monoacylglycerols or their corresponding ether analogues were added (33), which suggested that the monoacylglycerols might not only be serving as substrates for the synthesis of triacylglycerols but might also be inhibiting the acylation of glycerol-3-PO$_4$. Figure 5 shows the effect of increasing concentrations of 2-monooleoyl ether on the acylation of glycerol-3-PO$_4$ with intestinal microsomes used as the enzyme source. The ether analogue was employed since this bond is more resistant to hydrolytic cleavage. Previous studies have shown that the *sn*-3-ether analogue is utilized for the synthesis of higher glycerides via the same mechanisms as the *sn*-2-monoacylglycerols (32). As can be seen, with the increased concentrations of the *sn*-2-monooleoyl ether, acylation of glycerol-3-PO$_4$ decreased, reaching a maximum of about 80% inhibition. The inhibition is thought to be directed at the initial acylation step of glycerol-3-PO$_4$, since no evidence was obtained for the accumulation of lysophosphatidic acid. In order to ascertain whether the inhibition of glycerol-3-PO$_4$ by monoacylglycerols could be duplicated in whole-cell preparations, similar experiments were performed with intestinal slices. The fatty acids and 2-monoacylglycerols or alkylglycerols were added as taurodeoxycholate mixed micelles (33) and glycerol-3-PO$_4$ acylation was monitored by determining the amount of [^{14}C]glucose incorporated into glyceride-glycerol. The results of this study are shown in Figure 6. With increasing concentration of the *sn*-2-monooleoyl ether there was a significant decrease in the incorporation of labeled glucose into glyceride-glycerol. Whether or not the observed inhibition by monoacylglycerols is a direct inhibition of glycerol-3-PO$_4$ esterification cannot be clearly established with intact cells. However, the observed inhibition is consistent with the results obtained with intestinal microsomes.

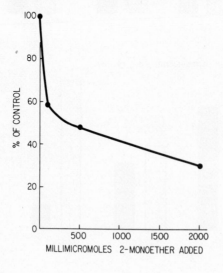

FIG. 5. Effect of addition of increasing concentrations of *sn*-2-monooleoyl ether on acylation of glycerol-3-PO$_4$ with intestinal microsomes used as the enzyme source.

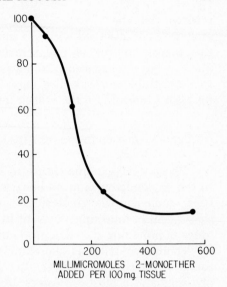

FIG. 6. Effect of addition of increasing concentrations of sn-2-monooleoyl ether on incorporation of labeled glucose into glyceride-glycerol with intestinal slices used as the enzyme source.

MILLIMICROMOLES 2-MONOETHER ADDED PER 100 mg. TISSUE

The specificity and nature of the inhibition of glycerol-3-PO$_4$ utilization by monoacylglycerols were examined further. Since monoacylglycerols may have some detergent properties and detergents are known to inhibit numerous enzymes, we examined the effect of monoacylglycerols or their ether analogues on the activity of two additional microsomal enzymes. No inhibition of the activity of NADPH and NADH cytochrome c reductases resulted when the monoalkylglycerol was added (33). These results suggest that the monoalkylglycerol is exerting a specific inhibition on glycerol-3-PO$_4$ utilization rather than a generalized inhibition of a number of microsomal enzymes. Experiments employing increasing concentrations of acyl-CoAs demonstrated that the inhibition of monoacylglycerols was a direct effect on the acylation of glycerol-3-PO$_4$ rather than a competition for available acyl-CoAs. Further support for this mechanism was provided by experiments in which the inhibition also could be observed when the sn-3-monoalkyl ether was employed. Previous in vitro and in vivo experiments had established that this isomer was not acylated to a significant extent (32).

These studies on the regulation of glyceride biosynthesis by the intestinal mucosa suggest a direct relationship between the acylation of glycerol-3-PO$_4$ and the available monoacylglycerols. If monoacylglycerols are present, they are utilized preferentially in the acylation of triacylglycerol biosynthesis, thus assuring that the cell synthesizes triacylglycerols by the most efficient pathway from an energetic viewpoint. The failure to completely inhibit glycerol-3-PO$_4$ acylation even at high concentrations would provide a mechanism for the synthesis of glycerophospholipid that would be necessary for chylomicron formation. Previous studies have shown that the glycerol-3-PO$_4$ pathway is utilized for both glycerophospholipid and triacylglycerol biosynthesis (18). In contrast, the monoacylglycerol pathway is almost exclusively utilized for triacylglycerol biosynthesis (18). Recently it has been reported that the inhibition of the glycerol-3-PO$_4$ pathway by monoacylglycerols was not observed with the micelle preparation and the everted sac as the enzyme source (3). The ratio of wet weight of tissue to micellar monoacylglycerol concentration was significantly lower in this study than in the intestinal mucosal slice experiments (33). Further investigations are necessary to evaluate the reason for the discrepancy between these results.

GLYCEROPHOSPHOLIPID BIOSYNTHESIS IN THE ENTEROCYTE

Phosphatidylcholine (lecithin) is the major glycerophospholipid present in the chylomicron, and its biosynthesis in relation to lipid absorption has been studied to the greatest extent. Although this component is a minor constituent of total lipids present in the chylomicron, it is of primary importance in providing the structural outer surface of the chylomicron. Phosphatidylcholine contributes approximately 50% of the membrane surface surrounding the chylomicron (47). In contrast, the neutral lipids such as triacylglycerols and cholesterol esters are dispersed in the so-called chylomicron core. The esterification reactions related to phosphatidylcholine biosynthesis in the enterocyte appear to be distinctly different from that of triacylglycerol biosynthesis. The first piece of evidence for this was the observation that the acyl groups of chylomicron phosphatidylcholine remain relatively constant despite larger variations in the composition of the dietary fatty acids (46). The explanation for this observation may reside in the fact that the intermediates of the glycerol-3-PO$_4$ and monoacylglycerol pathways do not equilibrate (19). In addition it appears that the intermediates of the glycerol-3-PO$_4$ pathway can be utilized for both glycerophospholipid and triacylglycerol biosynthesis. In contrast the monoacylglycerol pathway is utilized primarily for triacylglycerol biosynthesis (19).

It has been demonstrated that the enterocyte can synthesize lecithin either by the de novo pathway (12, 27) or by utilizing lysophosphatidylcholine (26, 40) as a precursor. The lyso derivative is produced by the action of pancreatic phospholipase A$_2$ in the intestinal lumen. The lysophosphatidylcholine acyltransferase is present in the endoplasmic reticulum of the enterocyte (24). Several investigations have attempted to quantitate the contribution of the lyso pathway and the de novo or CDP-choline pathway and the contribution of dietary, biliary, and plasma phosphatidylcholine to the phosphatidylcholine found in chylomicrons (24). Phosphatidylcholine synthesized by the de novo and the lyso pathways may be regulated by the availability of the substrates utilized by each of the pathways. Since the lyso pathway requires considerably less expenditure of energy for the synthesis of phosphatidylcholine, some relationship may exist between the two pathways based on availability of substrates similar to the relationship discussed for triacylglycerol biosynthesis. This mechanism would provide for the biosynthesis of phosphatidylcholine. Future investigations are needed to establish more direct proof for this postulated interrelationship.

CHOLESTEROL ESTERIFICATION IN THE ENTEROCYTE

A discussion of the esterification reactions of the intestinal mucosa should include some consideration of cholesterol absorption. Previous investigations have suggested that the mechanism of cholesterol esterification in the intestinal mucosa was the reversal of the enzyme cholesterol hydrolase (45). The enzyme present in the mucosal cell exhibited properties similar to the cholesterol hydrolase found in the pancreatic secretions. Since no requirement for ATP and CoA could be demonstrated (45), the reversal of the hydrolytic reaction was not an attractive mechanism from an energetic standpoint. Recently a mechanism has been suggested for the intracellular esterification of cholesterol that is more compatible with energetic considerations (13). The enzyme catalyzing the reaction has been shown to be of microsomal origin and the reaction is CoA dependent. Maximum activity was obtained in the intestinal mucosa subcellular fraction by the addition of long-chain acylcarnitines plus coenzyme A. The pH optimum of the enzyme was approximately 7.0 and it was demonstrated that the oleoylcarnitine is the preferred fatty acid for the acylation reaction. Cholesterol is the major cholesterol ester present in chylomicrons (47). The reaction was highest in the proximal duodenum, the location of triacylglycerol biosynthesis and chylomicron formation, and probably accounts for the higher capacity of this intestinal segment for the absorption of cholesterol. This mechanism for cholesterol esterification in the intestinal mucosa would be consistent with the esterification reaction in other tissues.

SUMMARY

The concepts discussed concerning the esterification reactions in the intestinal mucosa are summarized in Figure 7. In this reaction sequence the monoacylglycerol and fatty acids are taken up by the brush border of the mucosal cells and are rapidly translocated to the ER, possibly bound to the FABP. The monoacylglycerols and fatty acids, after their activation, are resynthesized into triacylglycerols. In addition, monoacylglycerols may serve as an inhibitor for the acylation of glycerol-3-PO_4. The activity of the monoacylglycerol pathway is much higher in the tip cells than in the crypt cells. The monoacylglycerol hydrolase specific activity is higher in the microsomes derived from the crypt cells. Thus, if monoacylglycerol concentration in the crypt cells is in excess of the available fatty acids for triacylglycerol biosynthesis, they could be hydrolyzed rapidly. The released fatty acids could be utilized for glycerolipid biosynthesis via the glycerol-3-PO_4 pathway. The presence of two pools of sn-1,2-diacylglycerols may be explained by the fact that the smooth endoplasmic reticulum (SER) and the rough endoplasmic reticulum (RER) have relatively greater amounts of the enzymes that esterify monoacylglycerols and glycerol-3-PO_4, respectively. Although this explanation has not been definitely established, a combined biochemical and

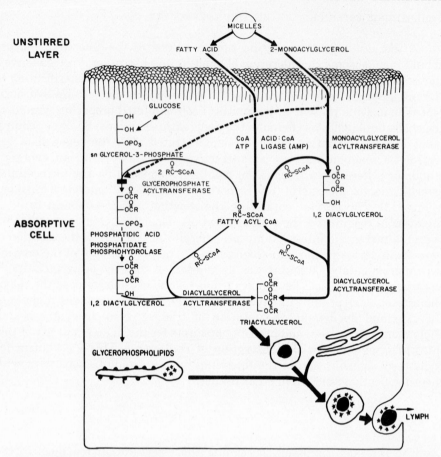

FIG. 7. Biosynthetic and regulatory pathways for triacylglycerol in the intestinal mucosal cell. Cooperation of various subcellular organelles in biosynthesis of chylomicrons is shown: triacylglycerol biosynthesis is via the monoacylglycerol pathway associated with the SER ⦿ and glycerophospholipid and protein biosynthesis forming the lipoprotein coat ⊛ in the RER; Golgi apparatus 〰️ is responsible for carbohydrate addition to the protein forming the glycoproteins found in chylomicrons.

morphological study on fat absorption suggested that the monoacylglycerol pathway was primarily associated with the SER and glycerol-3-PO$_4$ acylation was associated with the RER (14). Consistent with this view were other morphological and biochemical investigations that supported this concept (9). The newly synthesized triacylglycerols associated with the SER would migrate through the cisternae of the ER system to the RER, where the newly synthesized lipoprotein containing glycerophospholipids, cholesterol esters, and protein would be added to the developing prechylomicron. The prechylomicron would then be transported to the Golgi apparatus within the microtubule system, where the carbohydrate moiety of the glycoprotein would be added via the glycosylation reactions known to be associated with this subcellular fraction. The resulting chylomicron would leave the cell via a process of exocytosis. Recent investigations of Glickman et al. (11) seem to suggest that the microtubular system is involved in the latter process since they were able to demonstrate that the addition of certain plant alkyloids such as colchicine markedly inhibits the secretion of chylomicrons.

The author's work has been supported by Public Health Service Grant AM-03108 and by the Robert A. Welch Foundation, Houston, Texas.

REFERENCES

1. BAR-TANA, J., AND B. SHAPIRO. Studies on palmitoyl-coenzyme A synthetase. *Biochem. J.* 93: 533–538, 1964.
2. BORGSTRÖM, B. Fat digestion and absorption. *Biomembranes* 48: 556–620, 1974.
3. BRECKENRIDGE, W. C., AND A. KUKSIS. Diacylglycerol biosynthesis in everted sacs of rat intestinal mucosa. *Can. J. Biochem.* 53: 1170–1183, 1975.
4. BRINDLEY, D. N. The intracellular phase of fat absorption. *Biomembranes* 4B: 621–671, 1974.
5. BRINDLEY, D. N., AND G. HÜBSCHER. The effect of chain length on the activation and subsequent incorporation of fatty acids into glycerides by the small intestinal mucosa. *Biochim. Biophys. Acta* 125: 92–105, 1966.
6. BROWN, J. L., AND J. M. JOHNSTON. The mechanism of intestinal utilization of monoglycerides. *Biochim. Biophys. Acta* 84: 264–274, 1964.
7. CLARK, B., AND G. HÜBSCHER. Biosynthesis of glycerides in the mucosa of the small intestine. *Nature* 185: 35, 1960.
8. FORSTNER, G. G., E. M. RILEY, S. J. DANIELS, AND K. J. ISSELBACHER. Demonstration of glyceride synthesis by brush borders of intestinal epithelial cells. *Biochem. Biophys. Res. Commun.* 21: 83–88, 1965.
9. FRIEDMAN, H. I., AND R. R. CARDELL, JR. Alterations in the endoplasmic reticulum and Golgi complex of intestinal epithelial cells during fat absorption and after termination of this process: a morphological and morphometric study. *Anat. Record* 188: 77–102, 1977.
10. GALLO, L., AND C. R. TREADWELL. Localization of the monoglyceride pathway in subcellular fractions of rat intestinal mucosa. *Arch. Biochem. Biophys.* 141: 614–621, 1970.
11. GLICKMAN, R. M., J. L. PERROTTO, AND K. KIRSCH. Intestinal lipoprotein formation: effect of colchicine. *Gastroenterology* 70: 347–352, 1976.
12. GURR, M. I., W. F. R. POVER, J. N. HAWTHORNE, AND A. C. FRAZER. In: *Biochemical Problems of Lipids*, edited by A. C. Frazer. Amsterdam: Elsevier, 1963, p. 236–243.
13. HAUGEN, R., AND K. R. NORUM. Coenzyme-A-dependent esterification of cholesterol in rat intestinal mucosa. *Scand. J. Gastroenterol.* 11: 615–621, 1976.
14. HIGGINS, J. A., AND R. J. BARRNETT. Fine structural localization of acyltransferases: the monoglyceride and α-glycerophosphate pathways in intestinal absorptive cells. *J. Cell Biol.* 50: 102–120, 1971.
15. JOHNSTON, J. M. Triglyceride biosynthesis in the intestinal mucosa. In: *Biochemical and Clinical Aspects of Lipid Absorption*, edited by K. Rommil. Stuttgart: Schattauer, 1976, p. 38–42.
16. JOHNSTON, J. M. Gastrointestinal tissue. In: *Lipid Metabolism in Mammals I*, edited by F. Snyder. New York: Plenum, 1977, p. 151–188.
17. JOHNSTON, J. M., AND B. BORGSTRÖM. The intestinal absorption and metabolism of micellar solutions of lipids. *Biochim. Biophys. Acta* 84: 412–423, 1964.
18. JOHNSTON, J. M., F. PALTAUF, C. M. SCHILLER, AND L. D. SCHULTZ. The utilization of the α-glycerophosphate and monoglyceride pathways for phosphatidylcholine biosynthesis in the intestine. *Biochim. Biophys. Acta* 218: 124–133, 1970.
19. JOHNSTON, J. M., G. A. RAO, AND P. A. LOWE. The separation of the α-glycerophosphate and monoglyceride pathways in the intestinal biosynthesis of triglycerides. *Biochim. Biophys. Acta* 137: 578–580, 1967.
20. JOHNSTON, J. M., G. A. RAO, P. A. LOWE, AND B. E. SCHWARZ. The nature of the stimulatory role of the supernatant fraction on triglyceride synthesis by the α-glycerophosphate pathway. *Lipids* 2: 14–20, 1967.
21. KERN, F., AND B. BORGSTRÖM. Quantitative study of the pathways of triglyceride synthesis by hamster intestinal mucosa. *Biochim. Biophys. Acta* 98: 520–531, 1965.
22. LEVI, A. J., Z. GATMAITAN, AND I. M. ARIAS. Two hepatic cytoplasmic protein fractions, Y and Z, and their possible role in the hepatic uptake of bilirubin sulfobromophthalein, and other anions. *J. Clin. Invest.* 48: 2156–2167, 1969.
23. MANSBACH, C. M. II. Complex lipid synthesis in hamster intestine. *Biochim. Biophys. Acta* 296: 386–400, 1973.
24. MANSBACH, C. M. II. The origin of chylomicron phosphatidylcholine in the rat. *J. Clin. Invest.* 60: 411–420, 1977.
25. MATTSON, F. H., AND L. W. BECK. The specificity of pancreatic lipase or the primary hydroxyl groups of glycerides. *J. Biol. Chem.* 219: 735–740, 1956.
26. NILSSON, A. Intestinal absorption of lecithin and lysolecithin by lymph fistula rats. *Biochim. Biophys. Acta* 152: 379–390, 1968.
27. NOMA, A. Studies on the phospholipid metabolism of the intestinal mucosa during fat absorption. *J. Biochem.* 56: 522–532, 1964.
28. OCKNER, R. K., AND K. J. ISSELBACHER. Recent concepts of intestinal fat absorption. *Rev. Physiol. Biochem. Pharmacol.* 71: 107–146, 1974.
29. OCKNER, R. K., AND J. M. MANNING. Fatty acid binding protein in small intestine: identification, isolation and evidence for its role in cellular fatty acid transport. *J. Clin. Invest.* 54: 326–338, 1974.
30. OCKNER, R. K., J. M. MANNING, R. B. POPPENHAUSEN, AND W. K. L. HO. A binding protein for fatty acids in cytosol of intestinal mucosa, liver, myocardium, and other tissues. *Science* 177: 56–58, 1972.
31. O'DOHERTY, P. J. A., AND A. KUKSIS. Microsomal synthesis of di- and triacylglycerols in rat liver and Ehrlich ascites cells. *Can. J. Biochem.* 52: 514–524, 1974.
32. PALTAUF, F., AND J. M. JOHNSTON. The metabolism *in vitro* of enantiomeric 1-0-alkyl glycerols and 1,2- and 1,3-alkyl acylglycerols in the intestinal mucosa.

Biochim. Biophys. Acta 239: 47–56, 1971.

33. POLHEIM, D., J. S. K. DAVID, F. M. SCHULTZ, M. B. WYLIE, AND J. M. JOHNSTON. Regulation of triglyceride biosynthesis in adipose and intestinal tissue. *J. Lipid Res.* 14: 415–421, 1973.

34. RAO, G., AND J. M. JOHNSTON. Purification and properties of triglyceride synthetase from the intestinal mucosa. *Biochim. Biophys. Acta* 125: 465–473, 1966.

35. RAO, G. A., AND J. M. JOHNSTON. Studies of the formation and utilization of bound CoA in glyceride biosynthesis. *Biochim. Biophys. Acta* 144: 25–33, 1967.

36. RAO, G. A., M. F. SORRELS, AND R. REISER. Biosynthesis of triglycerides from triose phosphates by microsomes of intestinal mucosa. *Lipids* 5: 762–764, 1970.

37. ROBBINS, S. J., D. M. SMALL, AND R. M. DONALDSON. Triglyceride formation in intestinal microvillous membranes during fat absorption. *J. Clin. Invest.* 48: 69A, 1969.

38. ROBBINS, S. J., D. M. SMALL, J. S. TRIER, AND R. M. DONALDSON. Localization of fatty acid re-esterification in the brush border region of intestinal absorptive cells. *Biochim. Biophys. Acta* 233; 550–561, 1971.

39. SCHILLER, C. M., J. S. K. DAVID, AND J. M. JOHNSTON. The subcellular distribution of triglyceride synthetase in the intestinal mucosa. *Biochim. Biophys. Acta* 210: 489–491, 1970.

40. SCOW, R. O., Y. STEIN, AND O. STEIN. Incorporation of dietary lecithin and lysolecithin into lymph chylomicrons in the rat. *J. Biol. Chem.* 242: 4919–4925, 1967.

41. SMITH, M. E., B. SEDGWICK, D. N. BRINDLEY, AND G. HÜBSCHER. The role of phosphatidate phosphohydrolase in glyceride biosynthesis. *European J. Biochem.* 3: 70–77, 1967.

42. STEIN, Y., A. TIETZ, AND B. SHAPIRO. Glyceride synthesis of rat liver mitochondria. *Biochim. Biophys. Acta* 26: 286–293, 1957.

43. SUBBAIAH, P. V., S. S. RAGHAVAN, AND J. GANGULY. Further studies on the intestinal absorption of triglycerides and fatty acids in rats. *Indian J. Biochem.* 5: 147–152, 1968.

44. TAME, M. J., AND R. DILS. Fatty acid synthesis in intestinal mucosa of guinea pig. *Biochem. J.* 105: 709–716, 1967.

45. TREADWELL, C. R., AND G V. VAHOUNEY. Cholesterol absorption. In: *Handbook of Physiology. Alimentary Canal.* Washington, D. C.: Am. Physiol. Soc., sect. 6, vol. III, p. 1407–1438.

46. WHYTE, M., D. S. GOODMAN, AND A. KARMEN. Fatty acid esterification and chylomicron formation during fat absorption in rat: III. Positional relations in triglycerides and lecithin. *J. Lipid Res.* 6: 233–240, 1965.

47. ZILVERSMIT, D. B. The composition and structure of lymph chylomicrons in dog, rat, and man. *J. Clin. Invest.* 44: 1610–1622, 1965.

4

Assembly of Chylomicrons in the Intestinal Cell

DONALD B. ZILVERSMIT

Division of Nutritional Sciences and Section of Biochemistry, Molecular and Cell Biology, Division of Biological Sciences, Cornell University, Ithaca, New York

Preparation of Chylomicrons
Sizing of Chylomicrons
Structure of Chylomicrons
Surface-to-Volume Ratio
Intestinal Lipoprotein Biosynthesis
Transfer of Lipids and Proteins
Retinol as a Chylomicron Marker
Chylomicrons as a Major Determinant in Hypercholesterolemia
Chylomicron Remnants and Atherogenesis
Quantitation of Cholesterol Absorption with a Single Blood Sample
Conclusion

AFTER CONSIDERATION OF THE BIOCHEMISTRY of intestinal lipid biosynthesis, the next question might be how lipid and protein are combined to form intestinal lipoproteins, primarily chylomicrons and very-low-density lipoproteins (VLDL). The term "chylomicron" was coined by Gage in 1920 (15) in a short paper in the *Cornell Veterinarian*. He observed under dark-field illumination that blood taken several hours after a fatty meal was "literally alive with these dancing particles." For 20 or 30 years the microscope was the principal instrument for observation of chylomicrons, but more recently the electron microscope and the ultracentrifuge have served this purpose. Another technique that has materially aided the isolation and study of chylomicrons is lymph cannulation in laboratory animals such as the rat (6), rabbit (56), or dog (29).

PREPARATION OF CHYLOMICRONS

Normally thoracic duct lymph or intestinal lymph is collected in ethylenediaminetetraacetic acid (EDTA) or allowed to clot. Chylomicrons are removed by ultracentrifugation in an angle-head rotor at about 10^6 *g*/min. The buttery layer is easily removed, resuspended in 0.9% NaCl with or without added serum albumin, and recentrifuged. The process may be repeated a number of times. However, separation of chylomicrons in an angle-head rotor accomplishes relatively little washing of the particles even when the chyle is layered below a column of physiological saline (Fig. 1). Most of the particles travel through the chylous fluid to the inner wall of the centrifuge tube, where they form a viscous mass that rapidly slides to the top with a minimum amount of contact between individual chylomicrons and the washing solution. Better purification after the initial centrifugation probably can be accomplished by gel-permeation chromatography on agarose (19).

SIZING OF CHYLOMICRONS

Once isolated, the chylomicrons may be sized by electron microscopy (5, 12) or by centrifugation through a sucrose gradient (36). The latter procedure shows a particle size distribution between 80 and 500 nm (Fig. 2) for rat chylomicrons (58). The median of the distribution is close to 200 nm. A somewhat different impression is given when the diameter of the particles is plotted against the number of particles rather than their mass (Fig. 3). In this instance most of the chylomicrons are obviously smaller than 200 nm.

In chickens, fat absorption also results in the release of fat droplets from the intestine. The droplets, which resemble chylomicrons in composition, are released into the portal circulation. By analogy they have been named "portomicrons" (4).

STRUCTURE OF CHYLOMICRONS

Chylomicrons are considered to be droplets composed of apolar lipids surrounded by a monolayer of polar lipids and protein. Since there is no evidence of a bilayered membrane structure on the lipid surface (41), it seems likely that the vesicular membranes enclosing the chylomicrons fuse with the lateral portions of the plasma membranes and thus release their

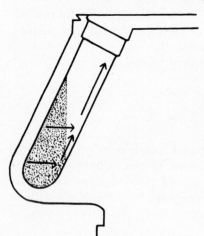

FIG. 1. Movement of lipid particles in Spinco 40 rotor. Initially, the bottom half is filled with chylomicron suspension (stippled area) and the top half with salt solution (clear area). During centrifugation the layers reorient themselves as shown. About half the particles strike the wall before encountering salt solution. [From Zilversmit (51).]

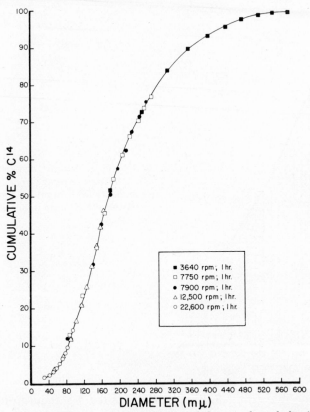

FIG. 2. Cumulative particle mass distribution of thoracic duct chylomicrons in whole defibrinated chyle from a rat fed cream containing [^{14}C]palmitate. Centrifugations in sucrose gradient for 1 h, 25°C in Spinco SW 25.1 rotor: ■ 3640 rpm; □ 7750 rpm; ● 7900 rpm; ○ 12,500 rpm; and △ 22,600 rpm. [From Zilversmit et al. (58).]

contents into the interstitial spaces from where the chylomicrons are carried to the lacteals.

Chylomicrons were disrupted by repeated freezing and thawing or by dehydration-rehydration cycles in order to study their structure (48, 50). The oil phase contained nearly all the triglyceride and cholesteryl ester and a portion of the unesterified cholesterol, whereas the surface film contained all the phospholipid and probably also the proteins (Table 1). Further evidence that the phospholipids are present on the surface of the droplet was obtained by analysis of different size classes (45), which showed that the ratio of phospholipid to triglyceride increased markedly as the size of the chylomicrons diminished (Table 2). Similar observations have been made on lymph chylomicrons from rabbits (12).

SURFACE-TO-VOLUME RATIO

The size distribution of chylomicrons may depend on fat load (13), degree of unsaturation of dietary fat (7, 10), and the protein-synthesizing

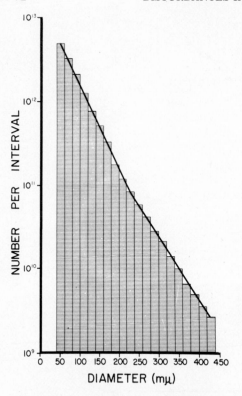

FIG. 3. Number distribution of lymph chylomicrons. Average from 2 rats fed cream and 2 rats fed corn oil. *Ordinate:* number of particles per 20-mμm interval. [Zilversmit et al. (58).]

capacity of the intestine (19, 21, 31). Rabbits fed a standard diet with 30% corn oil or butter make much larger chylomicrons than those fed a 5% fat diet (13). Chylomicron size shifts in a similar manner during different stages of fat absorption, being largest during peak absorption and smaller at the beginning and end of the absorptive period (13).

The effects of fatty acid composition of dietary fats on the size of chylomicrons have been studied with various results. Courel and Clément (10) reported that rat chylomicrons were larger after cream feeding than after corn oil feeding. In a later study from the same laboratory (7) no clear-cut differences in chylomicron particle sizes were seen when a variety of dietary fats were fed. No differences in chylomicron size distribution in thoracic duct lymph of rats fed corn oil and cream were reported by Zilversmit et al. (58). On the other hand Ockner and co-workers (31, 32) showed that in rats fed palmitate there were relatively more small particles (VLDL-like) in intestinal lymph than in animals fed oleate or linoleate. Subsequently these investigators showed that the absorption of palmitic acid required a greater length of intestine than the absorption of linoleic acid (33). A number of these findings about the relationship of dietary fat composition and dietary fat loads to chylomicron size distribution may be understood on the basis of the relative rates of triglyceride transport per mucosal cell and the synthetic rates of surface material (Fig. 4). At higher absorption rates the cell makes larger fat droplets because the amount of surface material synthesized by these cells becomes limiting. At lower absorption rates sufficient surface material is present to promote the packaging of relatively small fat droplets. The following summary illustrates this principle:

1) Lymph chylomicrons are larger during the absorption of high-fat meals than during lower fat loads.

2) Chylomicrons are relatively large during the peak of a given absorptive period and smaller before and after peak absorption.

3) Chylomicrons are larger during absorption of unsaturated fats than during absorption of saturated fat.

4) Chylomicrons are larger when protein synthesis is inhibited.

INTESTINAL LIPOPROTEIN BIOSYNTHESIS

Although the lymph chylomicrons contain relatively little protein, the observation that patients with abetalipoproteinemia do not secrete chylomicrons in response to a fat load (42) has focused attention on the role of protein biosynthesis in the assembly of chylomicrons.

TABLE 1. *Lymph chylomicron and oil and surface lipids from 2 dogs and 2 rats fed corn oil*

	Triglycerides, %	Phospholipids, %	Cholesterol, %		Protein, %
			Free	Esterified	
Dogs					
Chylomicron	95	4.3	0.62	0.21	0.6
Oil	99	0	0.27	0.24	0
Surface	23	70	7.3	0	4.4
Chylomicron	95	3.5	0.58	0.29	0.6
Oil	99	0	0.20	0.29	0
Surface	16	75	8.7	0	3.1
Rats					
Chylomicron	95	4.6	0.24	0.07	
Surface	11	87	3.0	0	
Chylomicron	96	3.7	0.25	0.07	
Surface	21	76	2.9	0	

Oil and membrane fractions prepared by freezing and thawing. Triglyceride phospholipid and cholesterol as percent of total lipid, protein as percent of total weight. [Adapted from Zilversmit (48).]

TABLE 2. *Composition of lymph chlyomicrons of various sizes*

Particle Size, nm	Triglyceride, %	Phospholipid, %	Cholesterol, %		Protein, %
			Free	Esterified	
>200	95	3.8	0.55	0.27	0.59
140–200	92	6.3	0.94	0.43	1.8
<140	88	9.1	1.45	0.68	2.3

Thoracic duct lymph from dogs fed cream. Percentages of total lipid for lipid fraction, of total weight for protein. [Adapted from Yokoyama and Zilversmit (45).]

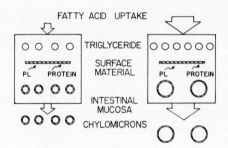

FIG. 4. Fat absorption and synthesis of surface material. On left, the rate of fat absorption is relatively low compared to the rate of surface material synthesis; resulting chylomicrons are small. On right, the fat absorption rate is higher but synthesis of surface material is the same; chylomicrons therefore are larger.

ApoB protein has been identified immunochemically in the $d < 1.006$ fraction present in rat intestinal Golgi vesicles (18, 28). The apoB concentration appears to be greater in large chylomicrons than in smaller ones, although as a class of lipoproteins the apoB concentration in VLDL exceeds that of chylomicrons (20).

Electron-microscopic studies (3) of rats treated with puromycin, ethionine, or cycloheximide showed that large numbers of chylomicrons were present in the extracellular spaces of the mucosal epithelium. However, fat droplets devoid of membranes appeared to accumulate within the cells while the Golgi membranes were strikingly diminished (14). It therefore seems that inhibition of protein biosynthesis may impede the intracellular transport of fat droplets from the endoplasmic reticulum to the Golgi vesicles. In biochemical studies, Glickman et al. (21) demonstrated a reduced lipid absorption after cycloheximide treatment, with an increase in the size of lymph chylomicrons. Although Redgrave and Zilversmit (39) demonstrated that puromycin treatment apparently slows down intestinal motility, which may in part account for the delay in fat absorption, most of the evidence seems to show that intestinal proteins play a key role in the assembly of chylomicrons. For example, Glickman and Kirsch (19) demonstrated that intestinal lymph chylomicrons of rats treated with acetoxycycloheximide contained only one-half of one of the major apoproteins normally present in chylomicrons. This apoprotein, which has a rapid rate of synthesis and shares antigenic determinants with high-density lipoproteins (HDL), seems likely to be identical to apoA-I (17). This apoprotein also has been identified as a major component of human chyle chylomicrons (27). In the studies by Glickman and Kirsch (19) neither apoB nor apoC proteins appeared to be decreased in the chylomicron fraction after the rats had been treated with the protein-synthesis inhibitor. Although apoB apparently is synthesized in the intestinal mucosa, the low-molecular-weight proteins, or apoC proteins, are not synthesized by the intestine (19, 44).

Evidently, however, puromycin interferes with the biosynthesis of other components of the chylomicron interface. For example, in isolated mucosal cells the synthesis of intestinal phosphatidylcholine was decreased by two-thirds under conditions in which the triglyceride biosynthesis was not altered (35). Moreover, there appears to be an interaction between phosphatidylcholine biosynthesis and the presence of polysomes in the intestinal cells. Whereas intestinal polyribosomes in bile-fistula rats are markedly decreased, the feeding of lysophosphatidylcholine resulted in restoration of the polysome profile along with lipoprotein biosynthesis and chylomicron release (46). In intact bile-fistula rats the impairment of chylomicron release can also be reversed by the feeding of phosphatidylcholine or choline (34).

The biosynthesis of apolipoprotein B by the intestinal cell during chylomicron formation has been demonstrated. Also, apoB protein can be demonstrated immunochemically in intestinal cells from fasted rats or from rats previously subjected to bile diversion for 3 days (18). The apoprotein apparently is concentrated in the endoplasmic reticulum and Golgi regions (18). The rapid increase in apparent apoB concentration and its localization after the onset of fat absorption suggest that apoB and chylomicron lipid are associated early in the assembly process. Such an early association is also suggested by the accumulation of fat droplets proximal to the Golgi region in the intestinal cells of abetalipoproteinemic patients. Microtubule involvement in the transport of lipids in the intestinal cells is suggested by the observation that lipid droplets accumulate after administration of colchicine (22).

Perhaps the assembly of intestinal chylomicrons proceeds in a manner similar to that of liver VLDL (2). In this instance, the triglyceride-rich particle appears to be synthesized in the smooth endoplasmic reticulum whereas the proteins originate in the rough endoplasmic reticulum. Apoproteins and lipid coalesce at the junctions of smooth and rough endoplasmic reticulum, whereupon the entire particle is transported via specialized tubules to the Golgi vesicles. The authors do not discuss how the synthesis and release of an apoprotein as hydrophobic as apolipoprotein B are accomplished without massive aggregation. Data derived from chylomicron composition studies suggest that the synthesis of surface proteins may be coupled to the synthesis of surface lipids, so that a complete lipoprotein is secreted into the intracisternal space of the endoplasmic reticulum. This lipoprotein may be similar to the low-density lipoproteins (LDL) of blood plasma with or without the addition of apoA-I. Indeed Glaumann et al. (16) observed that both rough and smooth endoplasmic reticulum of rat liver synthesize triglyceride and phospholipid of lipoproteins that appear to be more dense than plasma VLDL. In the intestine similar lipoproteins might, subsequent to their secretion, coat triglyceride droplets, thus unfolding and emptying their apolar lipids, primarily cholesteryl ester, into the core of the nascent chylomicrons. Such a phenomenon has been observed when serum lipoproteins form a monolayer at an oil-water interface (47). If such a sequence were taking place, it would account for the observation that the cholesteryl ester content of chylomicrons appears to vary with chylomicron size in approximately the same proportion as do protein, phospholipid, and unesterified cholesterol (45, 49). If the cholesteryl ester were initially layered on the surface of intracellular triglyceride droplets as part of a lipoprotein-complex, the amount of cholesteryl ester found in chylomicrons would be expected to be proportional to the surface area of the triglyceride droplet.

The fact that cholesteryl ester is found in the core of the mature chylomicron might reflect a subsequent step in which the cholesteryl ester is transferred from the chylomicron surface to its core.

TRANSFER OF LIPIDS AND PROTEINS

Once chylomicrons have left the intestinal cell they continue to undergo chemical transformations. Not only are surface components (phospholipids, unesterified cholesterol, and some of the proteins) readily exchangeable with other lipoproteins of the lymph and plasma, but net changes in lipid and protein composition take place (29). Thus when lymph chylomicrons are exposed to plasma in vitro, a net loss of chylomicron phospholipid and a net gain in unesterified cholesterol are seen (Fig. 5). Nascent chylomicrons appear to contain apolipoproteins A-I and B (17, 20). At a later stage C apolipoproteins are transferred from the high-density lipoproteins to the chylomicron surface (23). One of these apoproteins serves as an activator of lipoprotein lipase, an enzyme involved in one of the first steps of chylomicron catabolism. During degradation the C apolipoproteins are lost again by transfer back to the HDL fraction (23, 30).

RETINOL AS A CHYLOMICRON MARKER

Although the degradation of chylomicrons is discussed in detail by Fielding (chapt. 5) I should like to remark briefly here about a novel method for differentiating triglyceride-rich particles originating in the intestine from those derived from liver. Dietary retinol, present in a fat-containing

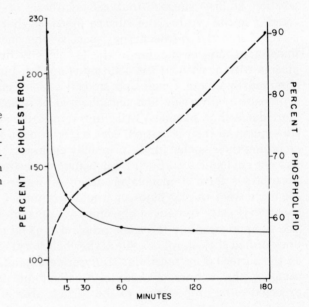

FIG. 5. Increase in percentage free cholesterol (-----) and decrease in percentage phospholipid (——●——●) of lymph chylomicrons during incubation in vitro with serum. [Adapted from Minari and Zilversmit (29).]

meal, is transported in the thoracic duct lymph largely in the form of chylomicrons. About 90% of the chylomicron retinol is esterified and remains with the chylomicron remnant after the bulk of the triglyceride has been removed by lipoprotein lipase. The glycerides and cholesterol contained in the chylomicron remnant are taken up by the liver parenchyma and are, at least in part, resecreted as VLDL. The retinol portion of the remnant is not resecreted as lipoprotein (Fig. 6) but appears in the plasma as a constituent of a retinol-binding protein-prealbumin complex (43). Thus, although the chylomicron remnants and liver VLDL have overlapping densities and particle size ranges, the presence or absence of retinol in a given particle differentiates between the lipoproteins originating in the intestine and those coming from the liver. With the use of chylomicrons labeled with radioactive cholesterol ester and retinol ester, we have been able to demonstrate in the cholesterol-fed rabbit an accumulation of chylomicron remnants in the plasma that accounts for most of the hypercholesterolemia (40, 55). By the same technique Hazzard and Bierman (24) demonstrated in patients with broad beta disease (type 3 hyperlipoproteinemia) that the efficiency of remnant removal from the bloodstream is diminished. Thus, the use of orally administered retinol, radioactively labeled or determined fluorometrically, appears to provide a relatively simple procedure for the study of the metabolism of chylomicrons and chylomicron remnants.

CHYLOMICRONS AS A MAJOR DETERMINANT IN HYPERCHOLESTEROLEMIA

In the rat, chylomicron remnants are removed rapidly from the bloodstream by hepatic mechanisms (38). Although chylomicrons transport a considerable amount of cholesterol when the diet contains high levels of this sterol, little or none of this cholesterol contributes directly to the plasma cholesterol concentration. Dietary cholesterol in the rat does contribute indirectly to plasma cholesterol as repackaged VLDL secreted by the liver. In the rabbit, however, it seems likely that a different sequence might prevail. For example, the addition of cholesterol to the rabbit's diet produces an immediate response of serum cholesterol in the $d < 1.006$ fraction. Figure 7 shows the plasma VLDL cholesterol in two rabbits fed 100 g of chow

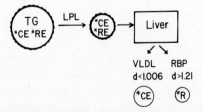

FIG. 6. Model for metabolism of chylomicron lipids. Chylomicron (left) is degraded to chylomicron remnant (middle), which is then taken up by liver (right). Liver subsequently secretes VLDL containing some of the labeled cholesterol of the chylomicron but none of the labeled retinol. [From Zilversmit (55).]

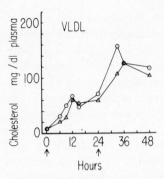

FIG. 7. Changes in rabbit plasma VLDL cholesterol concentrations on initiation of cholesterol feeding. Rabbits previously fed cholesterol-free chow diets were fed 100 g chow supplemented with 500 mg cholesterol and 2.7 g fat at 0 h and 24 h (↑). Nearly all food was consumed within 3 h. Data for 2 representative rabbits shown. [From Ross and Zilversmit (40).]

supplemented with 500 mg of cholesterol and 2.7 g of fat at the 0- and 24-h points. At both points the plasma cholesterol in this fraction responds with an upward phase followed 9–12 h later by a downswing. Such a profile would be compatible with the entry into the bloodstream of cholesterol-containing particles of dietary origin followed by a slow clearance of these particles.

We have used the retinol-labeling technique to determine whether the apparent delay in cholesterol clearance could be due to a rapid resecretion of repackaged cholesterol into the bloodstream by the liver (40). Figure 8 shows typical profiles of the conversion of retinol-labeled chylomicrons to higher density fractions. In the control rabbits (*panel A*) the chylomicrons, contained in the VLDL-1 fraction, are cleared rapidly and converted to lipoproteins with lower triglyceride contents (VLDL-2 and VLDL-3) and ultimately to LDL and HDL ($S_f < 20$). Except for the last fraction, the intermediates are cleared rapidly from the bloodstream. In contrast, the cholesterol-fed rabbits (*panel B*) show a much slower clearance pattern for the various intermediates. Apparently, the intermediates are cleared more slowly because of an impairment of liver function or because of an abnormal particle composition. Calculations based on the specific activities of cholesteryl ester in these intermediates, after injection with cholesterol-labeled chylomicrons, show that two-thirds or more of the cholesterol in VLDL is present in the form of partially degraded chylomicrons.

CHYLOMICRON REMNANTS AND ATHEROGENESIS

It may not be a coincidence that, in an animal as susceptible to cholesterol-induced atherosclerosis as the rabbit, a large portion of the circulating cholesterol is contained in chylomicron remnants. A causal link between circulating remnants and atherogenesis has been proposed by Hülsmann and Jansen (26). In a somewhat different scheme I suggested several years ago (53, 54) that chylomicron remnants might be formed at the arterial surface, quite analogous to the formation of remnants at the capillary surface. Some of these remnants might gain entrance into the arterial wall before the forces responsible for their release could return them to the circulation. Particularly if these remnants are enriched in cholesterol, as would be the case when the animal or person eats a cholesterol-rich meal, the direct uptake of dietary cholesterol by this pathway might be appreciable. Interestingly, the arterial wall contains lipoprotein lipase (11, 25) and the activity of lipoprotein lipase in rabbit aortas is increased when arterial lesions are developing (9). Thus, the mechanisms to degrade chylomicrons to remnants appear to be present in the larger arteries, and smooth muscle cells appear to incorporate efficiently the cholesterol in chylomicron remnants (1). If this sequence is quantitatively important, then dietary cholesterol may be atherogenic without necessarily raising the plasma cholesterol concentrations.

QUANTITATION OF CHOLESTEROL ABSORPTION WITH A
SINGLE BLOOD SAMPLE

The methodology for the measurement of cholesterol absorption from the digestive tract is cumbersome. A balance experiment is complicated by the fact that cholesterol is synthesized by the body and requires the use of isotopically labeled cholesterol as well as fecal collection for a period of a week or more (37). A novel approach is based on a single intravenous injection of labeled colloidal cholesterol at the same time at which an oral cholesterol dose with a different label is administered (52, 57). The intravenous dose is rapidly cleared by the Kupffer cells of the liver and released to the blood over approximately the same interval in which the oral dose is absorbed. Thus, the intravenous dose serves as an internal standard (100% absorption) for the oral dose, the absorption of which is to be measured. In other words, the isotope ratio in a single plasma sample, 48 h or more after the administration of the labeled cholesterols, is equal to the fraction of the orally administered cholesterol dose that is absorbed. Studies in our own laboratory have validated the procedure for rats. The method subsequently has been used in monkeys (8).

CONCLUSION

Chylomicrons are triglyceride-rich lipoproteins produced by the intestinal mucosa during periods of fat absorption. They are usually differentiated from very-low-density-lipoproteins by their flotation characteristics ($S_f >$ 400). Subfractionation and disruption procedure have shown that chylomi-

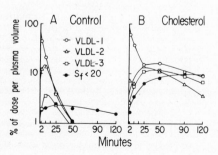

FIG. 8. [^{3}H]retinyl esters in plasma lipoprotein fractions of normal rabbits and rabbits fed cholesterol for 4 days. Lipoproteins were isolated by discontinuous gradient centrifugation. Very-low-density lipoprotein (VLDL-1) contains the larger particles, VLDL-3 the smallest ones. [From Ross and Zilversmit (40).]

crons contain a core of apolar lipids, triglyceride, and cholesteryl ester, surrounded by a mixed monolayer of phospholipid, unesterified cholesterol, and small amounts of partial glycerides and proteins. Chylomicron assembly appears to take place in the endoplasmic reticulum, followed by transfer to the Golgi vesicles and secretion into the extracellular spaces. Modifications of the chylomicron surface continue during transport into lymph and blood plasma. Apolipoproteins A-I and B are characteristic constituents of newly formed chylomicrons, whereas the apoC proteins appear to be added at a later stage. The use of dietary retinol as a marker for chylomicrons, intestinal VLDL, and their remnants helps to differentiate between these particles and the VLDL derived from liver. Apparently, most of the circulating VLDL cholesterol in the cholesterol-fed rabbit is composed of chylomicron remnants. This observation and the finding that chylomicron remnants are taken up by arterial smooth muscle cells in vitro support the hypothesis that chylomicron remnants enriched in cholesterol may be atherogenic. This in turn renews interest in the role of dietary cholesterol in atherogenesis of human beings and experimental animals. A new and convenient method for the measurement of cholesterol absorption in intact animals is likely to provide pertinent data about this relationship.

This investigation was supported by research grants (10933 and 10940) from the National Heart, Lung, and Blood Institute. D. B. Zilversmit is a Career Investigator of the American Heart Association.

REFERENCES

1. ALBERS, J. J., AND E. L. BIERMAN. The influence of lipoprotein composition on binding, uptake and degradation of different lipoprotein fractions by cultured human arterial smooth muscle cells. *Artery* 2: 337–348, 1976.

2. ALEXANDER, C. A., R. F. HAMILTON, AND R. J. HAVEL. Subcellular localization of B apoprotein of plasma lipoproteins in rat liver. *J. Cell Biol.* 69: 241–263, 1976.

3. ALLEN, C. H., P. S. GIBBS, AND R. A. JERSILD. Intestinal fat transport during inhibition of protein synthesis. An electron microscopic study. *Exptl. Mol. Pathol.* 14: 90–102, 1971.

4. BENSADOUN, A., AND A. ROTHFELD. The form of absorption of lipids in the chicken, *Gallus domesticus. Proc. Soc. Exptl. Biol. Med.* 141: 814–817, 1972.

5. BIERMAN, E. L., T. L. HAYES, J. N. HAWKINS, A. M. EWING, AND F. T. LINDGREN. Particle-size distribution of very low density plasma lipoproteins during fat absorption in man. *J. Lipid Res.* 7: 65–72, 1966.

6. BOLLMAN, J. L., J. C. CAIN, AND J. H. GRINDLAY. Techniques for the collection of lymph from the liver, small intestine, or thoracic duct of the rat. *J. Lab. Clin. Med.* 33: 1349–1352, 1948.

7. BOQUILLON, M., H. CARLIER, AND J. CLÉMENT. Effect of various dietary fats on the size and distribution of lymph fat particles in rat. *Digestion* 10: 255–266, 1974.

8. COREY, J. E., AND K. C. HAYES. Validation of the dual-isotope plasma ratio technique as a measure of cholesterol absorption in Old and New World monkeys. *Proc. Soc. Exptl. Biol. Med.* 148: 842–846, 1975.

9. COREY, J. E., AND D. B. ZILVERSMIT. Effect of cholesterol feeding on arterial lipolytic activity in the rabbit.

Atherosclerosis 27: 201–212, 1977.

10. COUREL, E., AND J. CLÉMENT. Influence de l'ingestion de crème sur le nombre et la taille des chylomicrons lymphatiques. *Compt. Rend. Soc. Biol.* 158: 715–718, 1964.

11. DiCORLETO, P. E., AND D. B. ZILVERSMIT. Lipoprotein lipase activity in bovine aorta. *Proc. Soc. Exptl. Biol. Med.* 148: 1101–1105, 1975.

12. FRASER, R. Size and lipid composition of chylomicrons of different Svedberg units of flotation. *J. Lipid Res.* 11: 60–65, 1970.

13. FRASER, R., W. J. CLIFF, AND F. C. COURTICE. The effect of dietary fat load on the size and composition of chylomicrons in thoracic duct lymph. *Quart. J. Exptl. Physiol.* 53: 390–398, 1968.

14. FRIEDMAN, H. I., AND R. R. CARDELL. Effects of puromycin on the structure of rat intestinal epithelial cells during fat absorption. *J. Cell Biol.* 52: 15–40, 1972.

15. GAGE, S. H. The free granules (chylomicrons) of the blood as shown by the dark-field microscope. *Cornell Vet.* 10: 154–155, 1920.

16. GLAUMANN, H., A. BERGSTRAND, AND J. L. E. ERICSSON. Studies on the synthesis and intracellular transport of lipoprotein particles in rat liver. *J. Cell Biol.* 64: 356–377, 1975.

17. GLICKMAN, R. M., AND P. H. R. GREEN. The intestine as a source of apolipoprotein A_1. *Proc. Natl. Acad. Sci. US* In press.

18. GLICKMAN, R. M., J. KHORANA, AND A. KILGORE. Localization of apolipoprotein B in intestinal epithelial cells. *Science* 193: 1254–1255, 1976.

19. GLICKMAN, R. M., AND K. KIRSCH. Lymph chylomicron formation during the inhibition of protein synthesis.

J. Clin. Invest. 52: 2910–2920, 1973.

20. GLICKMAN, R. M., AND K. KIRSCH. The apoproteins of various size classes of human chylous fluid lipoproteins. Biochim. Biophys. Acta 371: 255–266, 1974.

21. GLICKMAN, R. M., K. KIRSCH, AND K. J. ISSELBACHER. Fat absorption during inhibition of protein synthesis: studies of lymph chylomicrons. J. Clin. Invest. 51: 356–363, 1972.

22. GLICKMAN, R. M., J. L. PERROTTO, AND K. KIRSCH. Intestinal lipoprotein formation: effect of colchicine. Gastroenterology 70: 347–352, 1976.

23. HAVEL, R. J., J. P. KANE, AND M. L. KASHYAP. Interchange of apolipoproteins between chylomicrons and high density lipoproteins during alimentary lipemia in man. J. Clin. Invest. 52: 32–38, 1973.

24. HAZZARD, W. R., AND E. L. BIERMAN. Delayed clearance of chylomicron remnants following vitamin-A-containing oral fat loads in broad-β disease (type III hyperlipoproteinemia). Metabolism 25: 777–801, 1976.

25. HENSON, L. C., AND M. C. SCHOTZ. Detection and partial characterization of lipoprotein lipase in bovine aorta. Biochim. Biophys. Acta 409: 360–366, 1975.

26. HÜLSMANN, W. C., AND H. JANSEN. High lipoprotein lipase activity and cardiovascular disease. In: Energy, Regulation and Biosynthesis in Molecular Biology, edited by D. Richter. Berlin: Walter de Gruyter, 1974, p. 322–335.

27. KOSTNER, G., AND A. HOLASEK. Characterization and quantitation of the apolipoproteins from human chyle chylomicrons. Biochemistry 11: 1217–1223, 1972.

28. MAHLEY, R. W., B. D. BENNETT, D. J. MORRÈ, M. E. GRAY, W. THISTLETHWAITE, AND V. S. LEQUIRE. Lipoproteins associated with the Golgi apparatus isolated from epithelial cells of rat small intestine. Lab. Invest. 25: 435–444, 1971.

29. MINARI, O., AND D. B. ZILVERSMIT. Behavior of dog lymph chylomicron lipid constitutents during incubation with serum. J. Lipid Res. 4: 424–436, 1963.

30. MJØS, O. D., O. FAERGMAN, R. L. HAMILTON, AND R. J. HAVEL. Characterization of remnants produced during the metabolism of triglyceride-rich lipoproteins of blood plasma and intestinal lymph in the rat. J. Clin. Invest. 56: 603–615, 1975.

31. OCKNER, R. K., F. B. HUGHES, AND K. J. ISSELBACHER. Very low density lipoproteins in intestinal lymph: role in triglyceride and cholesterol transport during fat absorption. J. Clin. Invest. 48: 2367–2373, 1969.

32. OCKNER, R. K., AND A. L. JONES. An electron microscopic and functional study of very low density lipoproteins in intestinal lymph. J. Lipid Res. 11: 284–292, 1970.

33. OCKNER, R. K., J. P. PITTMAN, AND J. L. YAGER. Differences in the intestinal absorption of saturated and unsaturated long chain fatty acids. Gastroenterology 62: 981–992, 1972.

34. O'DOHERTY, P. J. A., G. KAKIS, AND A. KUKSIS. Role of luminal lecithin in intestinal fat absorption. Lipids 8: 249–255, 1973.

35. O'DOHERTY, P. J. A., I. M. YOUSEF, AND A. KUKSIS. Effect of puromycin on protein and glycerolipid biosynthesis in isolated mucosal cells. Arch. Biochem. Biophys. 156: 586–594, 1973.

36. PINTER, G. G., AND D. B. ZILVERSMIT. A gradient centrifugation method for the determination of particle size distribution of chylomicrons and of fat droplets in artificial fat emulsions. Biochim. Biophys. Acta 59: 116–127, 1962.

37. QUINTÁO, E., S. M. GRUNDY, AND E. H. AHRENS. An evaluation of four methods for measuring cholesterol

absorption by the intestine in man. J. Lipid Res. 12: 221–232, 1971.

38. REDGRAVE, T. G. Formation of cholesteryl ester-rich particulate lipid during metabolism of chylomicrons. J. Clin. Invest. 49: 465–471, 1970.

39. REDGRAVE, T. G., AND D. B. ZILVERSMIT. Does puromycin block release of chylomicrons from the intestine? Am. J. Physiol. 217: 336–340, 1969.

40. ROSS, A. C., AND D. B. ZILVERSMIT. Chylomicron remnant cholesteryl esters as the major constituent of very low density lipoproteins in plasma of cholesterol-fed rabbits. J. Lipid Res. 18: 169–181, 1977.

41. SALPETER, M. M., AND D. B. ZILVERSMIT. The surface coat of chylomicrons: electron microscopy. J. Lipid Res. 9: 187–192, 1968.

42. SALT, H. B., O. H. WOLFF, L. K. LLOYD, A. S. FOSBROOKE, A. H. CAMERON, AND D. V. HUBBLE. On having no beta-lipoprotein. Lancet 2: 325–329, 1960.

43. SMITH, J. E., Y. MUTO, P. O. MILCH, AND D. S. GOODMAN. The effects of chylomicron vitamin A on the metabolism of retinol-binding protein in the rat. J. Biol. Chem. 248: 1544–1549, 1973.

44. WINDMUELLER, H. G., P. N. HERBERT, AND R. I. LEVY. Biosynthesis of lymph and plasma lipoprotein apoproteins by isolated perfused rat liver and intestine. J. Lipid Res. 14: 215–223, 1973.

45. YOKOYAMA, A., AND D. B. ZILVERSMIT. Particle size and composition of dog lymph chylomicrons. J. Lipid Res. 6: 241–246, 1965.

46. YOUSEF, I. M., P. J. A. O'DOHERTY, E. F. WHITTER, AND A. KUKSIS. Ribosome structure and chylomicron formation in rat intestinal mucosa. Lab. Invest. 34: 256–262, 1976.

47. ZILVERSMIT, D. B. Extraction of cholesterol from human serum lipoprotein films. J. Lipid Res. 5: 300–306, 1964.

48. ZILVERSMIT, D. B. The composition and structure of lymph chylomicrons in dog, rat, and man. J. Clin. Invest. 44: 1610–1622, 1965.

49. ZILVERSMIT, D. B. Formation and transport of chylomicrons. Federation Proc. 26: 1599–1605, 1967.

50. ZILVERSMIT, D. B. The surface coat of chylomicrons: lipid chemistry. J. Lipid Res. 9: 180–186, 1968.

51. ZILVERSMIT, D. B. Chylomicrons. In: Structural and Functional Aspects of Lipoproteins in Living Systems. London: Academic, 1969, p. 329–368.

52. ZILVERSMIT, D. B. A single blood sample dual-isotope method for the measurement of cholesterol absorption in rats. Proc. Soc. Exptl. Biol. Med. 140: 862–865, 1972.

53. ZILVERSMIT, D. B. A proposal linking atherogenesis to the interaction of endothelial lipoprotein lipase with triglyceride-rich lipoproteins. Circulation Res. 33: 633–638, 1973.

54. ZILVERSMIT, D. B. Mechanisms of cholesterol accumulation in the arterial wall. Am. J. Cardiol. 35: 559–566, 1975.

55. ZILVERSMIT, D. B. Role of triglyceride-rich lipoproteins in atherogenesis. Ann. N. Y. Acad. Sci. 275: 138–144, 1976.

56. ZILVERSMIT, D. B., F. C. COURTICE, AND R. FRASER. Cholesterol transport in thoracic duct lymph of the rabbit. J. Atherosclerosis Res. 7: 319–329, 1967.

57. ZILVERSMIT, D. B., AND L. B. HUGHES. Validation of a dual-isotope plasma ratio method for measurement of cholesterol absorption in rats. J. Lipid Res. 15: 465–473, 1974.

58. ZILVERSMIT, D. B., P. H. SISCO, AND A. YOKOYAMA. Size distribution of thoracic duct lymph chylomicrons from rats fed cream and corn oil. Biochim. Biophys. Acta 125: 129–135, 1966.

5

Origin and Properties of Remnant Lipoproteins

CHRISTOPHER J. FIELDING

Cardiovascular Research Institute and Department of Physiology,
University of California, San Francisco, California

WHEN TRIGLYCERIDE-RICH LIPOPROTEINS are released into the plasma from intestinal lymph (as chylomicrons) or secreted from the liver [as very-low-density lipoproteins (VLDL)] the major part of their triglyceride content is hydrolyzed at the vascular surface of those tissues that use fatty acids for oxidative metabolism or storage. Lipoprotein lipase (LPL), the lipase active in this reaction, is functional at the vascular endothelial surface. This catabolic pathway leads to the formation of unesterified fatty acids and triglyceride-depleted lipoproteins (remnant particles). Only recently has information been obtained on the mechanism of formation and properties of these intermediates of plasma lipid metabolism. Under normal conditions they are not present to any significant extent in the plasma. However, their transient existence had been surmised from kinetic studies in vivo. The earliest information on the probable existence of circulating intermediates of triglyceride-rich lipoproteins came from studies on the fate of chylomicron cholesteryl ester, which showed that, while triglyceride from these particles was cleared in the extrahepatic tissues, cholesteryl ester was recovered from the liver (27, 37) and that after hepatectomy, while the triglyceride was removed as before, the cholesteryl ester was retained in the circulation (38). Later, it was shown that the lipoprotein product of LPL activity in the hepatectomized rat was a lipid-rich particle of intermediate flotation index that accumulated in the plasma but, after transfer to an intact animal, was cleared by the liver (42). Finally, in studies with VLDL labeled in the protein moiety, the transient appearance of radioactivity in the density zone between VLDL and low-density lipoproteins (LDL; $1.006 < d < 1.019$ g/cm^3) indicated not only a stepwise degradation of lipid from these particles but also the existence of these intermediates as free lipoprotein complexes in the plasma compartment (8).

Since that time, studies of remnant lipoproteins have been concerned primarily with the biochemical and kinetic properties of the particles that accumulate in the absence of the hepatic removal system. This chapter summarizes the information obtained in these experiments, adds some new information, and attempts to place available knowledge in the context of recent hypotheses on the nature and roles of remnant lipoproteins in plasma lipid metabolism. Because the properties of remnant particles intimately relate to those of the enzyme system that generates them, information is also presented on the substrate properties of lipoprotein lipase.

LIPOPROTEIN LIPASES

These form a well-defined enzyme group of neutral glyceride hydrolases whose primary reaction is at the lipid-water interface of triglyceride-rich lipid-protein complexes. Apart from a single report (24), all lipoprotein lipases are activated by a specific apoprotein (apoC-II) that is a component of the protein moiety of the natural lipoprotein substrates, chylomicrons and VLDL (23, 28, 30, 34, 40). Lipase activity with this property can be detected in most extrahepatic tissues and is released into solution by heparin. Lipoprotein lipases have been isolated from postheparin plasma (13, 14, 22, 23), from heart and adipose tissues (1, 4, 47), and from bovine milk (5, 32). The functional LPL from heart and possibly other muscle tissues has been reported to have a molecular weight of 34,000–37,000 and enzyme from adipose tissue has a molecular weight of 69,000–71,000. Both "big" and "little" LPL species can be recovered from plasma after the injection of heparin (23) and appear to represent the metabolically active species released from muscle and adipose tissues. Other, presumably precursor, forms have been identified in the parenchymal cells (25). Bovine milk LPL has a molecular weight (ca 55,000) intermediate between those of the heparin-released endothelial lipases (32), but also has uniquely high rates of reaction with micellar and soluble ester substrates and perhaps should be considered as a mixed esterase-lipase (6). Details of the molecular structure of the enzyme proteins are given in the original papers. Lipoprotein lipases also have the common property of inhibition by inorganic salts, a reaction that quantitatively reverses the activation obtained with the substrate apoprotein moiety (19) and specifically the apoC-II polypeptide. This reaction appears to be mediated via a single anion-binding site on the apoC-II protein although this has not yet been located in the detailed sequence of the protein. Activation of LPL involves the specific binding of a single apoC-II molecule with formation of a 1:1 molar complex with a dissociation constant of about 3 $\times$ 10^{-13} mol/cm^3 (20). The substrate properties of the various LPL species have received detailed investigation. Of most interest here is that all species studied so far appear to be reactive with both VLDL and chylomicron triglyceride, although the rate of reaction is about twofold greater with dietary (chylomicron) triglyceride (1, 17, 21). There is a significant difference in the apparent Michaelis constants of "big" (adipose tissue) and "little" (heart tissue) LPL species, at least in the rat. The former has an apparent K_m of about 0.25 mM chylomicron triglyceride and the latter has an apparent K_m of about 0.07 mM chylomicron triglyceride in terms of bulk substrate concentration; the values are somewhat lower for VLDL. These values apply for the purified enzymes in solution (Table 1). Since triglyceride occupies little or none of the particle surface in plasma lipoproteins (45) it seems inappropriate to consider substrate affinities for LPL in terms of substrate surface area, as has been proposed, for example, for pancreatic lipase. However, expressed in terms of particle number, for VLDL and chylomicrons of diameters 800 and 2000 Å, respectively, the K_m values for LPL from heart endothelium are approximately 4×10^{13} particles/cm^3 and 10^{11} particles/cm^3. In these terms LPL obviously has a much greater affinity for dietary triglyceride substrate. Similar specificity is shown by adipose tissue LPL (17).

LIPOPROTEIN LIPASE AT THE MEMBRANE SURFACE

The kinetic properties discussed above apply to the lipase in solution but permit the identification of areas of potential importance in any consideration of the LPL reaction at the vascular surface. First, the lipase reaction in muscle and adipose tissues may have different products, since the properties of the enzyme activities present are not the same. Second, since VLDL and chylomicrons have different sizes and properties their access to the membrane-supported lipase may differ from that observed in solution. Third, since both lipoproteins react with LPL, at least in solution, then as circulating levels of triglyceride rise these may become competing substrates at the lipolysis sites, with effects both on overall rates of catabolism and on the nature of the remnant particles produced. Obviously it is important to know whether the kinetic properties of LPL in solution correspond to those of the enzyme supported at its membrane site.

TABLE 1. *Kinetic constants of LPL functional in perfused heart and adipose tissues*

	Catalytic Constant (k_{cat}), s^{-1}		Apparent Michaelis Constant (K_m), mM TG	
	Chylomicrons	VLDL	Chylomicrons	VLDL
Adipose tissue				
Membrane supported	87	60	0.70*	0.45*
Solubilized	80	60	0.23	0.23
Heart tissue				
Membrane supported	57	30	0.08	0.06
Solubilized	47	34	0.08	0.05

Kinetic constants for solubilized LPL were obtained from activity isolated as described for each tissue after perfusion with heparin. * Apparent Michaelis constants for functional adipose tissue LPL at physiological flow rate (about 0.07 ml/g wet w per min) were 1.1 and 0.85 mM TG, respectively, for chylomicrons and VLDL. [Data taken in part from Fielding (17).]

In general, the kinetic properties of enzymes supported at membrane surfaces, or immobilized in sheets or fibers, differ significantly from those of the same enzyme species in free solution. There are several reasons to expect this to be so. The steric configuration of the enzyme is likely to be changed to some extent by attachment, and this in many cases will affect the active site. The steric configuration of the substrate may also be changed in the enzyme-substrate complex. The electrical properties of the membrane and its net charge often affect the reaction rate and particularly the hydrogen-ion dependence of the reaction. Substrate may be partitioned between the bulk phase and the local environment. Finally, the reaction at the membrane may be diffusion limited: i.e., the rate of reaction is determined, at least in part, by the diffusion of substrate to the active site. It can be readily shown that for membrane-supported enzymes the applicable equations have a form analogous to those of the Michaelis-Menten equation for soluble enzymes. These equations permit the calculation of Michaelis and catalytic constants for the immobilized enzyme. In view of the large substrates in the LPL system it is of interest to consider the effects caused by partition and diffusion-limited reaction. These will affect the apparent Michaelis constant but the catalytic constant, i.e., the maximal reaction velocity ($k_{cat}'E$), will be unchanged. Thus for substrate partition:

$$v = k_{cat}'Es_0/(K_m' + s_0')$$

where v is reaction velocity, k_{cat}' and K_m' are the catalytic and Michaelis constants for the enzyme, and s_0' is the substrate concentration at the membrane site.

$$s_0' = Ps_0$$

where s_0 is the bulk substrate concentration and P is the partition coefficient.

$$v = k_{cat}'E \, (s_0/P)/(K_m' + s_0/P)$$
$$v = k_{cat}'Es_0/(K_m'/P + s_0)$$

i.e., substrate partition increases the apparent Michaelis constant but is without effect on the maximal reaction velocity ($k_{cat}'E$). Since this equation does not include a term for the diffusion coefficient (D) the partition effect is independent of stirring or flow rate.

For diffusion-limited reaction at the membrane surface (assumed neutral) the following considerations apply:

The velocity of diffusion across the limiting layer (v_d) is given as

$$v_d = D(s_0 - s_i)x$$

where s_i is the substrate concentration at the membrane site, D is the diffusion coefficient, and x is the thickness of the limiting layer. The velocity of reaction at the enzyme site (v_r) is

$$v_r = k_{cat}'Es_i/(K_m' + s_i)$$

and at equilibrium:

$$v_d = v_r = v$$

Substituting in s_i:

$$vK_m' + \frac{vDs_o - v^2x}{D} = \frac{k_{cat}'EDs_o - k_{cat}'Evx}{D}$$

$$v^2 - v\left(k_{cat}'E + \frac{DK_m'}{x} + \frac{Ds_o}{x}\right) + k_{cat}'EDs_o = 0$$

which has the form

$$v^2 - va + b = 0$$

of which the roots are $v = b - a/b$ and $v = b/a$, where only the latter has real values.

$$v = b/a = \frac{k_{cat}'EDs_o}{x} \bigg/ \left(k_{cat}'E + \frac{DK_m'}{x} + \frac{Ds_o}{x}\right)$$

Multiplying by x/D:

$$v = k_{cat}'Es_o/(K_m' + s_o + k_c'Ex/D)$$

Thus, compared with the diffusion-independent reaction, the Michaelis constant is increased by a factor that is proportional to the maximal reaction velocity and thickness of the limiting layer and is inversely proportional to the diffusion constant. Since D in the reaction column is proportional to flow rate (33), in a diffusion-limited reaction K_m' will decrease as flow rate increases to a limiting value that is diffusion independent. It takes no account, however, of possible charge effects at the membrane surface although in general these will not be dependent on flow rate. A detailed analysis is given in a recent monograph (26).

The LPL system was analyzed by the equation derived by Lilly et al. (35):

$$(s_o - s_i) = k_{cat}'E/Q + K_m' \ln(s_o/s_i)$$

where s_o is the substrate concentration entering the system, s_i the concentration at the exit, and Q the flow rate. This approach has been applied to the case of LPL at the capillary surface of perfused tissues (17, 21). The plot of $(s_o - s_i)$ vs. ln (s_o/s_i) has a slope equal to K_m', the Michaelis constant for the immobilized enzyme; the intercept is $k_{cat}'E/Q$, and if Q is known the maximal reaction velocity is given (Fig. 1). The effect of flow rate on these parameters can be determined by varying Q for each set of substrate conditions, as described by the original authors.

The results obtained from a series of experiments, briefly summarized, have bearing both on the rate of production of remnant particles by LPL and on the type of particles produced. In the perfused heart, the kinetic constants of immobilized LPL functional at the membrane surface were found to be almost identical to those of the same enzyme in solution. Furthermore, the apparent Michaelis constant was independent of flow rate in the physiological range. These results, taken together with the extremely rapid release of the lipase by heparin perfused through the vascular bed, argue strongly for an extremely superficial binding site for this enzyme at the endothelial surface, where the approach of substrate particles is essentially unimpeded and the active-site geometry is unchanged by the binding process. On the other hand, in perfused epididymal adipose tissue, a quite different situation is indicated. The apparent Michaelis constant was found to be considerably greater for the membrane-supported lipase than for the enzyme in solution, for both chylomicrons and VLDL (Table 1). This parameter was flow dependent, decreasing with increasing flow to a minimum value that was about 2.5-fold greater than that obtained for the same enzyme in solution. It

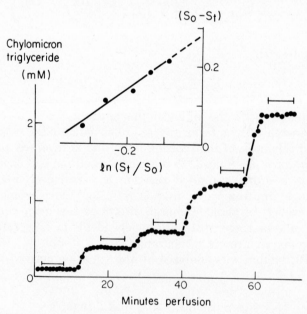

FIG. 1. Kinetics of triglyceride removal by perfused rat epididymal adipose tissue. Bars indicate input triglyceride concentration of 5 successive solutions of chylomicrons. [From Fielding (17).]

should be emphasized, however, that at physiological flow rates the K_m' was strongly flow dependent and approximately 5 times greater than for the soluble lipase. Thus, the kinetic data suggest a much less exposed site for LPL in perfused adipose tissue. Its release by heparin is also much slower (17). Although it has not yet been shown that other sources of adipose tissue, e.g., subcutaneous adipose tissue, have LPL with these properties, it seems relevant that in man, where adipose tissue is believed to supply most of the LPL released by heparin, the apparent K_m has been estimated from triglyceride tracer measurements to be approximately 1.0 mM (41). This is very similar to the value found for perfused rat adipose tissue LPL at physiological flow rates. Note that the effect of the changes induced by membrane binding on adipose tissue LPL is to strongly accentuate the differences in concentration dependence of saturation described for the soluble enzyme. Thus, at physiological flow rates, K_m' for membrane-bound adipose tissue LPL is about 20 times that for the membrane-bound enzyme functional in the heart.

These differences have considerable potential significance in relation to the levels of circulating triglyceride-rich lipoproteins. At normal levels of plasma triglyceride (0.2–2.0 mM), the enzyme functional at the endothelial surface of the heart will be highly saturated since its affinity for lipoprotein substrates is high (K_m' = 0.05–0.08 mM) and hence the rate of clearance by this tissue is substantially independent of substrate concentration. On the other hand, because of its low substrate affinity, the LPL species functional in adipose tissue (K_m' = 1.3 mM) will be highly unsaturated under normal conditions and hence the rate of clearance of triglyceride fatty acid into adipose tissue will be dependent on both enzyme concentration and substrate concentration. Thus overall the presence of the two LPL systems in the whole animal will ensure priority clearance of triglyceride fatty acid into utilizing tissues such as heart muscle at all triglyceride concentrations and will effect clearance into adipose tissue at a rate proportional to substrate concentration.

Superimposed on this regulation are factors that affect the level of enzyme functional at the endothelial surface. Numerous reports concerning the effects of a wide variety of hormones and hormone analogues on LPL have been reviewed recently (43). However, these agents generally have been delivered neither via the vascular route nor at levels as low as those found in vivo and the topic appears to warrant further investigation. The few data available on changes in heart muscle suggest that these changes are in a direction to reinforce the changes in clearance rate mandated by the effects of substrate concentration and the kinetic properties of the enzymes concerned. In any case, the variation in enzyme levels appears to be small compared with the changes in the concentration of circulating triglyceride.

PREPARATION OF REMNANT LIPOPROTEINS

Since triglyceride-rich lipoproteins (both VLDL and chylomicrons) contain, as secreted, many tens of thousands of triglyceride molecules per lipoprotein particle, and since LPL contains only a single active site per molecule (20), intermediates of lipolysis must exist, at least transiently, that are partially depleted of their triglyceride content. These intermediates are remnant lipoproteins. Issues raised in recent research on these particles have focused on the following major questions. First, are components other than triglyceride lost from lipoproteins in the course of reaction with LPL? These could include both potential alternative substrates for the lipase, such as cholesteryl esters and phospholipids, or other components transferred away to cells or to other lipoprotein classes. Second, does LPL release a spectrum of intermediates or is there a single final end product that is no longer a substrate for the enzyme, to which all particles are converted before clearance by the liver? Third, are the intermediates produced by lipase activity retained at the membrane surface for the course of their catabolism or are they released into the plasma compartment to compete there with newly secreted particles as substrates for further lipolysis? Three different techniques have been used to investigate these questions. All involve isolation of the peripheral LPL system from the hepatic removal mechanism to allow accumulation of remnant particles for isolation and analysis. In the functionally hepatectomized rat, large amounts of remnant lipoproteins can be produced readily (12, 36) and these have been analyzed in terms of the lipid and protein content. The principal disadvantages of this preparation are the presence of endogenous triglyceride-rich lipoproteins that contaminate remnants produced from injected chylomicrons and, for some purposes, catabolism by the mixed lipases present in the whole vascular bed. Obviously it cannot be used for studies of the roles of other lipoproteins in triglyceride catabolism. A second approach involves the use of isolated perfused organs, particularly heart and epididymal adipose tissues, that contain a single functional LPL system (17, 21, 39). This has the advantage of providing a well-defined enzyme and substrate system but the disadvantage that the amounts of remnant particles produced are very small because of the limited levels of functional LPL in these tissues compared with the whole animal. Other perfused organ systems, such as the lung and diaphragm, also seem suitable for this purpose. A third approach involves the use of solubilized LPL, either in whole postheparin plasma (9) or after purification (3), and incubated in vitro with purified chylomicrons or VLDL. This system has the advantage of producing large amounts of remnant particles quite easily. It has the disadvantage, in the case of whole postheparin plasma, that triglyceride hydrolysis is by a mixture of lipases including hepatic postheparin lipase; this lipase appears to play no direct role in remnant formation in vivo. In both soluble systems, fatty acid accumulates that can associate with the remnant particles, producing various irregular forms.

In all the systems described further factors deserve consideration. First, use of triglyceride concentrations greatly in excess of those occurring physiologically can lead to the production of abnormal remnant particles. Three factors contribute. The C apoprotein (and particularly apoC-II) content becomes rate limiting if the high-density lipoprotein (HDL) reservoir of these polypeptides becomes exhausted. The circulating half-life of the particles greatly exceeds that found in vivo and the time-dependent exchange of lipids (particularly free cholesterol) with other fractions can become significant. There is also evidence that a high concentration of triglyceride dispersions can itself release LPL (11). On the contrary, all available evidence suggests that under physiological conditions essentially all peripheral triglyceride hydrolysis occurs not in solution but at the membrane support (43).

A second consideration is the extremely low level of heparin required to release LPL into solution (44). Even small amounts of heparin used in animal preparations associate with both chylomicrons and VLDL. Factors such as low-Ca^{2+} medium also can release vascular cells, and their associated enzyme contents, into solution.

A third consideration relates to the purification of remnant lipoproteins. Since triglyceride-rich lipoproteins can be catabolized through the intermediate-density lipoprotein (IDL) range (8), flotation of remnants at a lower density than 1.019 g/cm^3 for purification purposes leads to preparation of an "end product" of lipolysis with a particle density obviously that of the chosen solvent density. Agarose gel chromatography has also been used and permits the recovery of the whole size range of product particles (31).

COMPOSITION OF REMNANT LIPOPROTEINS

In view of the observation that C apoproteins recycle between triglyceride-rich lipoproteins and the HDL fraction, remnant lipoproteins, in the course of their catabolism by LPL, would be expected to become depleted of these polypeptides. This has been demonstrated for remnants produced in the hepatectomized rat (36). The β-protein moiety and content of arginine-rich apoprotein appear to be retained.

Both cholesteryl esters and phospholipids are lipid esters and hence potential substrates for lipolysis. Cholesteryl ester is not a substrate for the lipase in either synthetic or natural lipoprotein form (Fielding, unpublished observations). On the other hand, chylomicron lecithin was hydrolyzed by purified bovine milk LPL (46) and also by both "big" and "little" LPL species isolated from postheparin plasma (23). Hydrolysis of both lecithin and phosphatidylethanolamine was observed, but sphingomyelin was not a substrate for LPL. Remnant particles thus become progressively enriched in sphingomyelin. Although the rates of phospholipase activity are not high compared with those found with neutral glycerides, they are significant when considered in terms of the surface-volume relationships of the lipoprotein, since phospholipid makes up most of the surface of these lipoproteins and triglyceride a large part of the core (45). Therefore LPL phospholipase activity could play a significant role in maintaining chylomicron and VLDL sphericity during triglyceride catabolism. Whether or not it does so in vivo remains an open question. Both studies cited were carried out with pure

LPL and chylomicrons in vitro. Although there is evidence that in whole postheparin plasma phospholipase contributes to loss of VLDL lecithin (10) this preparation also contains hepatic postheparin lipase, a distinct enzyme with major phospholipase activity (7) and without an apparent direct role in peripheral VLDL catabolism under physiological conditions. Additionally, transfer of phospholipid from triglyceride-rich lipoproteins to HDL has been demonstrated in the course of triglyceride hydrolysis in vivo (29). Whatever the mechanism involved, however, remnant particles are significantly depleted of phospholipid as well as protein and triglyceride (Table 2; 31, 36). Remnant particles produced from triglyceride-rich lipoproteins, on the contrary, retain most of their cholesterol content.

The presence of unesterified fatty acids and partial glycerides in remnant particles has been reported only in experiments where albumin was limited or totally lacking (3, 39), but such particles do not appear to correspond in structure to naturally occurring lipoproteins.

In summary, remnant particles generated from VLDL or chylomicrons in vivo or in perfused tissues in the presence of plasma proteins and albumin contain less triglyceride, protein, and phospholipid and become enriched, in relative terms, in arginine-rich apoprotein, sphingomyelin, and cholesterol.

MECHANISM OF FORMATION OF REMNANT LIPOPROTEINS

Two distinct mechanisms for production of remnant particles appear possible. Chylomicrons could be sequestered at endothelial lipase-binding sites for the course of their catabolism, at which time they would be released for clearance by the liver. Alternatively, the intermediate products of lipolysis can be considered in equilibrium with the intact (or newly secreted) lipoproteins in the plasma. In this latter case, catabolism can be envisaged as a succession of hydrolysis steps involving binding and release at the enzyme sites in the course of which all available substrate particles could be considered competitive (Fig. 2). These two models can be distinguished experimentally by the nature of the remnant products recovered in the plasma or perfusion medium. If the remnants were retained at the endothelium, lipoproteins of composition intermediate between intact particles and

TABLE 2. *Lipid and protein composition of intact and remnant lipoproteins*

	VLDL		Chylomicrons	
	Intact (1.0)	Remnant (0.25)	Intact (1.0)	Remnant (0.25)
Triglyceride	80.7	55.1	90.2	85.3
Phospholipid	8.5	11.8	3.9	7.0
Protein	7.3	18.5	2.4	8.2
Free cholesterol	1.7	3.8	0.3	0.8
Cholesteryl ester	1.7	10.8	0.5	1.5

Remnant particles (containing 25% of original triglyceride content) were prepared by recirculation in the isolated rat heart.   [Values taken from Higgins and Fielding (31).]

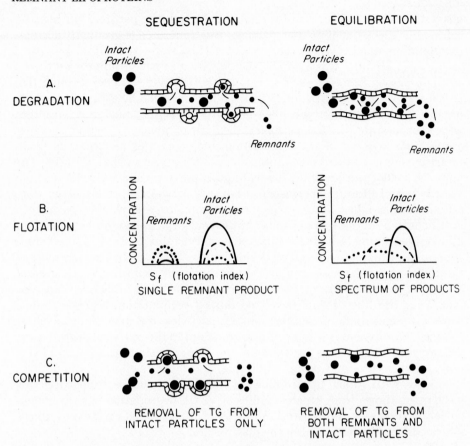

FIG. 2. Metabolic consequences of 2 mechanisms of remnant particle formation. *Left:* sequestration and retention of lipoproteins at the enzyme site in the course of their total catabolism. *Right:* equilibration of remnants and intact lipoproteins in the plasma compartment.

the remnant end product would not be released or recovered and any heterogeneity found in the medium population would result from the spread of particle size or composition in the original substrate population. Moreover, since at least 80–90% of triglyceride appears to be cleared in the peripheral tissues by the LPL mechanism (2), remnants recovered must contain no more than 10% of the triglyceride content of the original particles. This is a maximum value since it assumes no clearance of intact particles by the liver; however, this rate seems to be very small. Under these conditions chylomicron remnants would still be recovered in the density fraction for VLDL ($d < 1.006$ g/cm³), but VLDL remnants would have a minimum density of about 1.04 g/cm³. Several lines of evidence suggest that the intermediate products of catabolism of both chylomicrons and VLDL are not retained at the endothelium but are in equilibrium with the plasma lipoprotein population. First, when a subfraction of chylomicrons, quite homogeneous with respect to size, was recirculated through the perfused rat heart, a continuous spectrum of product particles was generated of gradually decreasing flotation index (31). Second, when VLDL were catabolized in vivo a spectrum of products was again recovered whose density gradually decreased as these passed from the density range for VLDL ($d < 1.006$) through IDL ($1.006 < d < 1.019$) to LDL ($d > 1.019$) (8). Thus in both cases intermediate products containing between 100% and 10% of original triglyceride content were demonstrated in the perfusion medium or plasma. Further evidence comes from analysis of the composition and properties of large and small intact chylomicrons and remnants generated from large chylomicrons. The large ($S_f > 400$) and small (S_f 100–400) intact particles had the same reaction velocity with LPL in the perfused rat heart (21), whereas, as discussed more fully below, smaller particles generated from large chylomicrons have a significantly reduced reaction rate. Moreover, large and small chylomicrons from fat-fed animals had the same cholesteryl ester content (21), whereas generated remnants from large chylomicrons (because they retain most of their cholesteryl ester as triglyceride is removed) contain a much greater content of cholesteryl ester than the same size of small intact chylomicrons (31). Thus the lipoproteins recovered during recirculation represent not a trace contamination of smaller, intact particles but true intermediates released from the enzyme sites into the medium in the course of degradation. These remain substrates for the enzyme. They continue to be degraded if replaced in circulation through the tissue, and they are effective competitive substrates with intact lipoproteins (31). Finally, evidence supporting this mechanism comes from kinetic studies of VLDL degradation in man, where modeling indicates the existence of a stepwise delipidation process whose intermediates are recovered in the plasma (48).

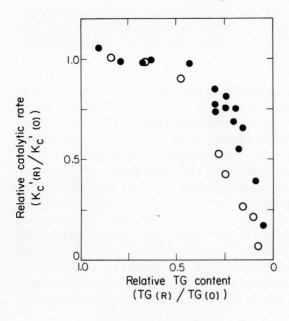

FIG. 3. Dependence of catalytic rate of LPL on the triglyceride content of remnant particles generated from chylomicrons (●) or VLDL (○). [From Higgins and Fielding (31).]

The kinetic properties of remnant particles generated from both VLDL and chylomicrons have been studied in the perfused heart. Initial triglyceride removal was not associated with a change in either apparent Michaelis constant or maximal reaction velocity with LPL (Fig. 3). However, after removal of 75–80% of initial triglyceride content of either VLDL or chylomicrons, further lipolysis was associated with a rapid decrease in lipolytic rate (31) such that particles with 10% of original triglyceride retain only 18% of maximal catalytic rate.

As discussed above the recycling of C apoproteins (including the apoprotein activator of LPL) between triglyceride-rich lipoproteins and HDL requires that as remnant particles are produced they become depleted in activator. Newly secreted chylomicrons entering the plasma bind an approximately fourfold excess of activator protein (18). The loss of reactivity of remnant particles has the same kinetic characteristics, in the opposite sense, as activation by apoC-II protein (16), i.e., remnant formation is limited to a decrease in catalytic constant, whereas activation is limited to an increase in the same constant. If the decrease in the rate of reaction of remnant particles with LPL is caused by loss of apoC-II, then activator should become rate limiting when about 75% of total activator has been lost from the original substrate; this should take place when 75–80% of triglyceride has been removed from the particle, since at this point the reactivity of the lipoprotein begins to steeply decline. This has been demonstrated for both VLDL and chylomicrons. This estimate correlates well with the data obtained with VLDL in postheparin plasma (9) where loss of 80% of original triglyceride content was associated with a decrease in apoC radioactivity from 35% to 8%. If this loss largely represents net transfer rather than exchange, as suggested by other studies of remnant apoprotein composition (36), then it appears likely that it is apoC-II content that limits the catabolism of remnant particles. However, as discussed above, remnant formation is associated with several other changes in composition, including those in the phospholipid and cholesterol content of the particles. These factors may also contribute, either by direct effects [such as the inhibition of LPL by free cholesterol observed in vitro (15)] or indirectly by affecting the binding of apoC-II to the remnant particle.

Both VLDL and chylomicrons are substrates for LPL and furthermore are competitive for the same population of enzyme sites (31). However, since the catalytic rate for chylomicrons is about twice that for VLDL and since the bulk apparent Michaelis concentration for chylomicrons is also about twice that for VLDL, the rate of production of triglyceride fatty acid from mixtures of these substrates will be in simple proportion to their relative concentrations in the medium. It was shown at the same time that the remnants generated from these substrates are also competitive substrates for the intact or newly secreted lipoproteins. Such competition will be without observable effect during the removal of the initial 75% of triglyceride content (when the catalytic rate of intact and remnant particles is the same), but a different situation arises for small remnants whose rate of reaction is significantly depressed. In this case, accumulation of remnant particles, even in the face of constant concentration of intact VLDL or chylomicrons, is associated with an overall decrease in the rate of triglyceride hydrolysis by the heart since the system is already highly saturated. In adipose tissue, where the system is highly unsaturated, such effects initially will be small and hence accumulation of remnants is associated with a shift in the balance of triglyceride clearance by the high- and low-affinity systems. In the face of a continuing entry of new intact particles into the system, remnant particles of increasingly large mean residual triglyceride content will accumulate in the system up to the point where their catalytic rate is the same as that of the intact, newly secreted particles. Beyond that point the intact and remnant particles are not discriminated. It follows that the most effective supply of fatty acids to the tissues from triglyceride-rich lipoproteins is achieved if remnant particles are selectively removed from the system at the point at which their catalytic rate as LPL substrates begins to decrease, i.e., when they retain about 20% of their initial triglyceride content. The optimal removal mechanism has a dependence on remnant triglyceride content that is a transform of that shown in the peripheral tissues by LPL: i.e., removal should rapidly become more efficient as the triglyceride content of the remnant particles decreases below 20% of its initial value.

This last observation points up the probable major function of the remnant lipoprotein mechanism and the associated specialized properties of LPL at the endothelium of different tissues. If LPL were to catabolize all of the triglyceride content of remnant particles then the overall efficiency of triglyceride clearance would be considerably impaired since the catalytic rate with these particles is reduced, probably because of loss of apoC-II activator content. If apoC-II were not removed into the HDL density reservoir during remnant formation it would not be available for the activation of chylomicrons newly entering the vascular compartment, and these particles are the best substrate for the enzyme. On the other hand, because the system is in constant equilibrium, with remnant and intact particles as competitors for the enzyme sites, it is constantly self-adjusting in a direction that maximizes the rate of triglyceride clearance. The price paid for this flexibility is the "futile synthesis" of triglyceride secreted by the liver and gut and returned to the liver without hydrolysis. However, since this only amounts to about 10% of the whole, the system seems to be highly efficient in maximizing triglyceride fatty acid supply and minimizing recirculation time, in the face of a constantly changing supply of substrate.

The author's personal research was supported by grants from the Public Health Service (Arteriosclerosis SCOR HL 14237 and HL 18705).

REFERENCES

1. BENSADOUN, A., C. ENHOLM, D. STEINBERG, AND W. V. BROWN. Purification and characterization of lipoprotein lipase from pig adipose tissue. *J. Biol. Chem.* 249: 2220–2227, 1974.

2. BERGMAN, E. N., R. J. HAVEL, AND T. BOHMER. Quantitative studies of the metabolism of chylomicron triglycerides and cholesterol by liver and extrahepatic tissues of sheep and dogs. *J. Clin. Invest.* 50: 1831–1839,

1971.

3. BLANCHETTE-MACKIE, E. J., AND R. O. SCOW. Retention of lipolytic products in chylomicrons incubated with lipoprotein lipase. Electron microscope study. *J. Lipid Res.* 17: 57-67, 1976.

4. CHUNG, J., AND A. M. SCANU. Lipoprotein lipase from rat heart: purification, molecular properties and kinetic parameters. *Circulation* 54, Suppl. II: 55, 1976.

5. EGELRUD, T., AND T. OLIVECRONA. The purification of a lipoprotein lipase from bovine skim milk. *J. Biol. Chem.* 247: 6212-6217, 1976.

6. EGELRUD, T., AND T. OLIVECRONA. Purified bovine milk (lipoprotein) lipase: activity against lipid substrates in the absence of exogenous serum factors. *Biochim. Biophys. Acta* 306: 115-127, 1975.

7. EHNHOLM, C., W. SHAW, H. GRETEN, AND W. V. BROWN. Purification from human plasma of a heparin-released lipase with activity against triglycerides and phospholipids. *J. Biol. Chem.* 250: 6756-6761, 1975.

8. EISENBERG, S., D. W. BILHEIMER, R. I. LEVY, AND F. T. LINDGREN. On the metabolic conversion of human plasma very low density lipoprotein to low density lipoprotein. *Biochim. Biophys. Acta* 326: 361-377, 1973.

9. EISENBERG, S., AND D. RACHMILEWITZ. Interaction of rat plasma very low density lipoprotein with lipoprotein lipase-rich (postheparin) plasma. *J. Lipid Res.* 16: 341-351, 1975.

10. EISENBERG, S., AND D. SCHURR. Phospholipid removal during degradation of rat plasma very low density lipoprotein *in vitro*. *J. Lipid Res.* 17: 578-587, 1976.

11. ENGELBERG, H. Human endogenous plasma lipemia clearing activity after intravenous fat emulsions. *J. Appl. Physiol.* 12: 292-296, 1958.

12. FELTS, J. M., H. ITAKURA, AND R. T. CRANE. Mechanism of assimilation of constituents of chylomicrons, very low density lipoproteins and remnants—a new theory. *Biochem. Biophys. Res. Commun.* 66: 1467-1475, 1975.

13. FIELDING, C. J. Purification of lipoprotein lipase from rat postheparin plasma. *Biochim. Biophys. Acta* 178: 499-507, 1969.

14. FIELDING, C. J. Human lipoprotein lipase. Purification and substrate specificity. *Biochim. Biophys. Acta* 206: 109-117, 1970.

15. FIELDING, C. J. Human lipoprotein lipase. Inhibition of activity by cholesterol. *Biochim. Biophys. Acta* 218: 221-226, 1970.

16. FIELDING, C. J. Kinetics of lipoprotein lipase: effects of the substrate apoprotein on reaction velocity. *Biochim. Biophys. Acta* 316: 66-75, 1973.

17. FIELDING, C. J. Lipoprotein lipase: evidence for high- and low-affinity enzyme sites. *Biochemistry* 15: 879-884, 1976.

18. FIELDING, C. J., AND P. E. FIELDING. Chylomicron protein content and the rate of lipoprotein lipase activity. *J. Lipid Res.* 17: 419-423, 1976.

19. FIELDING, C. J., AND P. E. FIELDING. Mechanism of salt-mediated inhibition of lipoprotein lipase. *J. Lipid Res.* 17: 248-256, 1976.

20. FIELDING, C. J., AND P. E. FIELDING. The activation of lipoprotein lipase by lipase co-protein (apo C-2). In: *Cholesterol Metabolism and Lipolytic Enzymes*, edited by J. Polonovski. New York: Masson, 1977, p. 165-172.

21. FIELDING, C. J., AND J. M. HIGGINS. Lipoprotein lipase: comparative properties of the membrane-supported and solubilized enzyme species. *Biochemistry* 13: 4324-4330, 1974.

22. FIELDING, P. E., V. G. SHORE, AND C. J. FIELDING. Lipoprotein lipase: properties of the enzyme isolated from postheparin plasma. *Biochemistry* 13: 4318-4324, 1974.

23. FIELDING, P. E., V. G. SHORE, AND C. J. FIELDING. Lipoprotein lipase. Isolation and characterization of a second enzyme species from postheparin plasma. *Biochemistry* 16: 1896-1900, 1977.

24. GANESAN, D., R. H. BRADFORD, P. ALAUPOVIC, AND W. J. McCONATHY. Differential activation of lipoprotein lipase from human postheparin plasma, milk and adipose tissue by polypeptides of serum apolipoprotein C. *Fed. European Biochem. Soc. Letters* 15: 205-208, 1971.

25. GARFINKEL, A. S., AND M. C. SCHOTZ. Sequential induction of two species of lipoprotein lipase. *Biochim. Biophys. Acta* 306: 128-133, 1973.

26. GOLDSTEIN, L. Kinetic behaviour of immobilized enzyme systems. *Methods Enzymol.* 44: 397-443, 1976.

27. GOODMAN, D. S. The metabolism of chylomicron cholesteryl ester in the rat. *J. Clin. Invest.* 41: 1886-1896, 1962.

28. HAVEL, R. J., C. J. FIELDING, T. OLIVECRONA, V. G. SHORE, P. E. FIELDING, AND T. EGELRUD. Cofactor activity of protein components of plasma very low density lipoprotein in the hydrolysis of triglycerides by lipoprotein lipase from different sources. *Biochemistry* 12: 1828-1833, 1973.

29. HAVEL, R. J., J. P. KANE, AND M. L. KASHYAP. Interchange of apolipoproteins between chylomicrons and high density lipoproteins during alimentary lipemia in man. *J. Clin. Invest.* 52: 32-38, 1973.

30. HAVEL, R. J., V. G. SHORE, B. SHORE, AND D. M. BIER. Role of specific glycopeptides of human serum lipoproteins in the activation of lipoprotein lipase. *Circulation Res.* 27: 595-600, 1970.

31. HIGGINS, J. M., AND C. J. FIELDING. Lipoprotein lipase. Mechanism of formation of triglyceride-rich remnant particles from very low density lipoproteins and chylomicrons. *Biochemistry* 14: 2288-2293, 1975.

32. IVERIUS, P., H., AND A. M. OSTLAND-LINDQVIST. Lipoprotein lipase from bovine milk. Isolation procedure, chemical characterization and molecular weight analysis. *J. Biol. Chem.* 251: 7791-7795, 1976.

33. KOBAYASHI, T., AND M. MOO-YOUNG. The kinetics of mass-transfer behaviour of immobilized invertase on ion-exchange resin beads. *Biotechnol. Bioeng.* 15: 47-68, 1974.

34. LaROSA, J. C., R. I. LEVY, P. HERBERT, S. E. LUX, AND D. S. FREDRICKSON. A specific apoprotein activator for lipoprotein lipase. *Biochem. Biophys. Res. Commun.* 41: 57-62, 1970.

35. LILLY, M. D., W. E. HORNBY, AND E. M. CROOK. The kinetics of carboxymethyl-cellulose-ficin in packed beds. *Biochem. J.* 100: 718-723, 1966.

36. MJØS, O. D., O. FAERGEMAN, R. L. HAMILTON, AND R. J. HAVEL. Characterization of remnants produced during metabolism of triglyceride-rich lipoproteins of blood plasma and intestinal lymph in rats. *J. Clin. Invest.* 56: 603-615, 1975.

37. NESTEL, P. J., R. J. HAVEL, AND A. BEZMAN. Sites of initial removal of chylomicron triglyceride fatty acids from the blood. *J. Clin. Invest.* 41: 1915-1921, 1962.

38. NESTEL, P. J., R. J. HAVEL, AND A. BEZMAN. Metabolism of constituent lipids of dog chylomicrons. *J. Clin. Invest.* 42: 1313-1321, 1963.

39. NOEL, S. P., P. J. DOLPHIN, AND D. RUBINSTEIN. An *in vitro* model for the catabolism of rat chylomicrons. *Biochem. Biophys. Res. Commun.* 63: 764-772, 1975.

40. OSTLAND-LINDQVIST, A. M., AND P. H. IVERIUS. Activation of highly-purified lipoprotein lipase from bovine milk. *Biochem. Biophys. Res. Commun.* 65: 1447-1455, 1975.

41. REAVEN, G. M., D. B. HILL, R. C. GROSS, AND J. W. FARQUHAR. Kinetics of triglyceride turnover of very

low density lipoproteins of human plasma. *J. Clin Invest.* 44: 1826–1833, 1965.

42. REDGRAVE, T. G. Formation of cholesteryl ester-rich particulate lipid during metabolism of chylomicrons. *J. Clin. Invest.* 49: 465–471, 1970.

43. ROBINSON, D. S. The function of the plasma triglycerides in fatty acid transport. In: *Comprehensive Biochemistry*, edited by M. Florkin and E. H. Stotz. Amsterdam: Elsevier, 1970, vol. 18, p. 51–116.

44. ROBINSON, D. S., G. H. JEFFRIES, AND J. C. F. POOLE. Further studies on the interaction of chyle and plasma in the rat. *Quart. J. Exptl. Physiol.* 40: 297–308, 1955.

45. SATA, T., R. J. HAVEL, AND A. L. JONES. Characterization of subfractions of triglyceride-rich lipoproteins separated by gel chromatography from blood plasma of normolipemic and hyperlipemic humans. *J. Lipid Res.* 13: 757–768, 1972.

46. SCOW, R. O., AND T. EGELRUD. Hydrolysis of chylomicron phosphatidyl choline *in vitro* by lipoprotein lipase, phospholipase A-2 and phospholipase C. *Biochim. Biophys. Acta* 431: 538–549, 1976.

47. TWU, J.-S., A. S. GARFINKEL, AND M. C. SCHOTZ. Rat heart lipoprotein lipase. *Atherosclerosis* 22: 463–472, 1975.

48. ZECH, L. A., S. M. GRUNDY, AND M. BERMAN. Triglyceride synthesis and metabolism in man: a model based on glycerol kinetics. *Circulation* 54, Suppl. II: 5, 1976.

6

Kinetic Characteristics of the Hepatic Transport of Chylomicron Remnants

BETTE C. SHERRILL

Department of Internal Medicine, University of Texas
Health Science Center, Dallas, Texas

Chylomicron Remnant Formation
Hepatic Uptake of Chylomicrons and Chylomicron Remnants
  Time dependency
  Concentration dependency
  Temperature effect
  Intact particle uptake
  Effect of physiological state of liver
Determinant(s) for Hepatic Recognition

FORMATION OF THE INTESTINAL CHYLOMICRONS and formation of the triglyceride-depleted intestinal chylomicrons (chylomicron remnants) by the action of lipoprotein lipases located in the capillary beds of extrahepatic tissues are the initial physiological steps performed to manage an exogenous, dietary load of lipid. It has been known for some time that the chylomicron remnants are the form of intestinal chylomicrons that are taken up preferentially by the liver (3, 13, 29–31). At some critical point during peripheral circulation the chylomicrons gain the necessary determinant(s) for the liver to recognize the chylomicron remnant particles and remove them from circulation. The liver then can metabolize chylomicron remnants and store or utilize the various components, namely, triglyceride, phospholipid, protein, and free and esterified cholesterol. At present the critical determinant(s) for hepatic recognition of chylomicron remnants are unknown. To gain insight into this area this chapter discusses the kinetic characteristics of the hepatic removal process for chylomicron remnants.

CHYLOMICRON REMNANT FORMATION

Several experimental methods are available for preparing triglyceride-depleted remnants from chylomicrons. Incubation of chylomicrons with postheparin plasma containing several heparin-releasable lipoprotein lipases is a common in vitro method (12, 13). Large quantities of remnants can be produced by this method but care must be exercised to prevent formation of abnormal particles containing excess free fatty acid (FFA) (6). Purified single lipoprotein lipase types extracted from heart (10, 37), milk (11, 19), or adipose tissue (2, 10) also can be used for in vitro formation of chylomicron remnants. High-density lipoproteins or serum must be present during in vitro incubations because the activator peptide, apoC-II, is required for the chylomicrons to become substrates for the lipoprotein lipase (2, 14–16, 37).

Another method for formation of remnants is the perfused-organ technique, which has the advantage of an organ-specific lipoprotein lipase but generally produces only small quantities of remnants. Organs that have been used include adipose tissue (32, 34), heart (17, 29), and mammary tissue (20, 21, 42).

Functionally hepatectomized rats (31) or the supradiaphragmatic portion of rats (4, 5) are two animal preparations that allow remnant formation from infused chylomicrons. Large quantities of remnants can be isolated from the animals, especially the functionally hepatectomized rats, because the remnants are maintained in the peripheral circulation separated from the hepatic removal mechanism. Since this method, in contrast to the other methods, more closely mimics the in vivo physiological situation for remnant formation, it was employed for preparation of remnants used to determine the kinetic characteristics of the hepatic transport process (35).

Intestinal lymph was collected by cannulation of the mesenteric lymph ducts of female Sprague-Dawley rats. Corn oil containing radioactive cholesterol and stearic acid was introduced into their stomach catheters so that in vivo doubly labeled chylomicrons were collected. In these fat-fed rats the chylomicrons ($S_f > 400$) ultracentrifugally separated from the lymph contained 60–70% of the cholesterol radioactive label in the free cholesterol fraction while the remainder was esterified cholesterol, findings similar to those with fat-fed dogs (18, 23, 41). The triglyceride core of the chylomicrons contained 80–90% of the stearic acid radioactive label. Thus, these doubly labeled chylomicrons contained a marker (stearic acid radioactive label) for the core and a marker (cholesterol radioactive label) for the outer monolayer.

The doubly labeled chylomicrons ($S_f > 400$) were infused into functionally hepatectomized rats and allowed to circulate for 3 h before isolation of the formed remnants by aortic puncture. The 3-h time interval was chosen based on results obtained in intact animal studies (26). Figure 1 illustrates the effect of time on serum cholesterol and hepatic cholesterol esters after injection of chylomicrons containing 6 mg total cholesterol/100 g rat wt. The serum cholesterol level rose in these intact animals immediately after infusion from 50 mg/100 ml to 200 mg/100 ml. Approximately 3 h after infusion of even the largest chylomicrons ($S_f > 8000$), which contained the greatest quantity of triglyceride core (approximately 850 mg total lipids/100 g rat wt), the serum cholesterols began to fall. Simultaneously the cholesterol esters in the livers of the intact animals began to rise as the serum cholesterol began decreasing, indicating that this period of time was sufficient for lipoprotein lipase activity to significantly alter the particles such that remnants were formed and were removed by the liver. Thus remnants for these transport studies were made by infusing functionally hepatectom-

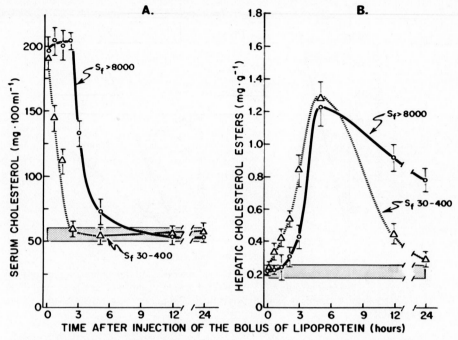

FIG. 1. Profiles of serum cholesterol levels (*A*) and hepatic cholesterol esters (*B*) in rats after bolus injections of chylomicrons, S_f 30–400 and $S_f > 8000$. [From Nervi et al. (26).]

ized rats with doubly labeled chylomicrons containing a maximum 4 mg total cholesterol and 800 mg total lipids/100 g rat wt and allowing 3 h of circulation before isolation.

HEPATIC UPTAKE OF CHYLOMICRONS AND CHYLOMICRON REMNANTS

Time Dependency

Solutions of chylomicrons and their remnants dissolved in oxygenated Krebs-Ringer-bicarbonate buffer (7, 33) were perfused in a nonrecirculating system entering through the portal vein and exiting out of the inferior vena cava of isolated rat livers (22, 25, 35). The perfusate solutions and perfused livers were maintained at 37°C. Duration of perfusions with the doubly labeled solutes varied from 1 to 15 min. As shown in Figure 2 uptake of both $S_f > 400$ chylomicrons and chylomicron remnants was linear per gram liver wet weight over the entire time course whether the uptake was monitored by the cholesterol marker or the stearic acid [fatty acid (FA)] marker. It is also obvious from these results that hepatic uptake of the chylomicron remnants occurs much more rapidly than uptake of the chylomicrons at any time period. Based on these linear time courses all subsequent liver perfusions were done in 4-min time periods.

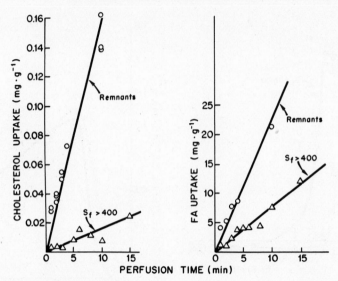

FIG. 2. Uptake time courses of $S_f > 400$ rat chylomicrons and their remnants in perfused liver preparation. Cholesterol uptake (left) as milligrams cholesterol per gram wet liver weight and fatty acid (FA) uptake as milligrams fatty acid per gram wet liver weight. [From Sherrill et al. (35).]

Concentration Dependency

Figure 3 demonstrates the effect of concentration on hepatic uptake of chylomicrons and remnants. Cholesterol uptake (mg cholesterol/g liver wet wt per min of perfusion) as a function of cholesterol perfusate concentration (mg/dl of remnants) and various sizes of chylomicrons is shown on the left. The right panel shows triglyceride FA uptake (mg/g per min) of the same lipoprotein particles as a function of total lipid perfusate concentration, which is essentially the triglyceride concentration since cholesterol is a minor fraction of the total lipids of these particles. The chylomicrons (closed triangles represent $S_f > 400$ and the closed circles $S_f < 400$) show only slight increases, if any, of uptake with increasing perfusate concentrations. The open triangles, which are $S_f > 400$ chylomicrons infused into functionally hepatectomized rats but removed immediately after the infusion period, demonstrate low uptake values just as the noninfused chylomicrons. There-fore, the 25-min infusion period for this load of chylomicrons (approximately 700 mg triglyceride/100 g rat wt) does not allow sufficient alteration of the chylomicrons such that hepatic flux is increased. The triglyceride core of the chylomicrons is only depleted 10–15% by the action of lipoprotein lipase during this infusion period (35, Table IV; Sherrill, unpublished observations).

In definite and striking contrast, the remnants (open circles) show not only markedly increased uptake at all concentrations but also a plateauing of uptake at high concentrations. These plateauing concentration curves for the chylomicron remnants suggest that hepatic uptake of remnants is by a specific saturable process and thus could involve a finite number of sites located on the sinusoidal membranes. Apparent kinetic constants for this high-capacity hepatic transport system can be determined from a Lineweaver-Burk plot as shown in Figure 4. Each point on this graph represents an individually perfused liver over a wide range of remnant-cholesterol perfusate concentrations. The intercepts of the linear regression curve give

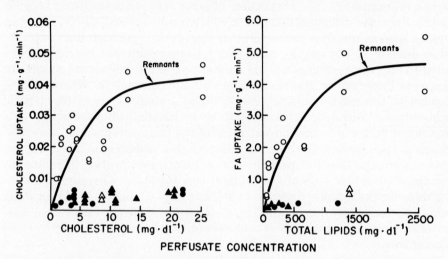

FIG. 3. Uptake concentration courses in perfused rat liver: (▲) $S_f > 400$ chylomicrons, (●) $S_f < 400$ chylomicrons, (○) 3-h remnants of $S_f > 400$ chylomicrons, and (△) $S_f < 400$ chylomicrons infused into functionally hepatectomized rats and isolated immediately after infusion. Cholesterol uptake in the left panel and fatty acid (FA) uptake in the right panel have dimensions of milligrams per gram liver wet weight per minute of perfusion. [From Sherrill et al. (35).]

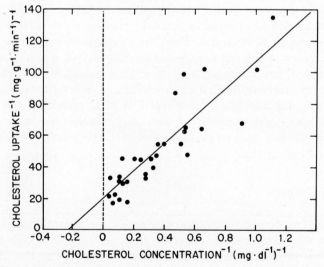

FIG. 4. Lineweaver-Burk plot of the rate of hepatic cholesterol uptake as a function of the perfusate concentration of chylomicron remnant-cholesterol in perfused livers. [From Sherrill et al. (35).]

an apparent maximum transport rate, in terms of the cholesterol carried in the remnant, of 0.052 mg/g per min and an apparent K_m of 4.5 mg/dl. Two possible sources of error exist in these calculations. If there were a significant diffusion barrier between the remnant particles of the perfusate in the sinusoidal space and the transport sites then both of these parameters would be overestimated (39, 40). This source of error does not seem likely because in the liver the diffusion distance could be only approximately 1 μm in length. Also in the time curves (Fig. 2) the linear regression lines extrapolated directly to the origin, indicating no major diffusion barrier existed between the transport sites and the remnant particles. The second possibility is a more likely source of error for these kinetic parameters. Where a finite number of transport sites are arrayed along a channel, as in the hepatic sinusoid, the Michaelis constant will be artifactually high if there is a significant decrease in the concentration of the transported solute along the length of the channel. In these experiments this situation occurred. At the lowest perfusate levels of particles the effluent concentration of remnants decreased 40–50% of that of the influent concentration. Therefore the true K_m value for the uptake of remnants is lower than 4.5 mg/dl, the lower limit being approximately 1.9 mg/dl. Thus, under physiological conditions, this system can achieve a high rate of transport at very low plasma concentrations of remnants.

Temperature Effect

There is a profound temperature effect on hepatic uptake of chylomicron remnants (35, 36). If the perfusate temperature is lowered to 27°C, the remnant uptake is decreased 4.5-fold. Under the same experimental conditions chylomicron uptake is only decreased twofold. The 4.5-fold decrease in remnant uptake per 10° decline in perfusing temperature corresponds to an activation energy of 27 kcal/mol. This large activation energy could be due to a phase change of the remnant particles themselves but if this were the case a similar large activation energy change would have been expected with the larger triglyceride-rich chylomicrons. A more likely possibility is that the sinusoidal membrane is affected at 27°C such that the transport sites are not functioning maximally. This suggests that the large activation energy results from a marked perturbation of the structure of the sinusoidal membrane during uptake.

Intact Particle Uptake

As stated previously (CHYLOMICRON REMNANT FORMATION), the doubly labeled $S_f > 400$ chylomicrons collected from mesenteric lymph ducts contained 60–70% of the cholesterol radioactive label in the free cholesterol component and 80–90% of the stearic acid radioactive label in the triglyceride component, thus allowing a marker for the outer monolayer and a marker for the inner core of the chylomicron. By monitoring the radioactive fatty acid:cholesterol ratio of the particles taken up by the perfused liver relative to the radioactive total lipids:cholesterol ratio of the particles in the perfusing solution, it was possible to determine if the hepatic uptakes reflected transport of the intact macromolecular structures or preferential uptake of specific components. Representative data shown in Figure 5 demonstrate that, from a series of remnants that had been metabolized by lipoprotein lipases in functionally hepatectomized animals to various sizes by varying the infusion loads and the circulation times, the slope is approximately unity, i.e., 0.98, indicating the macromolecular complexes are taken up by the perfused liver as intact structures. These chylomicron remnants varied from particles containing 90% of their original triglyceride core down to particles containing only 18% of their original triglyceride core. Thus regardless of the diameter of the chylomicron remnants they are capable of being transported across the liver sinusoidal membrane boundary as intact particles without prior hydrolysis at the sinusoidal surface.

Effect of Physiological State of Liver

Since hepatic uptake of chylomicron remnants is mediated by such a high-velocity transport mechanism and the remnants are taken up as intact macromolecular complexes, the question arises as to whether experimental manipulation of the liver can affect remnant uptake. Nilsson (28) has addressed this question by monitoring the effect colchicine, vinblastine, and cycloheximide had on hepatic uptake and hepatic metabolism of chylomicron remants. Colchicine, a microtubular inhibition agent, and vinblastine, a microfilament inhibition agent, were injected into intact rats prior to infusion of $S_f > 400$ chylomicrons to determine if intact microtubular functions were required by hepatocytes for transport and metabolism of the chylomicron remnant particles. The results demonstrated that neither colchicine nor vinblastine affected hepatic remnant uptake in control animals, although

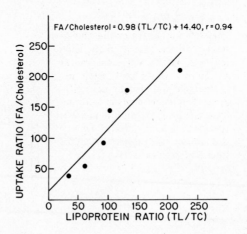

FIG. 5. Hepatic uptake ratio of fatty acid to cholesterol of chylomicron remnants relative to the perfusate lipoprotein ratio of total lipids to total cholesterol. [Adapted from Sherrill et al. (35, 36).]

both agents definitely delayed hepatic hydrolysis of the remnants after uptake. Livers of cycloheximide-treated animals showed no change in the rate of remnant uptake and no delay in hepatic hydrolysis of the remnant particles, indicating active protein synthesis was not necessary for hepatic transport or degradation of the remnants.

Another experimental manipulation done to affect the physiological state of the liver was to vary the hepatic de novo cholesterol synthetic rate over a 40-fold range (1). This was accomplished by subjecting rats to various experimental conditions such as 48-h fasting, cholesterol feeding, 48-h biliary obstructions, 48-h biliary diversions, and cholestyramine feeding. The rates of hepatic cholesterol synthesis varied from 56 nmol/g per h for 48-h-fasted animals to 2162 nmol/g per h for animals fed cholestyramine for 2 wk as shown in Figure 6. Cholesterol uptake from chylomicron remnants measured as a function of the rate of change in hepatic cholesterol ester content in these intact animals demonstrated constant uptake over the entire range of hepatic cholesterol synthetic rates. In a similar experiment livers from dietary-manipulated rats were perfused with doubly labeled chylomicron remnants and uptake was determined as described previously (*Concentration Dependency*). The hepatic cholesterol synthetic rates obtained were: 7 nmol/g per h for rats maintained on a 2% cholesterol diet for 2 wk, 94 nmol/g per h for 48-h-fasted animals, 890 nmol/g per h for control animals, and 2638 nmol/g per h for rats on a 2% cholestyramine diet for 2 wk. The remnant uptake rate in perfused livers from these animals was also a constant value independent of the cholesterol synthetic state of the liver (Sherrill, unpublished observation). These data from both the in vivo study and the in vitro perfused liver study demonstrate the remarkable clearance capacity of the liver to remove from blood circulation the chylomicron remnants independent of the de novo hepatic cholesterol synthetic rate. Physiologically, this independence of the hepatic remnant transport mechanism from the endoge-

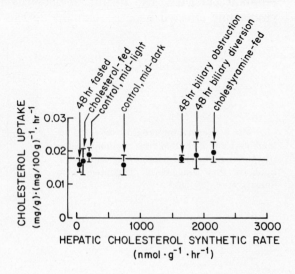

FIG. 6. Independence of chylomicron uptake from the cholesterol synthetic rate of livers. Chylomicron uptake was measured as milligrams cholesterol ester per gram liver wet weight per milligrams chylomicron-cholesterol infused per 100 g rat per h in animals that had various rates of hepatic cholesterol synthesis. [Adapted from Andersen et al. (1).]

nous rate of hepatic cholesterol synthesis is necessary for an organism to be able to handle its widely varying intestinal influxes of dietary lipids randomly ingested during any 24-h period. On the other hand, hepatic metabolism of the chylomicron remnants after uptake causes a decrease in the rate of hepatic endogenous cholesterol synthesis. This has been demonstrated in intact animals (9, 26, 27, 38) and in the perfused liver (8). This process is physiologically important to an organism for maintaining a delicate balance between rate of entry of exogenous cholesterol versus the rate of synthesis of endogenous cholesterol within the liver, while still allowing the hepatic transport mechanism for remnants to operate at maximum efficiency under all conditions.

DETERMINANT(S) FOR HEPATIC RECOGNITION

The key question that remains unanswered now is what are the specific determinant(s) of the chylomicrons that are altered, added, or deleted such that the liver now recognizes it as a chylomicron remnant and removes it from circulation? Several possibilities exist: *1*) size of the particle, *2*) lipid composition, *3*) a new component added to the particle, or *4*) apoprotein composition.

The size of the particle does not seem to be a major determinant because the perfused liver does not recognize small $S_f < 400$ chylomicrons and take them up with the saturable kinetics demonstrated for remnant uptake (Fig. 3). The diameter range of the small chylomicrons overlaps the diameter range for remnants formed from large chylomicrons (24); therefore the size of the particles is not a determinant for hepatic recognition.

Lipid composition of the remnant does not appear to be a determining factor of uptake either. In a representative experiment (35, Table IV) the total lipid:total cholesterol ratio of $S_f > 400$ was 192 and hepatic uptake was low, 0.004 mg cholesterol/g per min; the 3-h remnants formed from these chylomicrons had a total lipid:total cholesterol ratio of 105 and fivefold increased hepatic uptake of 0.022 mg cholesterol/g per min. In contrast the small $S_f < 400$ chylomicrons with an even lower total lipid:total cholesterol ratio of only 82 again demonstrated low hepatic uptake, 0.003 mg cholesterol/g per min. Thus from lipoprotein transport studies done in conjunction with lipid compositional analysis it appears that gross lipid compositional changes are not hepatic recognition factors. A more detailed compositional analysis comparing chylomicrons and remnants has been represented by Mjøs et al. (24, Table III). Although transport measurements were not made simultaneously, the analysis is of interest because comparison between the compositions of the small chylomicrons and remnants of large chylomicrons shows similar results. The small chylomicrons had the following composition: 77% triglyceride, 3.6% total cholesterol, 14.4% phospholipid, and 5.1% protein; the composition of the large chylomicron remnants was: 70% triglyceride, 11.3% total cholesterol, 10.4% phospholipid, and 8.9% protein. Therefore although the lipid compositional analyses are similar for small chylomicrons and large chylomicron remnants, the liver recognizes and removes only the remnants at a high velocity. Thus lipid composition of the lipoprotein particle alone does not seem to be a major determinant for hepatic removal.

The addition of lipoprotein lipase to the chylomicron during triglyceride metabolism has been postulated to be the hepatic removal determinant by Felts and co-workers (13). They demonstrated that both in vivo remnants made in a supradiaphragmatic rat preparation and in vitro remnants formed by incubating chylomicrons in rat postheparin serum contained 2 U of lipoprotein lipase activity/mg triglyceride whereas chylomicrons only contained 0.08 U of lipoprotein lipase activity/mg triglyceride. In a single-pass perfused liver 39% of the remnants were cleared by the liver. These results indicate that addition of lipoprotein lipase to the remnant may be a recognition factor, but whether this is a physiological determinant is not proven yet.

Apoprotein compositional changes on the surface of the chylomicrons may be the major determinant for hepatic recognition. The quantity of the C class of apoproteins is greatly reduced or absent from both small chylomicron remnants (24) and large chylomicron remnants (Sherrill, Catapano, Smith, Dietschy, and Gotto, unpublished observations). Further characterization of the distribution of the apoproteins on chylomicrons and remnants must be done simultaneously with transport studies to determine the precise relationship before this possibility can be established.

The author's personal research was supported by Public Health Service research grants (AM16386, HL 09610, and AM 19329).

REFERENCES

1. ANDERSEN, J. M., F. O. NERVI, AND J. M. DIETSCHY. Rate constants for the uptake of cholesterol from various intestinal and serum lipoprotein fractions by the liver of the rat in vivo. *Biochim. Biophys. Acta* 486: 298–307, 1977.
2. BENSADOUN, A., C. EHNHOLM, D. STEINBERG, AND W. V. BROWN. Purification and characterization of lipoprotein lipase from pig adipose tissue. *J. Biol. Chem.* 249: 2220–2227, 1974.
3. BERGMAN, E. N., R. J. HAVEL, B. M. WOLFE, AND T. BØHMER. Quantitative studies of the metabolism of chylomicron triglycerides and cholesterol by liver and extrahepatic tissues of sheep and dogs. *J. Clin. Invest.* 50: 1831–1839, 1971.
4. BEZMAN-TARCHER, A., S. OTWAY, AND D. S. ROBINSON. The removal of triglyceride fatty acids from the circulation of the supradiaphragmatic portion of the rat. *Proc. Roy. Soc., London, Ser. B* 162: 411–426, 1965.
5. BEZMAN-TARCHER, A., AND D. S. ROBINSON. A technique for the preparation of the functional supradiaphragmatic portion of the rat. *Proc. Roy. Soc., London, Ser. B* 162: 406–410, 1965.
6. BLANCHETTE-MACKIE, E. J., AND R. O. SCOW. Retention of lipolytic products in chylomicrons incubated with lipoprotein lipase. Electron microscope study. *J. Lipid Res.* 17: 57–67, 1976.
7. BLOXAM, D. L. Nutritional aspects of amino acid metabolism. 1. A rat liver perfusion method for the study of amino acid metabolism. *Brit. J. Nutr.* 26: 393–422, 1971.
8. COOPER, A. D. The metabolism of chylomicron remnants by isolated perfused rat liver. *Biochim. Biophys. Acta* 488: 464–474, 1977.
9. COOPER, A. D., AND R. K. OCKNER. Studies of hepatic cholesterol synthesis in experimental acute biliary obstruction. *Gastroenterology* 66: 586–595, 1974.
10. DOLPHIN, P. J., AND D. RUBINSTEIN. The metabolism of very low density lipoprotein and chylomicrons by purified lipoprotein lipase from rat heart and adipose tissue. *Biochem. Biophys. Res. Commun.* 57: 808–814, 1974.
11. EGELRUD, T., AND T. OLIVECRONA. The purification of a lipoprotein lipase from bovine skim milk. *J. Biol. Chem.* 247: 6212–6217, 1972.
12. EISENBERG, S., AND D. RACHMILOWITZ. Interaction of rat plasma very low density lipoprotein with lipoprotein lipase-rich (postheparin) plasma. *J. Lipid Res.* 16: 341–351, 1975.
13. FELTS, J. M., H. ITAKURA, AND R. T. CRANE. The mechanism of assimilation of constituents of chylomicrons, very low density lipoproteins and remnants— a new theory. *Biochem. Biophys. Res. Commun.* 66: 1467–1475, 1975.
14. FIELDING, C. J., AND P. E. FIELDING. Chylomicron protein content and the rate of lipoprotein lipase activity. *J. Lipid Res.* 17: 419–423, 1976.

15. FIELDING, C. J., AND P. E. FIELDING. The activation of lipoprotein lipase by lipase co-protein (apo C-2). In: *Cholesterol Metabolism and Lipolytic Enzymes,* edited by J. Polonovski. New York: Masson, 1977, p. 165–172.

16. HAVEL, R. J., J. P. KANE, AND M. L. KASHYAP. Interchange of apolipoproteins between chylomicrons and high density lipoproteins during alimentary lipemia in man. *J. Clin. Invest.* 52: 32–38, 1973.

17. HIGGINS, J. M., AND C. J. FIELDING. Lipoprotein lipase. Mechanism of formation of triglyceride-rich remnant particles from very low density lipoproteins and chylomicrons. *Biochemistry* 14: 2288–2293, 1975.

18. HILLYARD, L. A., I. L. CHAIKOFF, C. ENTENMAN, AND W. O. REINHARDT. Composition and concentration of lymph and serum lipoproteins during fat and cholesterol absorption in the dog. *J. Biol. Chem.* 233: 838–842, 1958.

19. IVERIUS, P. H., AND A. M. OSTLAND-LINDQVIST. Lipoprotein lipase from bovine milk. Isolation procedure, chemical characterization and molecular weight analysis. *J. Biol. Chem.* 251: 7791–7795, 1976.

20. McBRIDE, O. W., AND E. D. KORN. The uptake of doubly labeled chylomicrons by guinea pig mammary gland and liver. *J. Lipid Res.* 5: 459–467, 1964.

21. MENDELSON, C. R., AND R. O. SCOW. Uptake of chylomicron-triglyceride by perfused mammary tissue of lactating rats. *Am. J. Physiol.* 223: 1418–1423, 1972.

22. MILLER, L. L., C. G. BLY, M. L. WATSON, AND W. F. BALE. The dominant role of the liver in plasma protein synthesis. A direct study of the isolated perfused rat liver with aid of lysine-ϵ-C^{14}. *J. Exptl. Med.* 94: 431–453, 1951.

23. MINARI, O., AND D. B. ZILVERSMIT. Behavior of dog lymph chylomicron lipid constituents during incubation with serum. *J. Lipid Res.* 4: 424–436, 1963.

24. MJØS, O. D., O. FAERGEMAN, R. L. HAMILTON, AND R. J. HAVEL. Characterization of remnants produced during the metabolism of triglyceride-rich lipoproteins of blood plasma and intestinal lymph in the rat. *J. Clin. Invest.* 56: 603–615, 1975.

25. MORTIMORE, G. E. Effect of insulin on potassium transfer in isolated rat liver. *Am. J. Physiol.* 200: 1315–1319, 1961.

26. NERVI, F. O., AND J. M. DIETSCHY. Ability of six different lipoprotein fractions to regulate the rate of hepatic cholesterogenesis *in vivo. J. Biol. Chem.* 250: 8704–8711, 1975.

27. NERVI, F. O., H. J. WEIS, AND J. M. DIETSCHY. The kinetic characteristics of inhibition of hepatic cholesterogenesis by lipoproteins of intestinal origin. *J. Biol. Chem.* 250: 4145–4151, 1975.

28. NILSSON, A. Antimicrotubular agents inhibit the degradation of chyle cholesterol ester in vivo. *Biochem. Biophys. Res. Commun.* 66: 60–66, 1975.

29. NOEL, S., P. J. DOLPHIN, AND D. RUBINSTEIN. An in vitro model for the catabolism of rat chylomicrons. *Biochem. Biophys. Res. Commun.* 63: 764–772, 1975.

30. QUARFORDT, S. H., AND D. S. GOODMAN. Metabolism of doubly-labeled chylomicron cholesteryl esters in the rat. *J. Lipid Res.* 8: 264–273, 1967.

31. REDGRAVE, T. G. Formation of cholesteryl ester-rich particulate lipid during metabolism of chylomicrons. *J. Clin. Invest.* 49: 465–471, 1970.

32. RODBELL, M., AND R. O. SCOW. Metabolism of chylomicrons and triglyceride emulsions by perfused rat adipose tissue. *Am. J. Physiol.* 208: 106–114, 1965.

33. SCHOLZ, R., AND T. BUCHER. Hemoglobin-free perfusion of rat liver. In: *Control of Energy Metabolism,* edited by B. Chance, R. W. Estabrook, and J. R. Williamson. New York: Academic, 1965, p. 393–413.

34. SCOW, R. O., M. HAMOSH, E. J. BLANCHETTE-MACKIE, AND A. J. EVANS. Uptake of blood triglycerides by various tissues. *Lipids* 7: 497–505, 1972.

35. SHERRILL, B. C., AND J. M. DIETSCHY. Characterization of the sinusoidal transport process responsible for uptake of chylomicrons by the liver. *J. Biol. Chem.* In press.

36. SHERRILL, B. C., AND J. M. DIETSCHY. Uptake of lipoproteins of intestinal origin in the isolated perfused liver. *Circulation* 54, Suppl. II: 91, 1976.

37. TWU, J., A. S. GARFINKEL, AND M.C. SCHOTZ. Rat heart lipoprotein lipase. *Atherosclerosis* 22: 463–472, 1975.

38. WEIS, H. J., AND J. M. DIETSCHY. Failure of bile acids to control hepatic cholesterogenesis; evidence for endogenous cholesterol feedback. *J. Clin. Invest.* 48: 2398–2408, 1969.

39. WILSON, F. A., AND J. M. DIETSCHY. The intestinal unstirred layer: its surface area and effect on active transport kinetics. *Biochim. Biophys. Acta* 363: 112–126, 1974.

40. WINNE, D. Unstirred layer, source of biased Michaelis constant in membrane transport. *Biochim. Biophys. Acta* 298: 27–31, 1973.

41. YOKOYAMA, A., AND D. B. ZILVERSMIT. Particle size and composition of dog lymph chylomicrons. *J. Lipid Res.* 6: 241–246, 1965.

42. ZINDER, O., C. R. MENDELSON, E. J. BLANCHETTE-MACKIE, AND R. O. SCOW. Lipoprotein lipase and uptake of chylomicron triacylglycerol and cholesterol by perfused rat mammary tissue. *Biochim. Biophys. Acta* 431: 526–537, 1976.

7

Structure of Intact Human
Plasma Lipoproteins

WILLIAM A. BRADLEY AND ANTONIO M. GOTTO, JR.

*Division of Atherosclerosis and Lipoprotein Research, Department of Medicine,
Baylor College of Medicine and The Methodist Hospital, Houston, Texas*

THE QUEST FOR KNOWLEDGE has generated a vast literature concerning the structure and metabolism of the serum lipoproteins.[1] Although much has been learned about the components (i.e., apoproteins, phospholipids, etc.) of lipoproteins, reassembled species, and model systems, the most instructive information will be that revealing the structural interrelationships within the intact lipoprotein particle. Dynamic interchange of protein, lipid, and carbohydrate components may provide the key to understanding the function of these particles. Techniques such as electron microscopy and small-angle X-ray analysis allow us to examine the overall morphology of intact lipoproteins. Information about both whole lipoproteins and substructural interactions may be obtained by studies with nuclear magnetic resonance (NMR), thermal analysis [differential scanning calorimetry (DSC)], optical measurements [circular dichroism (CD), optical rotary dispersion (ORD), fluorescence spectroscopy, etc.], and hydrodynamic (ultracentrifugation) methods. Enzymatic and chemical modification studies have also provided some clues to the accessibility of the components of the intact lipoproteins. This chapter briefly reviews pertinent (but, of necessity, incomplete) information available on the structure of the intact lipoproteins. We consider separately the major

---

[1] This chapter considers studies *only* on human lipoproteins. Other animal lipoproteins have been studied and, in general, support the data discussed here.

classes of lipoproteins: high-density lipoproteins (HDL), low-density lipoproteins (LDL), very-low-density lipoproteins (VLDL), and the chylomicrons. Physicochemical properties of the lipoprotein proteins or apoproteins are summarized. Brief reference is made to abnormal lipoproteins (i.e., Lp-X), to the dynamics of lipoprotein exchange, and to current models of lipoprotein structure.

Obviously, structural data obtained from physical and chemical investigations should be consistent with what is known about the metabolic relationships among the lipoproteins. For this reason, a review of lipoprotein structure is germane to our interest in the formation, secretion, and metabolism of the major plasma lipoproteins.

NOMENCLATURE

The organization of knowledge about a subject begins with a system of classification. Based on the rate of flotation in salt solutions (144), the known human plasma lipoproteins have been traditionally divided into the following classes: HDL, d 1.063–1.210 g/ml; LDL, d 1.006–1.063 g/ml; VLDL, d 0.95–1.006 g/ml; and chylomicrons, $d < 0.95$ g/ml. Low-density lipoproteins have been subdivided into intermediate-density lipoproteins (IDL, d 1.006–1.019) and a redefined LDL fraction (d 1.019–1.063). Very-high-density lipoproteins (VHDL) refer to the density range of 1.210–1.250 g/ml.

Although a number of classification schemes have been applied to the apoproteins associated with the lipoprotein classes, the A, B, C designations are used here. ApoA, apoB, and apoC are used to represent groups of apoproteins rather than a discrete lipoprotein family.

STUDIES ON INTACT HUMAN PLASMA HIGH-DENSITY LIPOPROTEINS

Of all the plasma lipoproteins, the HDL have received the greatest attention in recent years by students of lipoprotein structure. The primary sequences of all the major protein components (apoA-I and apoA-II) have been elucidated (see APOLIPOPROTEINS) as well as several of the minor components (apoC-I, apoC-II, and apoC-III). Structures of the "arginine-rich" protein (ARP), also called apoE, and the "thin-line" proteins, referred to as apoD, have not been determined. In addition, the ability to reassemble the components of HDL into the "native" lipoproteins (115) makes it an attractive system to study.

Subclasses of HDL have been recognized by a number of techniques such as differential (22) and rate-zonal ultracentrifugation (97) and by analytical (79) and preparative gel electrofocusing (154). By analytical ultracentrifugation, the molecular weights of HDL$_2$ and HDL$_3$ are 3.4 × 10^5 and 1.75 × 10^5, respectively (144). Negatively stained HDL$_2$ (d 1.063–1.125 g/ml) appear in the electron microscope as circular particles of diameter 95–100 Å. The HDL$_3$ (d 1.125–1.12 g/ml) particles are smaller, of diameter 70–75

Å. Occasionally, a free-standing HDL particle can be seen to have a darker central core after being stained with phosphotungstate. This led to speculation that HDL contain subunit structure (36), but this finding has not been corroborated by other physical methods. Both the negative stain itself as well as focal perturbations lend themselves to artifacts.

Small-angle X-ray analysis (71, 72) of dilute solutions of monodispersed HDL_2 and HDL_3 shows that the particles are symmetrical spheres with two distinct regions of electron density. The central core, extending to 43 Å in HDL_2 and 37 Å in HDL_3, is electron deficient. An outer shell, radius 14 Å in HDL_2 and 11 Å in HDL_3, is electron rich. The best interpretation of these results is that the center of the spherical HDL contains the apolar lipids and that the outer shell at the hydrocarbon-water interface has the polar phospholipid head groups and the protein constituents.

The analysis of HDL by ^{13}C-NMR (8, 51, 52) reflects the liquidlike environment of both its lipid and protein moieties. The ^{13}C-spin-lattice relaxation times (T_1's) indicate that although the lipids are in a liquidlike environment they are relatively restricted compared with the same lipids in organic solvents. High-field (69.7 MHz) ^{13}C-NMR studies by Hamilton (49) have allowed resolution of heretofore unresolved resonances of cholesterol C-6 methine from the esterified form. With well-resolved spectral lines for C-3 and C-9 of the cholesteryl ester, there is the exciting possibility of studying the relative mobility of cholesterol and cholesteryl esters after various physiological processes, e.g., after interaction of the lipoproteins with lecithin:cholesterol acyltransferase (LCAT) or with lipoprotein lipase (LPL). Half-height resonances ($\nu_{1/2}$) in the high-field study lend further support to the restricted motion of the cholesteryl esters and the phospholipid glycerol backbone. Hamilton has speculated, from the values of $\nu_{1/2}$ and from the unequal intensities of the C'-1 and C'-3 of the glycerol backbone, the possibility that the C'-1 of the phospholipids interacts directly with the cholesterol.

Proton magnetic resonance (23, 150) detects no line-width broadening in HDL lipids compared with lipid dispersions and, in general, cannot discern the relative restricted motion of the lipid, unlike ^{13}C-NMR. This difference is probably due to the small percentage of protons involved in the protein-lipid interaction.

Electron paramagnetic resonance (EPR) spectra of HDL (40, 42) with the nitroxide radical 1-oxyl-2,2,6,6-tetramethyl-4-isothiocyanatopiperidine display both a broad and narrow component. The nitroxide radical is most likely attached to the ϵ-amino groups of the protein. The broad component is probably due to the apoprotein-lipid interaction, although this finding cannot at present be corroborated by other physical techniques.

The X-ray analysis of HDL indicates a region of high electron density, almost certainly containing the phospholipid and apoprotein in the periphery. Studies with ^{31}P-NMR have attempted to identify the location of the phospholipid. The use of the lanthanide shift reagent, Eu^{+3}, which supposedly differentiates externally located phospholipid (6, 21, 88), showed that both sphingomyelin and phosphatidylcholine are exclusively at the surface of the lipoprotein (9). Furthermore, $^{31}P\text{-}T_1$ analysis in native HDL, compared with sonicated lipid vesicles, showed no differences, a finding interpreted as evidence that the phospholipid head group is relatively unrestricted and does not interact with the apoprotein. The phospholipids of HDL_2 and HDL_3 also have been localized with the paramagnetic quenching reagent, Mn^{+2}, chelated to ethylenediaminetetraacetic acid (EDTA) in the ratio 1:2.2 (57). The chelated species have a larger molecular volume and are less able to penetrate the surface of the lipoprotein than the Eu^{+3} probe. Analysis of intensity measurements by ^{31}P-NMR, employing this probe [Mn^{+2} $(EDTA)_{2.2}$], demonstrated that 20% of the HDL_2 (17% for HDL_2) phosphates are inaccessible. Henderson et al. (57) have inferred that the inaccessible phospholipids are interacting with the apoprotein. They were unable to confirm the results with Eu^{+3} of Assmann et al. (9) and pointed out the complication that the lanthanide shift reagents precipitate phosphate-containing samples.

Evidence for the surface location of the phospholipid has also been provided by the kinetic analysis of the action of snake venom phospholipase A_2 with HDL_3 (99). All the preferred substrate (phosphatidylcholine and phosphatidylethanolamine) was hydrolyzed by the phospholipase, which shows that the phospholipid must be at, or in rapid equilibrium with, the surface of the lipoprotein. Interestingly, this phospholipid-depleted HDL is quite stable. It remains intact and has physical characteristics similar to those of the lipoprotein. These observations suggest that the integrity of the phosphatidylcholine and phosphatidylethanolamine is not necessary to preserve the overall skeletal stability of the lipoprotein.

The apoproteins of HDL are assigned to the outer electron-density shell based on the small-angle X-ray analysis (71, 72). Various experimental approaches support this assignment. The free amino groups of both HDL_2 and HDL_3 apoproteins are readily accessible to modification by succinic anhydride (124). The modified lipoprotein retains the hydrodynamic and optical properties (ultracentrifugal behavior and circular dichroism) of the native lipoproteins. Experiments of this type, although useful, are hampered by the lack of knowledge concerning solubilities of the chemical probe in the lipid matrix, i.e., hydrophobic environment. A more informative experiment in which the location of the chemical probe is known has been accomplished by iodination of the intact HDL protein with an immobilized enzyme, lactoperoxidase (112). Extensive iodination of apoHDL occurs, whereas in the intact lipoprotein only small amounts of apoA-I and apoA-II are iodinated. However, the apoC proteins react extensively even in intact HDL. The apoC components of HDL therefore are more accessible to surface-restricted reagents than are the apoA ones.

Antibodies raised against cyanogen bromide (CNBr) fragments from the NH_2- and COOH-terminal regions of apoA-I demonstrate that these regions are immunologically distinct and can be assayed independently (127). When these specific antibodies are used to probe the surface of intact HDL_2, the COOH-terminal region is immunologically more reactive by three- to fivefold on a molar basis than is the NH_2-terminal region. One point of view, then, is that the COOH terminal of apoA-I is more exposed and therefore less involved in lipid-lipid or lipid-protein interactions than is the NH_2 terminal. A point yet to be resolved is why the COOH terminal of apoA-I should be so accessible to a specific antibody whereas Tyr-239 in the COOH terminal does not react in the enzymic iodination. It is predicted that Tyr-239 is on the carboxy-terminal end of the helical segment 224–238 in the apoprotein (116), but may be included in an extended helical segment in the native lipoprotein. Thus, the antibody directed toward the carboxyl segment of apoA-I could be specific for the secondary structure (α-helix). One possible explanation is that Tyr-239 is located on the nonpolar face of an amphipathic helical structure (see MODELS OF LIPOPROTEIN STRUCTURE) and is protected from iodination by interaction with the lipid.

Mao et al. (80) postulate that all the apoA-II of intact HDL must lie on the surface of the particle. In radioimmunoassay, the quantity of apoA-II measured in HDL is 1.4 times greater than in apoHDL. The increased antigenicity in the whole particle compared with the apoHDL could reflect denaturation of the apoA-II by organic solvent delipidation (80). Interestingly, apoA-II reacts with its antibody on the surface of HDL but not with the immobilized lactoperoxidase-catalyzed iodination. This may be caused by the location of the tyrosine residues (14, 21, 41, 66) on the hydrophobic face of an amphipathic helix (58, 59), where they interact in a lipid environment and are not accessible to the immobilized enzyme.

Spectroscopic studies yield information concerning the secondary structure of the apoproteins in the HDL particle. Early results with ORD (114) have been confirmed by CD data (41, 120) and show that the protein of HDL is highly α-helical ($\sim 70\%$). Computer-aided spectral analyses of the CD data (78) allowed the following estimates of the 2° structure of the apoproteins in HDL: 70% α-helix; 5–15% β-structure; and 15–20% disordered. Infrared spectra of HDL display an amide I band at 1650 cm (41, 118) and 1540 cm consistent with the ORD and CD data, indicating high α-helicity.

The intrinsic fluorescence spectra (55) of HDL indicate that the Trp residues are located in a relatively polar environment as determined by the emission maximum, which is not shifted appreciably on delipidation. This is consistent with the protein (in this case apoA-I; apoA-II has no Trp) being at or located near the water-lipid interface.

With the advent of commercially available instruments to measure fluorescence depolarization, microviscosities of the lipoproteins can be obtained readily. Jonas (62) used 1,6-diphenyl-1,3,5-hexatriene (DPH) and perylene as probes to determine the microviscosity (η) for HDL, 5.0 ± 0.3 P. This compares to 2.0 ± 0.3 P for the extracted lipids of HDL. Jonas attributes this difference to the effect of the protein restricting the mobility of the lipids and concludes that the HDL lipids are in a fluid state, based on the value of η. Flow activation energies (obtained from a plot of log η vs. $1/T$) for HDL (7.9 ± 1.6 kcal/mol over the temperature range 0–40°C) are also consistent with the presence of anisotropic lipid domains.

Perturbations of the intact HDL by physicochemical (94) and thermal methods (156) and the use of denaturants such as Gdn·HCl (93) provide information about the relative interactions of the apoproteins and lipids of the lipoprotein. Dehydration by rotary evaporation disrupts the HDL structure (94). However, the denatured material may be resolubilized in aqueous buffers at pH 8.6 and fractionated by sequential ultracentrifugation through the various density ranges used to isolate lipoproteins. An interesting redistribution of the apoprotein occurs. The apoA-I combines with only very small amounts of lipid and is found almost exclusively in the $d > 1.21$ g/ml fraction. By contrast, apoA-II is found in association with phospholipid-rich products in d 1.006–1.063 g/ml and d 1.063–1.21 g/ml fractions. When HDL are exposed to 2–3 M Gdn·HCl (93) at 37°C, the amount of apoA-I associated with $d \leq 1.21$ g/ml decreases and, correspondingly, the apoA-I content in $d > 1.21$ g/ml increases. The dissociated apoA-I contains by weight about 1 part phospholipid per 100 parts protein. If the Gdn·HCl concentration is increased to 5–6 M, both apoA-I and apoA-II dissociate from the HDL. ApoA-II is found in the d 1.21 g/ml infranatant if, during the ultracentrifugation, Gdn·HCl is present. If Gdn·HCl is not present, the apoA-II is found with the phospholipid fractions. Although apoA-II appears to recombine with phospholipid preferentially in the absence of Gdn·HCl, this finding may be a function of the state of the association of the apoprotein and its ability to bind lipid. ApoA-II binds phospholipid preferentially in an oligomeric form (108). The process of repetitive heating and cooling to temperatures above 55°C also releases apoA-I from HDL (156). A reversible thermal transition of the lipid-free apoA-I denaturation occurs at 54°C (158) as observed with DSC. The fraction of apoA-I released is calculated from the enthalpy of the transition at 54°C. Heating at 70°C for 15 min increases by 5–15 times a lipid-free (i.e., contains <1% phospholipid) apoprotein in the d 1.21 g/ml infranatant. More than 90% of the lipid-free protein is apoA-I.

Incubation of HDL with multilamellar liposomes of dimyristoyl phosphatidylcholine (DMPC) (1:1.2, wt:wt) at 37°C for 12 h produces a broad transition with a maximum at 25.5°C detected by DSC (157). This is similar to that found when apoA-I–DMPC complexes are formed. Tall et al. (156) performed thermal analysis of HDL_2 and HDL_3 at temperatures above 60°C, where a broad, double-peak endotherm occurs. They attribute the first peak with a maximum at 71°C to the selective loss of apoA-I from the lipoprotein. Further general disruption of the HDL occurs when heated to higher temperatures. A second endothermic peak is observed at 90°C associated with the loss of cholesteryl esters and apoA-II. When the heat-disrupted HDL particle is rescanned, two new transitions are observed. One is a cholesteryl ester smectic-liquid transition at 23.5 ± 4.9°C and the second is a reversible denaturation of a lipid-free apoA-I at 54°C (see above). Since the cholesteryl ester transition is not observed until disruption of HDL, it is inferred that the cholesteryl ester may interact with the phospholipid-protein outer shell (156). This interaction inhibits the organization and cooperative transition of a lipid phase so that the transition associated with free cholesteryl ester is abolished. Another inference is that apoA-I is less important than apoA-II in the stabilization of the apolar lipids of HDL (156). Although selective release of apoA-I from HDL has been documented under various conditions as described above, none of these experiments have included a kinetic analysis of the phenomenon. In our opinion, any interpretation of the thermal phenomenon in terms of molecular events should be considered tentative, pending the outcome of a kinetic study. Interpretation of any kinetic studies is complicated by the fact that, once dissociated from the HDL particle, both apoA-I (106, 152) and apoA-II self-associate (152). However, apoA-II binds lipids preferentially as the oligomer whereas apoA-I binds only a highly dissociated form (107, 108). Therefore, both apoproteins might be released equally from the lipid matrix, but the inability of a self-associated apoA-I to return to the lipid matrix could make it appear that this apoprotein is selectively released.

The relationship between lipid and protein in the intact HDL and the general location of the protein have been the subjects of numerous investigations. The relationship of the proteins with respect to each other has received less attention. Scanu and co-workers (32, 117, 121) cross-linked the major apoproteins with dimethylsuberimidate

$$(CH_3—O—\overset{\overset{\displaystyle NH_2}{\|}}{C}—(CH_2)_6—\overset{\overset{\displaystyle NH_2}{\|}}{C}—OCH_3).$$ From the cross-linked derivatives, he concluded that HDL_2 contains two chains of apoA-I and four chains of apoA-II (two chains of the disulfide-linked protomers) per lipoprotein particle. Grow and Fried (46) used the bifunctional reagent 1,5-difluoro-2,4-dinitrobenzene (DFDNB), which allows cross-linking of groups less than 10 Å apart. In their system, *only* apoA-I is cross-linked to apoA-II in HDL_2 as detected on sodium dodecyl sulfate (SDS)-polyacrylamide gel electrophoresis (PAGE). Only one chain of the dimeric apoA-II is detected in the cross-linking. No intermolecular linkage is seen between the apoA and apoC proteins. These data preliminarily suggest that a close spatial relationship exists between apoA-I and apoA-II. On a cautionary note, kinetic analysis of the cross-linking experiments is necessary before a complete interpretation is possible.

STUDIES ON INTACT HUMAN PLASMA LOW-DENSITY LIPOPROTEINS

Structural studies of LDL have been limited to intact lipoproteins mainly due to the insolubility of the major apoprotein (apoB) in aqueous buffers (see APOLIPOPROTEINS; 115) and to the inability to perform reassembly experiments. Although two subclasses of LDL have been operationally defined as IDL or LDL_1 (d 1.006–1.019 g/ml) and LDL_2 (d 1.019–1.063 g/ml), our discussion is limited to LDL_2. For a complete compositional analysis of the LDL subfractions, the reader is referred to the compilation by Lee (74). By ultracentrifugation, LDL_2 has a molecular weight of 2.75×10^6 (115). However, the buoyant densities, sedimentation coefficients, and molecular weights can vary dramatically depending on the subject and dietary factors (1).

Overall geometry of LDL has been obtained by electron microscopy (36, 103) and small-angle X-ray scattering (70, 72, 84). Utilizing a negative staining technique, Forte and Nichols (36) visualized spherical particles and established a size range of 210–250 Å for LDL. Pollard and Devi (102) reported spherical particles of diameter 200 ± 5 Å. Each group has noticed substructural components at high magnification. Forte and Nichols describe this substructure as strandlike and forming a surface network. Pollard et al. (103), in contrast, interpret their micrographs as showing a set of globular subunits of 50-Å diameter, arranged in a dodecahedral array with overall icosahedral symmetry. Additional support for the dodecahedral arrangement is provided by image enhancement for construction of isodensity maps of the LDL particle (102). Small-angle X-ray scattering data are consistent with the above results bearing out the spherical symmetry and an overall radius of 100–120 Å (70, 72). The initial X-ray study of Mateu et al. (84), which depicts LDL as having a lipid bilayer structure with protein in the core of the particle, has been criticized (72) and revised (153, 159). The best current interpretation of the scattering data (70, 72) is that the lipoprotein is a spherical particle with protein and phospholipid at the polar interface and with the apolar lipids distributed in a central core.

Deckelbaum et al. (30) used X-ray and thermal analyses to show a broad reversible thermal transition for LDL between 20° and 45°C. The 36-Å fringe in the scattering curve is lost during the transition, a phenomenon ascribed to an order → disorder phase transition of the cholesteryl esters of LDL. This phenomenon is discussed in greater detail later in this section, but is introduced here to clarify the earlier interpretation of the X-ray data of Mateu et al. (84), which were collected below the phase-transition temperature. A complementary study of the small-angle X-ray work is the neutron scattering study of LDL by Stuhrmann et al. (153). From the radial scattering density function, LDL are seen as spheres having a radius of about 100–120 Å. They have a low-density core due to the hydrocarbon chains and a high-density outer shell due to protein. The spherical diameter of LDL is corroborated by the laser-homodyne spectroscopic technique [$D_{25,w} = 2.4 \pm 0.01 \times 10^{-1}$ cm²/s, diameter = 229 ± 10 Å (28)].

With the overall static shape of LDL established by X-ray and electron-micrographic studies, we now examine the interaction of the components of LDL with various spectroscopic techniques.

Steim et al. (150) have recorded the ¹H-NMR spectra of human LDL at low field (60 MHz) and have concluded that there is little difference between the intact particle and sonicated dispersions of the lipids. The narrowness of the observed resonances indicates that about 95% of the hydrocarbon protons are highly mobile. Leslie et al. (77) have confirmed the mobility of the lipids of LDL with a 100-MHz spectrometer. They also decribe an immobilization of the aromatic side chains of the protein, which is attributed to an unspecified type of apolar interaction with the lipids.

The natural-abundance ¹³C-NMR spectra for low-density lipoproteins

(51, 52), recorded at 36° and 15.18 MHz, reflect the liquidlike environment of the lipids and protein. However, analysis of the T_1 values indicates that the cholesterol ring system and the fatty acyl chains have a considerable degree of restriction of rotational mobility compared with model systems (cholesteryl oleate in $CHCl_3$, triolein in $CHCL_3$, and triolein alone). At high field, 67.88 MHz [63.41 kG (50)], higher anisotropy for rotation of the cholesteryl esters is observed in LDL compared with VLDL.

The ^{31}P-NMR spectra of LDL display two characteristic resonances for phosphatidylcholine (113.5 ppm from P_4O_6) and sphingomyelin (112.9 ppm) (9). Phosphatidylcholine comprises 60% and the sphingomyelin 40% of the total resonance area. The narrow band width of the phosphorus resonances is interpreted as evidence that the polar head groups are in relatively rapid motion (9, 38). Henderson et al. (57) have studied the quenching action of a $Mn^{+2}(EDTA)_{2.2}$ complex on the phosphorus resonance of LDL and have concluded that 50% of the phospholipid residues are accessible. Based on the X-ray data, discussed earlier, a plausible explanation of the result is that the inaccessible phospholipid is protected from quenching by interaction with the apoprotein. This interpretation is supported by the high-resolution ^{31}P-NMR analysis of a trypsin-treated LDL (166). In the native lipoprotein, two phospholipid environments are observed: approximately 80% of the phospholipid resonance is narrow while 20% is somewhat broadened. The latter finding indicates immobilization. In the trypsin-treated LDL ^{31}P-NMR spectra, no broad resonance component is apparent: i.e., all the phospholipid resonances are highly mobile.

The ESR data also provide evidence for the interaction of the apoprotein with lipid. Spin labeling of the apoprotein of LDL (40) with isothiocyanate or maleimide derivatives of the nitroxide radical N-(1-oxyl-2,2,6,6,-4-tetramethylpiperidine) produces spectra with two types of signal. One type is consistent with a free and the other with a constrained environment for the probe. Experiments with a series of lipid-soluble spin labels (e.g., nitroxide derivatives of cholesteryl stearate, and cholesterol) indicate that the lipid components have at least three distinct environments (64). The lipid environment with the highest mobility appears to be at the water-lipid interface and the spin label is readily accessible to reduction by ascorbic acid.

Microviscosities of the hydrophobic lipids of the plasma lipoproteins have been measured by fluorescence depolarization with DPH and perylene (62). Low-density lipoproteins have the highest microviscosity of all the lipoproteins, with a value of 6.1 ± 0.9 P, at 25°C. The absolute viscosity of the extracted LDL lipids is 2.4 ± 0.3 P; that of intact VLDL is 1.3 ± 0.2 P. Therefore, by comparison the lipid constituents of LDL are relatively highly constrained.

Examination of pyrene eximer-monomer fluorescence intensity of LDL from subjects on different diets (saturated vs. polyunsaturated fats) suggests that the lipid fluidity is also a function of the saturation of the phospholipid fatty acid chains (91). The higher the degree of unsaturation the greater the mobility of the lipid matrix (91). Other fluorescence techniques have been used to probe the relationship of sterol to protein. Smith and Green (147) measured the proximity of an incorporated cholesta-5,7,9(11)-trien-3β-ol and its oleate ester to the apoprotein of LDL by observing the efficiency of quenching the tryptophan of the protein. Although both lipids quenched inefficiently, the energy-transfer efficiency was higher in the cholesterol derivative. From this result, it is suggested that cholesterol is in closer proximity to the protein than the cholesteryl ester. Morrisett et al. (89) have advised caution in this interpretation due to the large number of tryptophans in LDL ($\sim$20).

Enzymatic probes, such as phospholipase A_2 and phospholipase C, have been useful alternative tools to investigate the location of the phospholipid of LDL. Snake venom phospholipase A_2 (2) hydrolyzes all the phosphatidyl-choline and phosphatidylethanolamine with first-order kinetics and produces an LDL particle remarkably similar to the native lipoprotein. Phospholipase C (24), which cleaves the choline head group, hydrolyzes about 60% of the phospholipid residues rapidly and about 30% slowly. This result is consistent with the interpretation of the NMR and EPR data that a portion of the phospholipid is less available because of interactions with the apoprotein.

In a series of experiments to probe the structure of the apolar core of LDL, Small and his co-workers (10, 20, 30, 129) have demonstrated that the liquid-crystalline phase transition present in the X-ray, DSC, NMR, and polarizing-microscopy experiments is due to the cholesteryl esters (see MODELS OF LIPOPROTEIN STRUCTURE).

Attempts to characterize the role of the apoproteins in the LDL particle have been frustrating. Shackled by the limited knowledge concerning the chemical properties of the protein, little information about apoB-lipid inter-action exists. Efforts to characterize the apoprotein have continued nonethe-less (15, 68, 100; see below).

Chemical modification of the functional groups of the apoproteins in the intact LDL as a probe of the topology has been reviewed by Margolis (82) and Scanu and Wisdom (125). These experiments provide a good deal of information that unfortunately cannot be adequately interpreted until the sequence of apoB is known.

Enzymatic digestion of intact LDL with trypsin or pronase (83) releases only a small fraction of the hydrolyzable peptide linkages. It is concluded that either the peptide-susceptible linkages are protected in the lipid environ-ment or the protease is unable to react with a peptide linkage in its native conformation. Margolis and Langdon (83) observed that the released peptides of LDL are distinct and differ from either intact apoB or the remaining large tryptic fragment. Bernfeld and Kelley (13) have obtained different results, however, and Rudman et al. (111) report that only 10% of the apoprotein is cleaved by trypsin with peptides in the molecular weight range of 2000. The remaining material is soluble in SDS and is reported to have a molecular weight of 15,000–20,000.

The secondary structure of the apoprotein in intact LDL appears to contain a considerable amount of β-structure, as demonstrated by CD (43, 45), ORD (43), and infrared (IR) (43, 45) spectra. Dearborn and Wetlaufer (27) confirm the above findings and add that the amount of each type of secondary structure is a function of temperature. The greater the lipid content of the subfraction of LDL and the higher the temperature, the more β-pleated sheet present. Scanu and co-workers (118, 119) have found α-helical structure in LDL at room temperature. With the variation in the content of β-structure reported from various laboratories and the evidence that the conformation of the protein in LDL is temperature dependent (27, 122), it would seem advantageous to reexamine the CD, ORD, and IR data in light of the cholesteryl ester phase transition (30). The crucial point is whether measurements are made above or below the cholesteryl ester phase-transition temperature. The carotenoid component of LDL also contributes to the optical activity (ORD and CD) of LDL; its contribution is constrained by environmental conditions below 37°C, probably due to an organized lipid phase (26).

In summary, intact LDL can be described as a quasispherical particle of 250 Å with a molecular weight of 2.75×10^6. The phospholipid and protein are situated at the surface of the particle with portions of the apoprotein buried deeper in the lipid environment, perhaps interacting with some cholesterol. The protein contains β-pleated sheet, disordered structure, and α-helical structure. The carbohydrate of the glycoprotein is also near the surface as evidenced by its ability to bind concanavalin A (ConA) (54, 86) and by the release of about 90% of the sialic acid with exposure to neuraminidase (83). An apolar core 140–150 Å in diameter is rich in cholesteryl ester and exhibits liquid-crystalline melting behavior (30). Both DSC and X-ray scattering indicate a cooperative, reversible thermal transition in LDL in the temperature range 15–45°C (30). The ^{13}C-NMR spectra demonstrate the same temperature dependency and suggest (from line-broadening considerations) that the cholesteryl esters of LDL are selectively less restricted in going from below the phase-transition temperature to above it (129), but that the ester remains motionally restricted compared with an isotropic solution. The peak of the transition temperature appears to be influenced mainly by the content of triglycerides. Increased TG content lowers the transition temperature and eventually abolishes it at a sufficiently high concentration (29). Additional factors such as boundary constraints due to the size of LDL or interaction with the phospholipid and/or protein must also influence the cholesteryl esters in the intact particle compared with the lipids removed from the particle (29). In the intact lipoprotein, a relatively large cholesteryl ester domain must exist—i.e., larger than 70 Å (29)—in order to allow for the observed thermal behavior. With these structural features, LDL particles circulate in the bloodstream, transporting cholesterol, influencing cholesterol metabolism in tissues, and, under the right circumstances, contributing to pathological changes within the arterial wall.

STUDIES ON INTACT HUMAN VERY-LOW-DENSITY LIPOPROTEINS AND CHYLOMICRONS

Very-low-density lipoproteins and chylomicrons are discussed in the same section because of their similarities and the paucity of structural information available. They remain future challenges for the students of lipoprotein structure. Operationally, we have distinguished VLDL and chylomicrons by their density ranges, $d = 0.95$–1.006 g/ml, $d \leq 0.95$ g/ml, respectively. Both particles are rapidly, and probably continuously, being acted on by apoC-II-activated LPL (14), which is present in peripheral tissues. In this process, the lipoproteins become triglyceride poor and cholesteryl ester enriched and are transformed into structures called remnants. (Remnant catabolism is discussed in chapt. 6)

In the electron microscope, the spherical VLDL particles have a grayish halo at the periphery and a diameter ranging from 300 to 900 Å (36). The halo may be an artifact of the negative staining. Chylomicrons are also spherical and have a range of diameters from 1200 to 11,000 Å. The molecular weight ranges are 3–128×10^6 and 500–$430,000 \times 10^6$ (115) for VLDL and chylomicrons, respectively.

Results with ^{13}C-NMR indicate that the lipids of VLDL have spin-lattice relaxation times much shorter than LDL but still longer than the extracted lipids (50). Fluorescence depolarization studies of Jonas (62) with DPH also suggest that the lipids are in a relatively fluid, isotropic state. The microviscosity value of the VLDL is 1.3 ± 0.27 P and for chylomicrons is 1.0 ± 0.2 P at 25°C. In contrast to the results with HDL and LDL, the extracted lipids from VLDL and chylomicrons have virtually the same microviscosity values as the native lipoproteins.

Using X-ray, DSC, and polarizing light microscopy, Deckelbaum et al. (31) have shown that VLDL do not have the reversible thermal transition associated with a cholesteryl ester-rich domain. These findings contrast with those in LDL (29) and reflect the higher triglyceride content in the core of VLDL.

The rate of VLDL catabolism appears to be related to the microscopic fluidity of its constituent fatty acids. Pyrene fluorescence experiments suggest that unsaturated triglycerides are hydrolyzed by lipoprotein lipase more rapidly than saturated triglycerides (145).

Both the apoproteins and the polar lipids appear localized on the surface of the VLDL and chylomicrons. They rapidly equilibrate with components from the other lipoproteins (33, 109, 110, 128), e.g., HDL, both in vitro and in vivo. They are accessible to proteases (82, 83) and phospholipases (82). Neuraminidase treatment of VLDL releases about 95% of its sialic acid (163), whereas ConA-Sepharose treatment binds VLDL (86). Both results are consistent with a surface location of the glycopeptide portion of the apoprotein.

STUDIES ON INTACT ABNORMAL HUMAN LIPOPROTEINS
AND LIPOPROTEIN DYNAMICS

Characterization of abnormal lipoproteins may allow a better understanding of the structure-function relationships in the major classes of normal human lipoproteins. Much less information is available concerning the abnormal particles compared with the normal ones.

The best characterized abnormal lipoprotein is Lp-X. It is found in patients with advanced obstructive liver or LCAT-deficiency diseases (3, 37). It floats in the ultracentrifuge in the density range d 1.006–1.063 g/ml and contains 65% phospholipid, 25% cholesterol, 2% triglyceride, 3% cholesteryl ester, and 5% protein (96). ApoB is absent (134). Unlike normal lipoproteins, serum albumin is a major protein component (134). Lp-X has cathodic migration on agar electrophoresis (133). Patsch et al. (96) have isolated three Lp-X subpopulations, Lp-X$_1$, Lp-X$_2$, and Lp-X$_3$, by Cohn fractionation and zonal ultracentrifugation. The Stokes radii (96) of Lp-X$_1$, Lp-X$_2$, and Lp-X$_3$ are 339 ± 6 Å, 343 ± 5 Å, and 294 ± 4 Å, respectively, as determined by quasi-electric light scattering or gel filtration. The calculated molecular weight (M_r) for Lp-X$_1$ is 22.2×10^{-6} and for Lp-X$_2$ is 15.3×10^6.

Negatively stained preparations of Lp-X appear as rouleaux as viewed by electron microscopy (53, 132, 162). The physical characteristics of Lp-X are not changed by acylation with succinic anhydride (53). Hydrodynamic data suggest that Lp-X is a spherical structure in solution, in contrast to the negatively stained preparations.

The lipids of Lp-X are relatively immobile compared with normal lipoproteins, as measured in 2,2,6,6-tetramethylpiperidine-1-oxyl (TEMPO)-EPR studies (16, 96) and by high-field (63.4 kG) ^{13}C-NMR (16). The value of $\nu_{1/2}$ of the olefinic and methylene resonances of the fatty acyl chains and the failure to observe the C'-1 and C'-2 resonances of the glycerol backbone of the phospholipids suggest that the lipid environment is extremely rigid in comparison with normal lipoproteins (16). This abnormal rigidity is a possible explanation for the depressed activity of Lp-X with LCAT (98). In contrast to these results, fluorescence depolarization with DPH shows that LDL lipids are more rigid than Lp-X. The DPH probe does not shows the order $\rightarrow$ disorder phase transition (30) in LDL and may be reflecting a selective solubility in the LDL particle that is not representative of its true fluidity.

A lipid bilayer structure containing an aqueous compartment has been proposed for Lp-X based on X-ray and electron-microscopy studies (53). Results with ^{31}P-NMR, employing a Pr^{+3} shift reagent, are in agreement with this hypothesis. The ratio of phospholipid in the lipid bilayer of Lp-X is estimated at about 70:30, outer:inner (J. D. Morrisett, personal communication). The bilamellar lipid structure of Lp-X has not been detected in normal lipoproteins.

Mahley, in chapter 11, discusses the abnormal lipoprotein HDL$_c$, induced in man by cholesterol feeding. HDL$_c$ (d = 1.095–1.21 g/ml) contains apoE, but lacks the apoB protein. No structural information is yet available.

Lipoprotein Exchange and Transfer

Human plasma lipoproteins are dynamic systems that continuously are being secreted and catabolized and are exchanging their constituents with themselves, other lipoproteins, and cell components. These transfer and exchange phenomena make studies of the kinetics of the lipoproteins difficult. Jackson et al. (59) and Pownall et al. (104) have summarized this topic in recent reviews and our discussion here is therefore abbreviated.

Phospholipid (69), triglyceride (92, 95, 105), and free cholesterol (12), but not cholesteryl ester, transfer relatively rapidly to other lipoproteins. Charlton et al. (25) have suggested that the lipid transfer is a function of the solubility of the lipid in the aqueous compartment. Proteins, whose role is to facilitate transfer of lipids, have been reported for phospholipid (165) and cholesterol precursors (113), although these proteins are not necessary for such transfer.

The in vitro transfer of apoC from VLDL to HDL, and vice versa, is known (33, 109, 110). The transfer of apoC-II to chylomicrons and VLDL is probably important to their attack by lipoprotein lipase. The mechanism of the transfer remains to be clarified.

The apoproteins of HDL_2 and HDL_3 appear to exchange readily (47). The transfer of ^{125}I-labeled apoHDL from one subclass to the other occurs with no loss of protein. ApoC and apoA proteins are exchanged. The cross-linking reagent DFDNB prevents this exchange. Therefore, it is speculated that the apoproteins transfer separately, not as a unit, or that cross-linking prevents a conformational change in the apoprotein necessary before exchange. Whether lipid is involved in this transfer is open to question.

APOLIPOPROTEINS

The voluminous information available on the chemical and physical properties of the apoproteins has been reviewed recently (59, 89, 90, 139). Only a brief sketch is presented here with highlights of some recent developments.

ApoA-I, the major apoprotein of HDL, is a single polypeptide chain and has a molecular weight of 28,331. The amino acid sequence has been established (11). ApoA-I can self-associate, a property that greatly affects its ability to bind lipid (107). It is highly helical, containing 55% α-helix, 8% β-structure, and 37% disordered structure (78). On binding lipid (egg yolk phosphatidylcholine) (78), the α-helical content of apoA-I is increased to 69% in the isolated complex. A blue shift occurs in the tryptophan fluorescence (336.5 → 334.0 nm) spectrum (90), indicating that the indole ring is shifted to a more hydrophobic environment in the lipid-protein complex. ApoA-I stimulates lecithin:cholesterol acyltransferase (37, 148).

ApoA-II is the other major apoprotein of HDL (~25% of the total protein). It contains two identical chains of 77 amino acids linked at cystine-6 (17) and self-associates to form a dimer of 34,000 mol wt (48, 152). Recently, Ritter and Scanu (108) found that apoA-II, unlike apoA-I, binds phospholipid preferentially in the oligomeric form. Mao et al. (81), using native and synthetic fragments of apoA-II, have defined a phospholipid-binding region between residues 47 and 77. On incubation with dimyristoyl phosphatidylcholine (DMPC), fragment 47-77 shows a marked increase in α-helix from 25 to

48%. A phospholipid-protein complex is formed and may be isolated by KBr-density ultracentrifugation between d 1.07 and 1.10 g/ml. No physiological role is known at present for apoA-II; it is reported to reduce LCAT activity in the presence of apoA-I (35, 148).

The apoC proteins have been most extensively studied in connection with VLDL; the larger the VLDL the higher the apoC content relative to apoB (34). ApoC-I and apoC-II have known physiological roles; apoC-III does not as yet.

The sequence of apoC-I is known (61, 141). It contains 57 residues and has a calculated molecular weight of 6530. Total synthesis has been achieved by solid-phase techniques (142). The synthetic protein binds phospholipid and activates LCAT similarly to the apoprotein isolated from VLDL (142).

ApoC-II is probably the physiological activator of LPL (14, 56, 73). The apoprotein is a single polypeptide chain of 78 amino acid residues and it contains no cystine, cysteine, or histidine (58). Its sequence recently has been completed (58). Because of its potential importance in triglyceride metabolism, it is of interest that the structural component of apoC-II needed for binding and activation of LPL has recently been elucidated (65). The COOH-terminal CNBr fragment, residues 60–78, activates LPL about 50% as much as the whole apoprotein. The synthetic COOH-terminal fragment (residues 55–78) enhances lipolysis to 90% of that of the intact apolipoprotein. It also appears that the COOH-terminal sequence Gly-Glu-Glu is necessary for the binding of C-II to the lipase.

ApoC-III has been the subject of numerous investigations because of its relative abundance and facility in binding phospholipid (90). It is a single polypeptide chain of 79 amino acid residues (18). Polymorphism on PAGE is due to varied amounts of sialic acid, from 0 to 2 mol/mol of apoprotein (18, 20). The polypeptide is cleaved into two halves (between Arg-40 and Gly-41) by the action of thrombin (149). The carboxyl-terminal half of the molecule readily binds phospholipid whereas the amino-terminal half does not (149).

The major apoprotein of LDL, apoB, has been implicated in the metabolism of cellular cholesterol (19) in various tissues (i.e., fibroblasts, smooth muscle, adrenal, etc.) and it is the major transport vehicle for plasma cholesterol. Although of great importance in the understanding of atherogenesis, the apoprotein remains an enigma. Characterization is hampered by its insolubility in aqueous environments. For example, the range of molecular weights reported for the apoprotein is 8000–275,000 (84, 103, 123, 146). The apoprotein maintains a high proportion of its β-structure relative to the native lipoprotein (39, 44) and shows a tryptophan fluorescence maximum at 334 nm (101) only slightly red shifted from that of the intact LDL at 330 nm. ApoB contains 5–9% carbohydrate including galactose, mannose, fucose, glucosamine, and sialic acid (76, 155). The sequence of the carbohydrate moiety of two thermolytic glycopeptides constituting 50% of the carbohydrate has been established (155). One of the two glycopeptides has a terminal mannose, a finding consistent with the binding of LDL to ConA (54, 86).

The thin-line protein (5), isolated from HDL, is also called apoA-III (67) or apoD (85, 87). The protein has been found in HDL_3 (85), LDL (75), and VLDL (4). It has a molecular weight of 20,000 (67) and contains glucosamine and COOH-terminal serine (67). The dual designation apoA-III or apoD arises from the controversy over whether this protein is associated with the apoA group of proteins from HDL (67) or whether it represents a fourth class of lipoproteins (85, 87), namely, lipoprotein D. It is possible that apoA-III and apoD are different proteins, especially in view of the differences in their amino acid compositions (67, 87). Kostner's (66) report that apoD activates LCAT has not been confirmed by other investigators (148).

The arginine-rich protein or apoE was first isolated as a minor component of normal VLDL (137). It has a molecular weight of about 33,000 (135), a high helical content (138), and lacks cysteine and cystine. The carboxy-terminal sequence is Leu-Ser-Ala and the amino terminal is lysine (135). Subsequently, it has been found to be associated with cholesterol-rich particles and to be induced by cholesterol feeding (see chapter 11). Its concentration is increased in patients with diseases such as type 3 hyperlipidemia (56, 140), hypothyroidism (140), LCAT deficiency (161, 162), and alcoholic hepatitis (106). Utermann (160) has reported three polymorphic forms of apoE, one of which is reportedly absent in patients with type III hyperlipidemia. It is a highly insoluble protein that aggregates readily (unpublished observations).

MODELS OF LIPOPROTEIN STRUCTURE

Structural models for the classes of lipoproteins have been presented to represent available chemical, compositional and physical data. Recent reviews have summarized most of this information (59, 90, 116, 125).

HDL Models

Based on both ^{31}P- and ^{13}C-NMR studies, Assmann and Brewer (7) propose a spherical assembly of protein and lipid resembling the Singer and Nicolson model (143) of proteins ("icebergs") swimming in a "sea" of lipid (Fig. 1). Interaction of protein with lipid is thought to be predominantly due to hydrophobic forces and there is little or no interaction between the phospholipid choline head groups and the ionic charges of the protein. This conclusion is supported by the ^{31}P-NMR results, which show that all the phospholipids are titrated (phosphorous resonances shifted and broadened) with increasing concentrations of Eu^{+3}. In this model, all constituent polar groups (phospholipid and proteins) are located at the surface of a sphere whose nucleus contains the apolar moieties (cholesteryl ester and triglyceride; cholesterol). The protein molecules are located parallel to the long axes of the fatty acid chains of the phospholipid. This model requires that the protein be oriented so as to reduce charge-apolar interactions.

Stoffel and co-workers (151) present a model of HDL that also excludes strong interactions between the phospholipid head group and the apopro-teins. Their interpretations are based on NMR experiments with ^{13}C-enriched phospholipid and cholesteryl esters, reconstituted HDL liposomes. The mea-sured ^{13}C-spin relaxation time (T_1) for the choline head group in liposomes and mixed liposomes (including apoproteins) indicate no significant head group-apoprotein interaction. A decrease in T_1 values for C-14 of linoleic acid of phosphatidylcholine and C-11 of oleic acid in sphingomyelin when combined with apoHDL is interpreted as direct evidence for the hydrophobic interaction between these constituents. Reassembly experiments suggest that the distribution of sphingomyelin with A-II and phosphatidylcholine with A-I is not random. The model (Fig. 2) assigns the phospholipid to a monolayer, which, with cholesterol, covers one-half the surface of the particle. The other half of the surface is occupied by the hydrated hydrophilic areas of the apoproteins. Cholesteryl esters are interiorly located with some of the fatty acyl chains oriented toward the surface of the particle to facilitate hydrophobic interaction with the phospholipid and apoprotein. Note that this model is based on evidence obtained from a reassembled HDL particle that is 2.5 times the size of the native HDL_2.

Compositional analysis (130, 164) of *native* HDL raises a problem in packing the cholesteryl esters if they are oriented with their fatty acid chains toward the surface or toward the core of the particle. An outward orientation of the cholesteryl ester sterol moiety is suggested by calculations with a freedom-of-motion parameter (130), f, and compositional and size considerations (164). The Verdery-Nichols model (164), based on size and composition, requires not only that the cholesteryl ester sterol be outwardly directed but that in HDL_3 the fatty acyl chains must be folded over the steroid nucleus (Fig. 3, *A* and *B*) in a large percentage of the cholesteryl ester.

Segrest et al. (131) and Jackson et al. (60) have proposed a model for HDL (Fig. 4) based on a lipid-protein interaction hypothesis, known as the

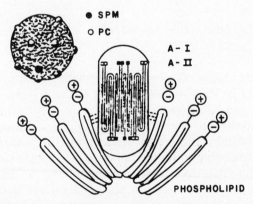

FIG. 1. Schematic model of high-density lipoprotein as described by Assmann and Brewer (7).

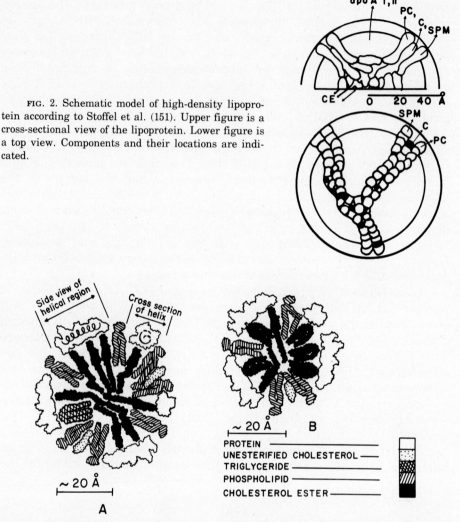

FIG. 2. Schematic model of high-density lipoprotein according to Stoffel et al. (151). Upper figure is a cross-sectional view of the lipoprotein. Lower figure is a top view. Components and their locations are indicated.

FIG. 3. Schematic models of HDL$_2$ (A) and HDL$_3$ (B) based on compositional and packing considerations as described by Verdery and Nichols (164).

amphipathic-helix theory. This model is consistent with the X-ray scattering data. An increase in the α-helical content of the protein occurs (104) when apoproteins are incubated with phospholipids. On examination of space-filling models of the apoprotein, an outstanding feature of the α-helical segments of the protein is that they are amphipathic. One face of the α-helix is extremely hydrophobic while the opposite face is hydrophilic and contains 1, 2 and 1, 4 Glu (Asp)-Lys (Arg) ion pairs (Fig. 5). In the amphipathic model, the fatty acyl chains of the phospholipid are perpendicular to the helical apoprotein on the surfaces. The hydrophobic face of the helix interacts with carbons C_2–C_4 of the phospholipid fatty acids. The ion pairs of amino

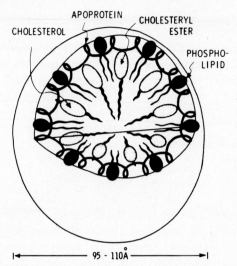

FIG. 4. Model of HDL structure with amphipathic helix as hypothesized by Jackson et al. (60).

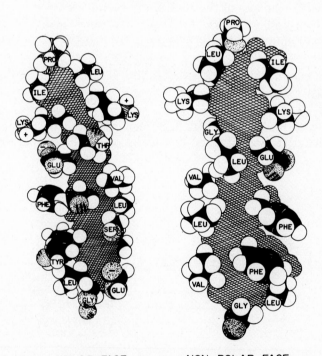

POLAR FACE   NON-POLAR FACE

FIG. 5. Corey-Pauling-Kendrew (CPK) space-filling model of residues 51–71 of apoA-II in an amphipathic-helix conformation taken from Mao et al. (81). Figure on the left shows the polar face of the helix; figure on the right shows the highly hydrophobic residues found on the nonpolar face. The Lys residues are located at the edges of the polar and nonpolar faces of the helix.

acids are oriented toward the aqueous surface on the hydrophilic face. No direct interaction of the charged phospholipid head groups with the zwitter-ionic amino acids has been demonstrated. It may be speculated that the alternating pairs of amino acids orient the phospholipids in their binding to the apoprotein. Detailed accounts of the model are available (59, 131). Also, a functional regulatory role for the amphipathic-helix structure of apoprotein has been proposed by Segrest (130). Exchange of phospholipid and/or choles-terol is suggested to be modulated by the extent of dissociation of amphipathic helix from the lipoprotein surface.

LDL Models

Models of LDL are micellar with the exception of a bilayer proposal (84) that has been revised (153, 159) and discussed above. A currently accepted view places the apoprotein and phospholipid near the periphery of the LDL in a polar outer shell. An apolar inner core contains cholesteryl esters and triglyceride (Fig. 6). The model also allows for a cooperative interaction involving a part of the cholesteryl esters to account for the liquid-crystalline melt observed by the loss of the 36-Å X-ray scattering fringe and the phase transition measured at 28.5°C by DSC (Fig. 6, A and B). Unesterified cholesterol is assigned to an intermediate position between cholesteryl esters and the outer periphery.

VLDL Models

A lipid-core model for VLDL has been advanced by Schneider et al. (126). Quantitative and detailed consideration of the geometric factor in

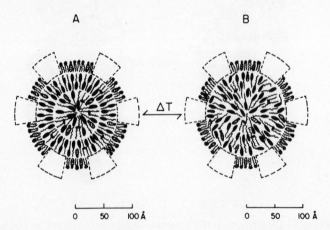

FIG. 6. Schematic diagram of LDL as presented by Decklebaum et al. (29). ●∿∿ phospholipids; ◖▥▷ cholesterol; ∿∿● cholesteryl ester; ∿∿∿ triglyceride. A: cholesteryl ester in an ordered arrangement of 2 concentric layers with 36-Å periodicity at 10°C. B: cholesteryl ester above the phase-transition temperature, at 45°C in a disordered arrangement.

relation to the lipid packing at a curved surface allows calculation of the maximum lipid that can be accommodated at the surface of a sphere of given size. Morrisett et al. (90) describe a composite VLDL model based on available compositional, enzymatic, and physical evidence (Fig. 7). It is a spherical one in which an outer polar shell of about 20 Å contains apoB and apoC proteins, phospholipids, and cholesterol. Triglyceride and a small amount of cholesteryl ester (~10%) are distributed throughout the apolar core.

Shen et al. (136) have proposed a general structural model for all circulating lipoproteins inferred from compositional data. The hydrophobic core consists of triglycerides and cholesteryl esters and is surrounded by a 20-Å-thick monolayer of protein, phospholipid, and cholesterol. Phospholipid and protein compete for space on the surface of the lipoprotein. Cholesterol interacts directly with the protein and phospholipid but is not directly exposed to the aqueous environment. This is the first model that attempts to consider all the lipoproteins with a common structure (Fig. 8).

CONCLUSIONS

The labors of many investigators to elucidate the structure of the human plasma lipoproteins are beginning to bear fruit. Although the exact

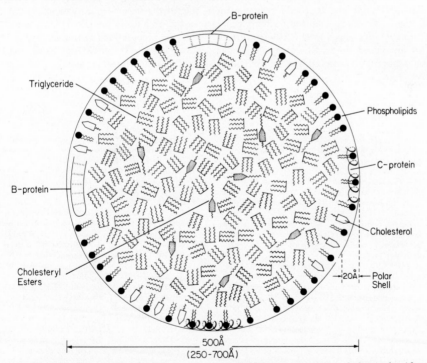

FIG. 7. Composite VLDL model based on compositional, enzymatic, and physical evidence. [From Morrisett et al. (90).]

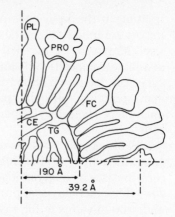

FIG. 8. Model of general structure of lipoprotein, with HDL$_3$ as an example, as illustrated by Shen et al. (136). Outer monolayer of 20 Å, containing phospholipid (PL) and protein (PRO), surrounds the apolar core of triglyceride (TG) and cholesteryl ester (CE). Cholesterol (C) is seen as part of the outer monolayer interacting with the PRO and PL, but not with the water.

intricacies of the multicomponent lipoproteins are not yet known, substantial information is now available to allow testing of structure-function relationships. A concept of the general structure of a lipoprotein (apolar core, outer polar monolayer) seems to be consistent with the data from many physico-chemical techniques and reinforces a sometimes forgotten goal of science — the unification of thought. As illustrated by LDL and HDL structures, there may, however, be a number of variations of the basic pattern.

We thank Drs. J. T. Sparrow, J. R. Patsch, H. J. Pownall, J. D. Morrisett, M. F. Rohde, and in particular Dr. R. L. Jackson for their helpful discussions and criticisms. We are indebted to Ms. Debbie Mason for her excellence in the preparation of this manuscript. This material was developed by the Atherosclerosis, Lipids and Lipoproteins section of the National Heart and Blood Vessel Research and Demonstration Center, Baylor College of Medicine, a grant-supported research project of the National Heart, Lung, and Blood Institute, Grant HL 17269.

REFERENCES

1. ADAM, G. H., AND V. N. SHUMAKER. Polydispersity of human low density lipoproteins. *Ann. N.Y. Acad. Sci.* 164: 130–146, 1969.

2. AGGERBECK, L. P., F. J., KÉZDY, AND A. M. SCANU. Enzymatic probes of lipoprotein structure. Hydrolysis of human serum low density lipoprotein-2 by phospholipase A$_2$. *J. Biol. Chem.* 251: 3823–3830, 1976.

3. AHRENS, E. H., and H. G. KUNKEL. The relationship between serum lipid and skin xanthomas in eighteen patients with primary biliary cirrhosis. *J. Clin. Invest.* 28: 1565–1574, 1949.

4. ALAUPOVIC, P., S. S. SANBAR, R. H. FURMAN, M. L. SULLIVAN, AND S. L. WALRAVEN. Studies of the composition and structure of serum lipoproteins. Isolation and characterization of very high density lipoproteins of human serum. *Biochemistry* 5: 4044–4053, 1966.

5. ALAUPOVIC, P. C., D. M. LEE, AND W. J. Mc-CONATHY. Studies on the composition and structure of plasma lipoproteins. Distribution of lipoprotein families in major density classes of normal human plasma lipoproteins. *Biochim. Biophys. Acta* 260: 689–707, 1972.

6. ANDREWS, S. B., J. W. FALLER, J. M. GILLIAM, AND R. J. BARRNETT. Lanthanide ion-induced iso-tropic shifts and broadening for nuclear magnetic resonance structural analysis of model membranes. *Proc. Natl. Acad. Sci. US* 70: 1814–1818, 1973.

7. ASSMANN, G., AND H. B. BREWER, JR. A molecular model of high density lipoproteins. *Proc. Natl. Acad. Sci. US* 71: 1534–1538, 1974.

8. ASSMANN, G., R. J. HIGHET, E. A. SOKOLOSKI, AND H. B. BREWER, JR. ^{13}C nuclear magnetic resonance spectroscopy of native and recombined lipoproteins. *Proc. Natl. Acad. Sci. US* 71: 3701–3705, 1974.

9. ASSMANN, G., E. A. SOKOLOSKI, AND H. B. BREWER, JR. ^{31}P nuclear magnetic resonance spectroscopy of native and recombined lipoproteins. *Proc. Natl. Acad. Sci. US* 71: 549–553, 1974.

10. ATKINSON, D., R. J. DECKELBAUM, D. M. SMALL, AND G. G. SHIPLEY. Structure of human plasma low-density lipoproteins: molecular organization of the central core. *Proc. Natl. Acad. Sci. US* 74: 1042–1046, 1977.

11. BAKER, H. N., T. DELAHUNTY, A. M. GOTTO, JR., AND R. L. JACKSON. The primary structure of human plasma high density apolipoprotein glutamine I (apoA-I). *Proc. Natl. Acad. Sci. US* 71: 3631–3634, 1974.

12. BASFORD, J. M., J. GLOVER, AND C. GREEN. Exchange of cholesterol between human β-lipoproteins

and erythrocytes. *Biochim. Biophys. Acta* 84: 764–766, 1964.

13. BERNFELD, P., AND T. F. KELLEY. Proteolysis of human serum β-lipoprotein. *J. Biol. Chem.* 239: 3341–3346, 1964.

14. BIER, D. M., AND R. J. HAVEL. Activation of lipoprotein lipase by lipoprotein fractions of human serum. *J. Lipid Res.* 11: 565–570, 1970.

15. BRADLEY, W. A., M. F. ROHDE, R. L. JACKSON, AND A. M. GOTTO, JR. Aggregation states of the cyanogen bromide peptides of human low density lipoproteins (abstr. 2942). *Federation Proc.* 36: 829, 1977.

16. BRAINARD, J. R., J. A. HAMILTON, E. H. CORDES, J. R. PATSCH, A. M. GOTTO, AND J. D. MORRISETT. EPR and NMR studies of an abnormal lipoprotein (LP-X) (abstr.). In: *Proc. VI Intern. Symp. Magnetic Resonance in Biological Systems, Banff, Canada, 1977.*

17. BREWER, H. B., JR., S. E. LUX, R. RONAN, AND K. M. JOHN. Amino acid sequence of human apoLP-Gln-II, an apolipoprotein isolated from the high density lipoprotein complex. *Proc. Natl. Acad. Sci. US* 69: 1304–1308, 1972.

18. BREWER, H. B., JR., R. SHULMAN, P. HERBERT, R. RONAN, AND K. WEHRLY. The complete amino acid sequence of alanine apolipoprotein (apoC-III), an apolipoprotein from human plasma very low density lipoproteins. *J. Biol. Chem.* 249: 4975–4984, 1974.

19. BROWN, M. S., AND J. L. GOLDSTEIN. Familial hypercholesterolemia: defective binding of lipoproteins to cultured fibroblasts associated with impaired regulation of 3-hydroxy-3-methylglutaryl coenzyme A reductase activity. *Proc. Natl. Acad. Sci. US* 71: 788–792, 1974.

20. BROWN, W. V., R. I. LEVY, AND D. S. FREDRICKSON. Further characterization of apolipoproteins from the human plasma very low density lipoproteins. *J. Biol. Chem.* 245: 6588–6594, 1970.

21. BYSTROV, V. F., N. I. DUBROVINA, L. I. BARSCIHOV, AND L. D. BERGELSON. NMR differentiation of the internal and external phospholipid membrane surface using paramagnetic Mn^{+2} and Eu^{+3} ions. *Chem. Phys. Lipids* 6: 343–350, 1971.

22. CAMEJO, G., V. MUÑOZ, AND E. AVILA. The size and chemical characteristics of six fractions obtained by differential centrifugation from human high density lipoprotein. *Acta Cient. Venezolana* 22: 45–48, 1971.

23. CHAPMAN, D., R. B. LESLIE, R. HERZ, AND A. M. SCANU. High-resolution NMR spectra of high-density serum lipoproteins. *Biochim. Biophys. Acta* 176: 524–536, 1969.

24. CHAPMAN, M. J., AND S. GOLDSTEIN. Human serum low-density lipoprotein: structural studies with phospholipase C (abstr. 962). *Federation Proc.* 35: 379, 1976.

25. CHARLTON, S. C., J. S. OLSON, K.-Y. HONG, H. J. POWNALL, D. D. LOUIE, AND L. C. SMITH. Stopped flow kinetics of pyrene transfer between human high density lipoproteins. *J. Biol. Chem.* 251: 7952–7955, 1976.

26. CHEN, G. C., AND J. P. KANE. Contribution of carotenoids to the optical activity of human serum low-density lipoprotein. *Biochemistry* 13: 3330–3335, 1974.

27. DEARBORN, D. G., AND D. B. WETLAUFER. Reversible thermal conformation changes in human serum low-density lipoprotein. *Proc. Natl. Acad. Sci. US* 62: 179–185, 1969.

28. DEBLOIS, R. W., E. E. UZGIRIS, S. K. DEVI, AND A. M. GOTTO, JR. Application of laser self-beat spectroscopic technique to the study of solutions of human plasma low-density lipoproteins. *Biochemistry* 12: 2645–2649, 1973.

29. DECKELBAUM, R. J., G. G. SHIPLEY, AND D. M. SMALL. Structure and interactions of lipids in human plasma low density lipoproteins. *J. Biol. Chem.* 252: 744–754, 1977.

30. DECKELBAUM, R. J., G. G. SHIPLEY, D. M. SMALL, R. S. LEES, AND P. K. GEORGE. Thermal transitions in human plasma low density lipoproteins. *Science* 190: 392–394, 1975.

31. DECKELBAUM, R. J., A. R. TALL, AND D. M. SMALL. Interaction of cholesterol ester and triglyceride in human plasma very low density lipoprotein. *J. Lipid Res.* 18: 164–168, 1977.

32. EDELSTEIN, C., C. T. LIM, AND A. M. SCANU. On the subunit structure of the protein of human serum high density lipoprotein. I. A study of its major polypeptide component (Sephadex, fraction III). *J. Biol. Chem.* 247: 5842–5849, 1972.

33. EISENBERG, S., D. W. BILHEIMER, AND R. I. LEVY. The metabolism of very low density lipoproteins. II. Studies on the transfer of apoproteins between plasma lipoproteins. *Biochim. Biophys. Acta* 280: 94–104, 1972.

34. EISENBERG, S., D. W. BILHEIMER, F. LINDGREN, AND R. I. LEVY. On the apoprotein composition of human plasma very low density lipoprotein subfraction. *Biochim. Biophys. Acta* 260: 329–333, 1972.

35. FIELDING, C. J., V. G. SHORE, AND P. E. FIELDING. A protein cofactor of lecithin:cholesterol acyltransferase. *Biochem. Biophys. Res. Commun.* 46: 1493–1498, 1972.

36. FORTE, T., AND A. V. NICHOLS. Application of electron microscopy to the study of plasma lipoprotein structure. *Advan. Lipid Res.* 10: 1–41, 1972.

37. GLOMSET, J. A. Plasma lecithin:cholesterol acyltransferase. In: *Blood Lipids and Lipoproteins: Quantitation, Composition, and Metabolism,* edited by G. J. Nelson. New York: Wiley, 1972, p. 745–787.

38. GLONEK, T., T. O. HENDERSON, A. W. KRUSKI, AND A. M. SCANU. ^{31}P nuclear magnetic resonance: application to the study of human serum high density lipoproteins. *Biochim. Biophys. Acta* 348: 155–161, 1974.

39. GOTTO, A. M., JR. Recent studies on the structure of human serum low- and high-density lipoproteins. *Proc. Natl. Acad. Sci. US* 64: 1119–1127, 1969.

40. GOTTO, A. M., AND H. KON. Application of electron spin resonance to the study of the structure of human serum lipoproteins. *Biochem. Biophys. Res. Commun.* 37: 444–450, 1969.

41. GOTTO, A. M., AND H. KON. Observations on the conformation of human serum high-density lipoproteins using infrared spectroscopy, circular dichroism, and electron spin resonance. *Biochemistry* 9: 4276–4282, 1970.

42. GOTTO, A. M., H. KON, AND M. E. BIRNBAUMER. Electron spin resonance studies of lipid-protein interaction in human serum lipoproteins. *Proc. Natl. Acad. Sci. US* 65: 145–157, 1969.

43. GOTTO, A. M., R. I. LEVY, AND D. S. FREDRICKSON. Observations on the conformation of human beta lipoprotein: evidence for the occurrence of beta structure. *Proc. Natl. Acad. Sci. US* 60: 1436–1441, 1968.

44. GOTTO, A. M., JR., R. I. LEVY, S. E. LUX, M. E. BIRNBAUMER, AND D. S. FREDRICKSON. A comparative study of the effects of chemical modification on the immunochemical and optical properties of human plasma low-density lipoprotein(s) and apoproteins. *Biochem. J.* 133: 369–382, 1973.

45. GOTTO, A. M., R. I. LEVY, A. S. ROSENTHAL, M. E. BIRNBAUMER, AND D. S. FREDRICKSON. The

structure and properties of human beta-lipoprotein and beta-apoprotein. *Biochem. Biophys. Res. Commun.* 31: 699–705, 1968.

46. GROW, T. E., AND M. FRIED. Lipoprotein geometry. I. Spatial relationships of human HDL apoproteins studied with a bifunctional reagent. *Biochem. Biophys. Res. Commun.* 66: 352–356, 1975.

47. GROW, T. E., AND M. FRIED. Lipoprotein geometry. II. Apoprotein exchange in human plasma high density lipoprotein. *Biochem. Biophys. Res. Commun.* 75: 117–124, 1977.

48. GWYNNE, J., G. PALUMBO, J. C. OSBORNE, H. B. BREWER, AND H. EDELHOCH. The self-association of apoA-II, an apoprotein of the human high density lipoprotein complex. *Arch. Biochem. Biophys.* 170: 204–212, 1975.

49. HAMILTON, J. A. ^{13}C-NMR studies of human plasma high-density lipoproteins. Observations of new lipid resonances at high magnetic field (abstr. 2945). *Federation Proc.* 36: 829, 1977.

50. HAMILTON, J. A., N. J. OPPENHEIMER, R. ADDLEMAN, A. O. CLOUSE, E. H. CORDES, P. M. STEINER, AND C. J. GLUECK. High-field ^{13}C NMR studies of certain normal and abnormal human plasma lipoproteins. *Science* 194: 1424–1427, 1976.

51. HAMILTON, J. A., C. TALKOWSKI, R. F. CHILDERS, E. WILLIAMS, A. ALLERHAND, AND E. H. CORDES. Rotational and segmental motions in the lipids of human plasma lipoproteins. *J. Biol. Chem.* 249: 4872–4878, 1974.

52. HAMILTON, J. A., C. TALKOWSKI, E. WILLIAMS, E. M. AVILA, A. ALLERHAND, E. H. CORDES, AND G. CAMEJO. Natural abundance carbon-13 nuclear magnetic resonance spectra of human serum lipoproteins. *Science* 180: 193–195, 1975.

53. HAMILTON, R. L., R. J. HAVEL, J. P. KANE, A. E. BLAUROCK, AND T. SATA. Cholestasis: lamellar structure of the abnormal human serum lipoprotein. *Science* 172: 478, 1971.

54. HARMONY, J. A. K., AND E. H. CORDES. Interaction of human plasma low density lipoprotein with concanavalin A and with ricin. *J. Biol. Chem.* 250: 8614–8617, 1975.

55. HART, C. J., R. B. LESLIE, AND A. M. SCANU. Fluorescence studies of a high density serum lipoprotein. *Chem. Phys. Lipids* 4: 367–374, 1970.

56. HAVEL, R. J., AND J. P. KANE. Primary dysbetalipoproteinemia: predominance of a specific apoprotein species in triglyceride-rich lipoproteins. *Proc. Natl. Acad. Sci. US* 70: 2015–2019, 1973.

57. HENDERSON, T. O., A. W. KRUSKI, L. G. DAVIS, T. GLONEK, AND A. M. SCANU. ^{31}P nuclear magnetic resonance studies on serum low and high density lipoproteins: effect of paramagnetic ion. *Biochemistry* 14: 1915–1920, 1975.

58. JACKSON, R. L., H. N. BAKER, E. B. GILLIAM, AND A. M. GOTTO, JR. Primary structure of very low density apolipoprotein C-II of human plasma. *Proc. Natl. Acad. Sci. US* 74: 1942–1945, 1977.

59. JACKSON, R. L., J. D. MORRISETT, AND A. M. GOTTO, JR. Lipoprotein structure and metabolism. *Physiol. Rev.* 56: 259–316, 1976.

60. JACKSON, R. L., J. D. MORRISETT, A. M. GOTTO, AND J. P. SEGREST. The mechanism of lipid-binding by plasma lipoproteins. *Mol. Cell. Biochem.* 6: 43–50, 1975.

61. JACKSON, R. L., J. T. SPARROW, H. N. BAKER, J. D. MORRISETT, O. D. TAUNTON, AND A. M. GOTTO, JR. The primary structure of apolipoprotein-serine. *J.*

Biol. Chem. 249: 5308–5313, 1974.

62. JONAS, A. Microviscosity of lipid domains in human serum lipoproteins. *Biochim. Biophys. Acta* 486: 10–22, 1977.

63. JONAS, A., AND D. SEIDEL. Properties of the abnormal human plasma lipoprotein (LP-X) characteristic of cholestasis after chemical modification with succinic anhydride. *Arch. Biochem. Biophys.* 163: 200–210, 1974.

64. KEITH, A. D., R. J. MEHLHORN, N. K. FREEMAN, AND A. V. NICHOLS. Spin labeled lipid probes in serum lipoproteins. *Chem. Phys. Lipids* 10: 223–236, 1973.

65. KINNUNEN, P. K. J., R. L. JACKSON, L. C. SMITH, A. M. GOTTO, JR., AND J. T. SPARROW. Activation of lipoprotein lipase by native and synthetic fragments of human plasma apoC-II. *Proc. Natl. Acad. Sci. US* In press.

66. KOSTNER, G. Studies on the cofactor requirement for lecithin:cholesterol acyltransferase. *Scand. J. Clin. Lab. Invest.* 33, Suppl. 137: 19–21, 1974.

67. KOSTNER, G. M. Studies of the composition and structure of human serum lipoproteins. Isolation and partial characterization of apolipoprotein AIII. *Biochim. Biophys. Acta* 336: 383–395, 1974.

68. KUEHL, D. S., L. E. RAMM, AND R. G. LANGDON. Chemical evidence for subunit structure of low density lipoprotein (abstr. 2941). *Federation Proc.* 36: 828, 1977.

69. KUNKEL, H. G., AND A. G. BEARN. Phospholipid studies of different serum lipoproteins employing p^{32}. *Proc. Soc. Exptl. Biol. Med.* 86: 887–891, 1954.

70. LAGGNER, P. Physicochemical characterization of low density lipoproteins. In: *Low Density Lipoproteins*, edited by C. E. Day and R. S. Levy. New York: Plenum, 1976, p. 49–69.

71. LAGGNER, P., K. MÜLLER, O. KRATKY, G. KOSTNER, AND A. HOLASEK. Studies on the structure of lipoprotein A of human high density lipoprotein HDL$_3$: the spherically averaged electron density distribution. *Fed. European Biochem. Soc. Letters* 33: 77–80, 1973.

72. LAGGNER, P., K. MÜLLER, O. KRATKY, G. KOSTNER, AND A. HOLASEK. X-ray small angle scattering on human plasma lipoproteins. *J. Colloid Interface Sci.* 55: 102–108, 1976.

73. LaROSA, J. C., R. I. LEVY, R. HERBERT, S. E. LUX, AND D. S. FREDRICKSON. A specific apoprotein activator for lipoprotein lipase. *Biochem. Biophys. Res. Commun.* 41: 57–62, 1970.

74. LEE, D. Isolation and characterization of low density lipoproteins. In: *Low Density Lipoproteins*, edited by C. E. Day and R. S. Levy. New York: Plenum, 1976, p. 3–47.

75. LEE, D. M., AND P. ALAUPOVIC. Composition and concentration of apolipoproteins in very-low- and low-density lipoproteins of normal human plasma. *Atherosclerosis* 19: 501–520, 1974.

76. LEE, P., AND W. C. BRECKENRIDGE. Isolation and carbohydrate composition of glycopeptides of human apo low-density lipoprotein from normal and type II hyperlipoproteinemic subjects. *Can. J. Biochem.* 54: 829–832, 1976.

77. LESLIE, R. B., D. CHAPMAN, AND A. M. SCANU. Nuclear magnetic resonance of serum low density lipoproteins (LDL$_2$). *Chem. Phys. Lipids* 3: 152–158, 1969.

78. LUX, S. E., R. HIRZ, R. I. SHRAGER, AND A. M. GOTTO. The influence of lipid on the conformation of human plasma high density apolipoproteins. *J. Biol. Chem.* 247: 2598–2606, 1972.

79. MACKENZIE, S. L., G. S. SUNDARAM, AND H. S.

SODHI. Heterogeneity of human serum high-density lipoprotein (HDL$_2$). *Clin. Chim. Acta* 43: 223–229, 1973.

80. MAO, S. J. T., A. M. GOTTO, JR., AND R. L. JACKSON. Immunochemistry of human plasma high density lipoproteins. Radioimmunoassay of apolipoprotein A-II. *Biochemistry* 14: 4127–4131, 1975.

81. MAO, S. J. T., J. T. SPARROW, E. B. GILLIAM, A. M. GOTTO, JR., AND R. L. JACKSON. Mechanism of lipid-protein interaction in the plasma lipoproteins: the lipid-binding properties of synthetic fragments of apolipoprotein A-II. *Biochemistry* 16: 4150–4156, 1977.

82. MARGOLIS, S. Structure of very low and low density lipoproteins. In: *Structural and Functional Aspects of Lipoproteins in Living Systems*, edited by E. Tria and A. M. Scanu. New York: Academic, 1969, p. 369–424.

83. MARGOLIS, S., AND R. G. LANGDON. Studies on human serum β_1-lipoprotein. III. Enzymatic modifications. *J. Biol. Chem.* 241: 485–493, 1966.

84. MATEU, L., A. TARDIEU, V. LUZZATI, L. AGGERBECK, AND A. M. SCANU. On the structure of human serum low density lipoprotein. *J. Mol. Biol.* 70: 105–116, 1972.

85. McCONATHY, W. J., AND P. ALAUPOVIC. Isolation and partial characterization of apolipoprotein D: a new protein moiety of the human plasma lipoprotein system. *Fed. European Biochem. Soc. Letters* 37: 178–182, 1973.

86. McCONATHY, W. J., AND P. ALAUPOVIC. Studies on the interaction of concanavalin A with major density classes of human plasma lipoproteins: evidence for the specific binding of lipoprotein B in its associated and free forms. *Fed. European Biochem. Soc. Letters* 41: 174–177, 1974.

87. McCONATHY, W. J., AND P. ALAUPOVIC. Studies on the isolation and partial characterization of apolipoprotein D and lipoprotein D of human plasma. *Biochemistry* 15: 515–520, 1976.

88. MICHAELSON, D. M., A. F. HORWITZ, AND M. P. KLEIN. Transbilayer asymmetry and surface heterogeneity of mixed phospholipids in cosonicated vesicles. *Biochemistry* 12: 2637–2645, 1973.

89. MORRISETT, J. D., R. L. JACKSON, AND A. M. GOTTO, JR. Lipoproteins: structure and function. *Ann. Rev. Biochem.* 44: 183–207, 1975.

90. MORRISETT, J. D., R. L. JACKSON, AND A. M. GOTTO, JR. Lipid-protein interactions in the plasma lipoproteins. *Biochim. Biophys. Acta* 472: 93–133, 1977.

91. MORRISETT, J. D., H. J. POWNALL, R. L. JACKSON, R. SEGURA, A. M. GOTTO, JR., AND O. D. TAUNTON. Effects of polyunsaturated and saturated fat diets on the chemical composition and thermotropic properties of human plasma lipoproteins. In: *Polyunsaturated Fatty Acids*, edited by R. T. Holman and W.-H. Kunau. Champaign, Ill.: A.O.C.S. Publ., 1977, p. 139–161.

92. NICHOLS, A. V., E. L. COGGIOLA, L. C. JENSEN, AND E. H. YOKOYAMA. Physical-chemical changes in serum lipoproteins during incubation of human serum. *Biochim. Biophys. Acta* 168: 87–94, 1968.

93. NICHOLS, A. V., E. L. GONG, P. J. BLANCHE, T. M. FORTE, AND D. W. ANDERSON. Effects of guanidine hydrochloride on human plasma high density lipoproteins. *Biochim. Biophys. Acta* 466: 226–239, 1976.

94. NICHOLS, A. V., S. LUX, T. FORTE, E. GONG, AND R. I. LEVY. Degradation products from human serum high density lipoproteins following dehydration by rotary evaporation and solubilization. *Biochim. Biophys. Acta* 270: 132–148, 1972.

95. NICHOLS, A. V., AND L. SMITH. Effect of very low density lipoproteins on lipid transfer in incubated serum. *J. Lipid Res.* 6: 206–210, 1975.

96. PATSCH, J. R., K. C. AUNE, A. M. GOTTO, JR., AND J. D. MORRISETT. Isolation, chemical characterization, and biophysical properties of three different abnormal lipoproteins: LP-X$_1$, LP-X$_2$, and LP-X$_3$. *J. Biol. Chem.* 252: 2113–2120, 1977.

97. PATSCH, J. R., S. SAILER, G. KOSTNER, F. SANDHOFER, A. HOLASEK, AND H. BRAUNSTEINER. Separation of the main lipoprotein density classes from human plasma by rate-zonal ultracentrifugation. *J. Lipid Res.* 15: 356–366, 1974.

98. PATSCH, J. R., A. K. SOUTAR, J. D. MORRISETT, A. M. GOTTO, AND L. C. SMITH. Lipoprotein-X: a substrate for lecithin:cholesterol acyltransferase. *European J. Clin. Invest.* 7: 213–217, 1977.

99. PATTNAIK, N. M., F. J. KÉZDY, AND A. M. SCANU. Kinetic study of the action of snake venom phospholipase A$_2$ on human serum high density lipoprotein 3. *J. Biol. Chem.* 251: 1984–1990, 1976.

100. PINON, J.-C. Insolubility of the protein moiety of human plasma low-density lipoproteins. In: *Lipid-Protein Complexes*, edited by H. Peeters and J. P. Massue. Ghent, Belgium: European Press, 1977, p. 14–25.

101. POLLARD, H. B., AND R. F. CHEN. Fluorescence and circular dichroism studies on human serum low density lipoprotein particles and lipid-depleted derivatives. *J. Supramol. Struct.* 2: 177–184, 1973.

102. POLLARD, H. B., AND S. K. DEVI. Construction of a three-dimensional iso-density map of the low-density lipoprotein particle from human serum. *Biochem. Biophys. Res. Commun.* 44: 593–599, 1971.

103. POLLARD, H., A. M. SCANU, AND E. W. TAYLOR. On the geometrical arrangement of the protein subunits of human serum low density lipoprotein: evidence for a dodecahedral model. *Proc. Natl. Acad. Sci. US* 64: 304–310, 1969.

104. POWNALL, H. J., R. L. JACKSON, J. D. MORRISETT, AND A. M. GOTTO, JR. Structure and dynamics of reassembled plasma lipoproteins. In: *Atherosclerosis*, edited by A. M. Scanu, R. W. Wissler, and G. S. Getz. New York: Dekker, in press.

105. QUARFORDT, S. H., F. BOSTON, AND H. HILDERMAN. Transfer of triglyceride between isolated human lipoproteins. *Biochim. Biophys. Acta* 231: 290–294, 1971.

106. RAGLAND, J. B., H. L. HAWKINS, AND S. M. SABESIN. Arginine rich protein (ARP) in nascent high density lipoprotein of alcoholic hepatitis (AH): a model to study lipoprotein metabolism (abstr. 0100). *Circulation* 54: II-27, 1976.

107. RITTER, M. C., AND A. M. SCANU. Role of apolipoprotein A-I in the structure of human serum high density lipoproteins. *J. Biol. Chem.* 252: 1208–1216, 1977.

108. RITTER, M. C., AND A. M. SCANU. Human apolipoprotein A-II (apoA-II): self-association and lipid binding in aqueous solutions (abstr. 2944). *Federation Proc.* 36: 829, 1977.

109. RUBINSTEIN, B., AND D. RUBINSTEIN. Interrelationship between rat serum very low density and high density lipoproteins. *J. Lipid Res.* 13: 317–324, 1972.

110. RUBINSTEIN, B., AND D. RUBINSTEIN. Comparison of the metabolic behavior *in vitro* of the apoproteins of rat serum high density lipoprotein$_2$ and high density lipoprotein$_3$. *J. Lipid Res.* 14: 357–363, 1973.

111. RUDMAN, D., L. A. GARCIA, L. L. ABELL, AND S. AKGUN. Observation on the protein components of human plasma high- and low-density lipoproteins. *Biochemistry* 7: 3136–3148, 1968.

112. SAE, S. W., B. SHORE, AND V. SHORE. Surface exposed proteins of human plasma high density lipopro-

teins (abstr. 963). *Federation Proc.* 35: 380, 1976.

113. SCALLEN, T. J., M. V. SCHUSTER, AND A. K. DHAR. Evidence for a noncatalytic carrier protein in cholesterol biosynthesis. *J. Biol. Chem.* 246: 224–230, 1971.

114. SCANU, A. Studies on the conformation of human serum high-density lipoprotein, HDL_2 and HDL_3. *Proc. Natl. Acad. Sci. US* 54: 1699–1705, 1965.

115. SCANU, A. M. Structural studies on serum lipoproteins. *Biochim. Biophys. Acta* 265: 471–508, 1972.

116. SCANU, A. M., C. EDELSTEIN, AND P. KEIM. Serum lipoproteins. In: *The Plasma Proteins: Structure, Function and Genetic Control*, edited by F. W. Putnam. New York: Academic, 1975, p. 318–391.

117. SCANU, A. M., C. EDELSTEIN, AND C. T. LIM. Subunit structure of serum HDL studies by cross-linking agent suberimidate. *Federation Proc.* 31: abstr. 829, 1972.

118. SCANU, A., AND J. L. GRANDA. Comparative optical properties of human serum low- and high-density lipoproteins before and after delipidation. *Progr. Biochem. Pharmacol.* 4: 153–158, 1968.

119. SCANU, A., AND R. HIRZ. Human serum low-density lipoprotein protein: its conformation studied by circular dichroism. *Nature* 218: 200–201, 1968.

120. SCANU, A., AND R. HIRZ. On the structure of human serum high density lipoproteins. Studies by the technique of circular dichroism. *Proc. Natl. Acad. Sci. US* 59: 890–894, 1968.

121. SCANU, A. M., C. T. LIM, AND C. EDELSTEIN. On the subunit structure of the protein of human serum high density lipoprotein. II. A study of Sephadex fraction IV. *J. Biol. Chem.* 247: 5850–5855, 1972.

122. SCANU, A., H. POLLARD, R. HIRZ, AND K. KOTHARY. On the conformational instability of human serum low-density lipoprotein: effect of temperature. *Proc. Natl. Acad. Sci. US* 62: 171–178, 1969.

123. SCANU, A., H. POLLARD, AND W. READER. Properties of human serum low density lipoproteins after modification by succinic anhydride. *J. Lipid Res.* 9: 342–348, 1968.

124. SCANU, A., W. READER, AND C. EDELSTEIN. Molecular weight and subunit structure of human serum high density lipoprotein after chemical modification by succinic anhydride. *Biochim. Biophys. Acta* 160: 32–45, 1968.

125. SCANU, A. M., AND C. WISDOM. Serum lipoproteins structure and function. *Ann. Rev. Biochem.* 41: 703–730, 1972.

126. SCHNEIDER, H., R. S. MORROD, J. R. COLVIN, AND N. H. TATTRIE. The lipid core model of lipoproteins. *Chem. Phys. Lipids* 10: 328–353, 1973.

127. SCHONFELD, G., R. A. BRADSHAW, AND J.-S. CHEN. Structure of high density lipoprotein. The immunologic reactivities of the COOH- and NH_2-terminal regions of apolipoprotein A-I. *J. Biol. Chem.* 251: 3921–3926, 1976.

128. SCHUMAKER, V. N., AND G. H. ADAMS. Circulating lipoproteins. *Ann. Rev. Biochem.* 38: 113–136, 1969.

129. SEARS, B., R. J. DECKELBAUM, M. J. JANIAK, G. G. SHIPLEY, AND D. M. SMALL. Temperature-dependent ^{13}C nuclear magnetic resonance studies of human serum low density lipoproteins. *Biochemistry* 15: 4151–4157, 1976.

130. SEGREST, J. P. Molecular packing of high density lipoproteins: a postulated functional code. *Fed. European Biochem. Soc. Letters* 69: 111–115, 1976.

131. SEGREST, J. P., JACKSON, R. L., J. D. MORRISETT, AND A. M. GOTTO, JR. A molecular theory of lipid-protein interactions in the plasma lipoproteins. *Fed.*

European Biochem. Soc. Letters 38: 247–253, 1974.

132. SEIDEL, D., B. AGOSTINI, AND P. MÜLLER. Structure of an abnormal plasma lipoprotein (LP-X) characterizing obstructive jaundice. *Biochim. Biophys. Acta* 260: 146–152, 1972.

133. SEIDEL, D., P. ALAUPOVIC, AND R. H. FURMAN. A lipoprotein characterizing obstructive jaundice. I. Method for quantitative separation and identification of lipoproteins in jaundiced subjects. *J. Clin. Invest.* 48: 1211–1223, 1969.

134. SEIDEL, D., P. ALAUPOVIC, R. H. FURMAN, AND W. J. McCONATHY. A lipoprotein characterizing obstructive jaundice. II. Isolation and partial characterization of the protein moieties of low density lipoprotein. *J. Clin. Invest.* 49: 2396–2407, 1970.

135. SHELBURNE, F. A., AND S. H., QUARFORDT. A new apoprotein of human plasma very low density lipoproteins. *J. Biol. Chem.* 249: 1428–1433, 1974.

136. SHEN, B. W., A. M. SCANU, AND F. J. KÉZDY. Structure of human serum lipoproteins inferred from compositional analysis. *Proc. Natl. Acad. Sci. US* 74: 837–841, 1977.

137. SHORE, B., AND V. SHORE. Isolation and characterization of polypeptides of human serum lipoproteins. *Biochemistry* 8: 4510–4516, 1969.

138. SHORE, B., AND V. SHORE. An apolipoprotein preferentially enriched in cholesteryl ester-rich very low density lipoproteins. *Biochem. Biophys. Res. Commun.* 58: 1–7, 1974.

139. SHORE, V. G., AND B. SHORE. The apolipoproteins: their structure and functional roles in human-serum lipoproteins. In: *Blood Lipids and Lipoproteins: Quantitation, Composition, and Metabolism*, edited by G. J. Nelson. New York: Wiley, 1972, p. 789–824.

140. SHORE, V. G., AND B. SHORE. Heterogeneity of human plasma very low density lipoproteins. Separation of species differing in protein components. *Biochemistry* 12: 502–507, 1973.

141. SHULMAN, R. S., P. N. HERBERT, K. WEHRLY, AND D. S. FREDRICKSON. The complete amino acid sequence of C-I (apoLP-Ser), an apolipoprotein from human very low density lipoproteins. *J. Biol. Chem.* 250: 182–190, 1975.

142. SIGLER, G. F., A. K. SOUTAR, L. C. SMITH, A. M. GOTTO, JR., AND J. T. SPARROW. The solid phase synthesis of a protein activator for lecithin-cholesterol acyltransferase corresponding to human plasma apoC-I. *Proc. Natl. Acad. Sci. US* 73: 1422–1426, 1976.

143. SINGER, S. J., AND G. L. NICOLSON. The fluid mosaic model of the structure of cell membranes. *Science* 175: 720–731, 1972.

144. SKIPSKI, V. P. Lipid composition of lipoproteins in normal and diseased states. In: *Blood Lipids and Lipoproteins: Quantitation, Composition and Metabolism*, edited by G. J. Nelson. New York: Wiley, 1972, p. 471–583.

145. SMITH, L. C., A. L. MILLER, O. D. TAUNTON, A. S. HU, AND H. J. POWNALL. Effect of post-heparin lipolytic activity on microviscosity of the hydrocarbon region of plasma lipids in type IV hyperlipoproteinemia. *Circulation* VII-VIII, Suppl. IV: abstr. 445, 1973.

146. SMITH, R., J. R. DAWSON, AND C. TANFORD. The size and number of polypeptide chains in human serum low density lipoprotein. *J. Biol. Chem.* 247: 3376–3381, 1972.

147. SMITH, R. J. M., AND C. GREEN. Fluorescence studies of protein-sterol relationships in human plasma lipoproteins. *Biochem. J.* 137: 413–415, 1974.

148. SOUTAR, A., C. GARNER, H. N. BAKER, J. T.

SPARROW, R. L. JACKSON, A. M. GOTTO, AND L. C. SMITH. The effects of plasma apolipoproteins on lecithin:cholesterol acyltransferase. *Biochemistry* 14: 3057–3064, 1975.

149. SPARROW, J. T., H. J. POWNALL, F.-H. HSU, AND A. M. GOTTO. Lipid binding by fragments of apolipoprotein C-III-1 obtained by thrombin cleavage. *Biochemistry* In press.

150. STEIM, J. M., O. J. EDNER, AND F.-G. BARGOOT. Structure of human serum lipoproteins: NMR supports a micellar model. *Science* 162: 909–911, 1968.

151. STOFFEL, W., O. ZIERENBERG, B. TUNGGAL, AND E. SCHREIBER. ^{13}C nuclear magnetic resonance spectroscopic evidence for hydrophobic lipid-protein interactions in human high density lipoproteins. *Proc. Natl. Acad. Sci. US* 71: 3696–3700, 1974.

152. STONE, W. L., AND J. A. REYNOLDS. The self-association of the apo-Gln-I and apo-Gln-II polypeptides of human high density serum lipoproteins. *J. Biol. Chem.* 250: 8045–8048, 1975.

153. STUHRMANN, H. B., A. TARDIEU, L. MATEU, C. SARDET, V. LUZZATI, L. AGGERBECK, AND A. M. SCANU. Neutron scattering study of human serum low density lipoprotein. *Proc. Natl. Acad. Sci. US* 72: 2270–2273, 1975.

154. SUNDARAM, G. S., S. L. MACKENZIE, AND H. S. SODHI. Preparative isoelectric focusing of human serum high-density lipoprotein (HDL$_3$). *Biochim. Biophys. Acta* 337: 196–203, 1974.

155. SWAMINATHAN, N., AND F. ALADJEM. The monosaccharide composition and sequence of the carbohydrate moiety of human serum low density lipoproteins. *Biochemistry* 15: 1516–1522, 1976.

156. TALL, A. R., R. J. DECKELBAUM, D. M. SMALL, AND G. G. SHIPLEY. Thermal behavior of human plasma high density lipoprotein. *Biochim. Biophys. Acta* 487: 145–153, 1977.

157. TALL, A. R., AND D. M. SMALL. Solubilisation of phospholipid membranes by human plasma high density lipoproteins. *Nature* 265: 163–164, 1977.

158. TALL, A. R., D. M. SMALL, G. G. SHIPLEY, AND R. S. LEES. Apoprotein stability and lipid-protein interactions in human plasma high density lipoproteins. *Proc. Natl. Acad. Sci. US* 72: 4940–4942, 1975.

159. TARDIEU, A., L. MATEU, C. SARDET, B. WEISS, V. LUZZATI, L. AGGERBECK, AND A. M. SCANU. Structure of human serum lipoprotein in solution. II. Small angle x-ray scattering of HDL$_3$ and LDL. *J. Mol. Biol.* 101: 129–153, 1976.

160. UTERMANN, G. Isolation and partial characterization of an arginine-rich apolipoprotein from human plasma very-low-density lipoproteins: apolipoprotein E. *Hoppe-Seyler's Z. Physiol. Chem.* 356: 1113–1121, 1975.

161. UTERMANN, G., H. J. MENZEL, AND K. H. LANGER. On the polypeptide composition of an abnormal high density lipoprotein (LP-E) occurring in LCAT-deficient plasma. *Fed. European Biochem. Soc. Letters* 45: 29–32, 1974.

162. UTERMANN, G., W. SCHOENBORN, K. H. LANGER, AND P. DIEKER. Lipoproteins in LCAT-deficiency. *Humangenetik* 16: 295–306, 1972.

163. VAN DER BIJL, P., AND F. C. REMAN. Human very low density lipoproteins: loss of electrophoretic mobility on enzymatic removal of sialic acid residues. *Clin. Chim. Acta* 60: 191–195, 1975.

164. VERDERY, R. B. III, AND A. V. NICHOLS. Arrangement of lipid and protein in human serum high density lipoproteins: a proposed model. *Chem. Phys. Lipids* 14: 123–134, 1975.

165. WIRTZ, K. W. A. Transfer of phospholipids between membranes. *Biochim. Biophys. Acta* 344: 95–117, 1974.

166. YEAGLE, P. L., R. B. MARTIN, AND R. G. LANGDON. Phospholipid-protein interactions in human low density lipoprotein. *Biophys. J.* 17: 107a, 1977.

8

Hormonal Regulation of Lipoprotein Synthesis

RICHARD L. JACKSON, LAWRENCE CHAN, L. DALE SNOW,
AND ANTHONY R. MEANS

*Departments of Cell Biology and Medicine, Baylor College of Medicine,
Houston, Texas*

Specificity of Estrogen Action
Characterization and Properties of VLDL Proteins
Effects of Estrogen on ApoproteinVLDL-II Synthesis
Effects of Progesterone on VLDL Synthesis
Interaction of Estrogen with Liver Nuclei
Discussion

ORAL CONTRACEPTIVE PREPARATIONS have now been in worldwide use for
over 15 years (7). Although estrogens have proved valuable in preventing
conception, there are a number of adverse side effects in women taking
these drugs. These include hypertension, depression, weight gain, throm-
boembolic disease, and hypertriglyceridemia. A number of investigators (25,
47, 50, 53) have shown that women taking estrogens have elevated fasting
plasma triglycerides. Most of the increase in triglycerides is due to increased
pre-β-lipoprotein or very-low-density lipoprotein (VLDL) levels. Although
the significance of a moderate increase in plasma triglycerides observed in
women taking oral contraceptives remains unclear, long-term estrogen
therapy may lead to an increase in premature cardiovascular disease (40,
52). The marked effects of oral contraceptives on plasma triglyceride levels
have led to increased interest in the mechanism of hormone action and in
the factors that regulate VLDL synthesis and catabolism. Both the intestine
and the liver synthesize VLDL. A number of hormonal and dietary factors,
reviewed elsewhere (17, 30), regulate plasma VLDL levels. Clearly, in the
steady-state condition, the concentration of VLDL is maintained by equal
rates of input and output. The fact that estrogen increases the plasma levels
of VLDL means that there is either increased synthesis of VLDL proteins
and lipids or a decreased catabolism or a combination of both.

A number of studies (18, 23, 31, 34) have suggested that estrogen
therapy results in increased triglyceride synthesis. Kissebah et al. (34)
determined plasma free fatty acid (FFA) and triglyceride turnover rates in
premenopausal women on either estrogen and progesterone alone or on a
combination preparation containing both hormones. In women on the combined preparation or the individual drugs, mean fasting plasma FFA concen-

139

tration and FFA turnover rate were not significantly different from values in control women. However, the rate of triglyceride turnover or influx into the plasma was significantly different. For the control group, the rate of influx was 16 μmol/kg per h compared with 35 μmol/kg per h in the women on the combined preparation. A similar increase in triglyceride turnover rate was found in the women taking estrogen alone. However, progesterone taken alone had little effect on turnover. Since there was no change in FFA turnover, Kissebah et al. (34) suggest that estrogen increases the fraction of FFA converted into triglycerides. Hazzard et al. (23, 25), Glueck et al. (18), and Kekki and Nikkila (31) also have reported increased triglyceride production in women on estrogen therapy. One possible reason for the hypertriglyceridemia is that estrogen causes an elevation of fasting insulin levels and diminishes glucose tolerance (20, 25, 44, 45). Spellacy et al. (45) have proposed that estrogens also cause elevated growth hormone levels that may give rise to the hyperinsulinemia.

A second possible mechanism of action of the estrogen-induced hypertriglyceridemia is an effect on VLDL catabolism. The first step in the catabolism of VLDL is the hydrolysis of triglycerides by extrahepatic lipoprotein lipase (30). As a result of this hydrolysis, intermediate-density lipoproteins (IDL) are formed that are then further catabolized, presumably in the liver, to form low-density lipoproteins (LDL). A specific decrease in lipoprotein lipase activity by estrogen could reduce VLDL catabolism and account for the hypertriglyceridemia. Lipoprotein lipase activity is usually measured after heparin injection and is referred to as plasma postheparin lipolytic activity (PHLA); the activity consists of both a hepatic triglyceride lipase and an extrahepatic lipoprotein lipase. Studies in humans (3, 19, 42) and rats (21, 33) consistently have demonstrated a decrease in plasma PHLA with estrogen therapy. In the study of Kissebah et al. (34), PHLA activity was 295 μeq triglyceride hydrolyzed/h for control women compared to 118 μeq/h on estrogen. On the other hand, treatment with a combined preparation of both estrogen and progesterone gave no significant difference in PHLA activity from controls; progesterone alone produced an increase in PHLA (410 μeq/ h). Hazzard et al. (23, 25), Rossner et al. (42), and Glueck et al. (19) also have reported decreased PHLA in women during oral estrogen contraceptive therapy; Hamosh and Hamosh (21) and Kim and Kalkhoff (33) have reported similar findings in rats. Despite the depressed PHLA during estrogen treatment, the in vivo clearance of triglycerides remains normal (24, 37, 42). Appelbaum et al. (3) have attempted to clarify this apparent dichotomy of reduced PHLA and normal triglyceride clearance and have reported that the decrease in PHLA during estrogen results from a selective decline in the hepatic triglyceride lipase while the extrahepatic lipoprotein lipase activity is not significantly changed with estrogens. Since plasma triglycerides increase with estrogen therapy, Ehnholm et al. (16) have suggested that the hepatic lipoprotein lipase probably does not play a major physiologic role in triglyceride removal. Taken together, these studies support the notion that estrogens increase plasma triglycerides by augmenting hepatic triglyceride production rates. Since triglycerides are transported in VLDL, it also suggests that the level of VLDL apoproteins is enhanced with estrogens. To understand the molecular mechanism for the enhanced hepatic VLDL apoprotein production by estrogen, we have used the model system (36) of the estrogen-treated cockerel. The cockerel was chosen because normally they only have small amounts of VLDL. However, after administration of estrogen, there is a dramatic increase in plasma VLDL (26, 39). The studies described here are concerned with the cellular events of VLDL synthesis and the hormonal regulation of this class of lipoproteins by estrogen.

SPECIFICITY OF ESTROGEN ACTION

To determine the specificity of estrogen in the cockerel, four plasma proteins were measured both before and after hormone treatment. The proteins include the VLDL, high-density lipoproteins (HDL), vitellogenin, and albumin.

As shown in Figure 1, the concentration of VLDL triglycerides in cockerels is 75 mg/dl. After a single injection of diethylstilbestrol (DES), there is an initial consistent drop in plasma triglycerides followed by an increase in plasma VLDL protein and triglycerides (9). With this dose, the maximum amount of the VLDL components occurred between 24 and 48 h after DES injection and returned to base-line values by 72 h. At the maximal accumulation, VLDL protein increased fivefold and triglyceride sevenfold.

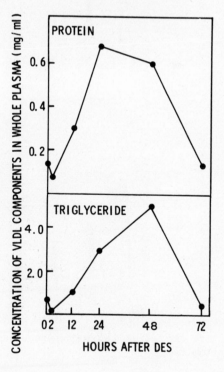

FIG. 1. Effects of estrogen on plasma VLDL protein and lipids. Groups of four cockerels were treated with a single injection of DES (2.5 mg) subcutaneously. Animals were decapitated at indicated times, and VLDL were isolated and protein and triglyceride determined as described previously (9).

Cockerel HDL is similar to human HDL in that it contains one major protein, designated apoprotein A-I (apoA-I). The protein has a molecular weight of 25,000 and preliminary amino acid sequence studies (27) suggest that it is similar to the human apoprotein. Antisera prepared against chicken apoA-I were specific for the apoprotein and did not react with the VLDL proteins. The concentration of apoA-I was determined on delipidated plasma by the technique of rocket immunoelectrophoresis as described by Laurell (38). As shown in Figure 2, a single injection of estradiol had little effect on the concentration of apoA-I. Thus, for the lipoproteins, estrogen is specific and causes the accumulation of plasma VLDL but not HDL.

Vitellogenin is a nonlipoprotein induced by estrogen that is normally absent in nonlaying hens. However, after the onset of egg laying, the levels

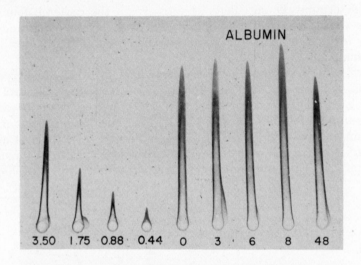

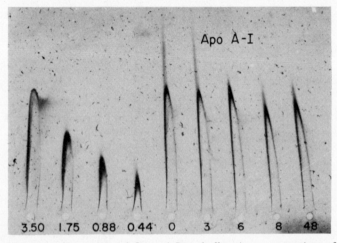

FIG. 2. Plasma apolipoproteins A-I (apoA-I) and albumin concentrations after estradiol treatment.

of this phosphoprotein dramatically increase. The phosphoprotein consists of 3% phosphorus and has a molecular weight of 240,000 (12). Deeley et al. (12) have shown that vitellogenin is a single polypeptide chain consisting of two molecules of phosvitin and one of lipovitellin; the order of these polypeptide chains in the primary structure of vitellogenin is not known. Vitellogenin is transported as an intact protein to the ovary, where it is cleaved by some unknown mechanism to yield phosvitin and lipovitellin. We have measured the levels of plasma vitellogenin in delipidated plasma by immunoprecipitation techniques using antisera prepared against the isolated egg yolk phosvitin (29). The phosvitin antiserum was specific for vitellogenin and did not react with any of the other plasma proteins studied. As shown in Figure 3, after a 2.5-mg injection of DES there was a marked increase in the plasma levels of vitellogenin; the concentration increased within 5 h of hormone treatment and was maximal at 25 h. Furthermore, the accumulation of vitellogenin appeared to parallel that of plasma triglycerides. However, although the triglyceride levels dropped to base-line values by 48 h, the vitellogenin level remained elevated.

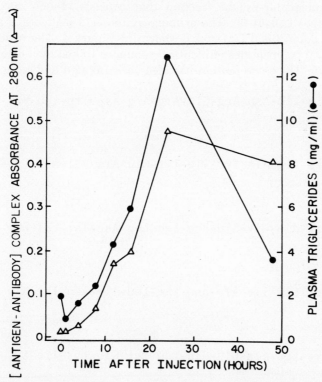

FIG. 3. Effects of DES on plasma triglyceride and vitellogenin. Groups of three cockerels were treated with a single injection of DES (2.5 mg) subcutaneously. Animals were decapitated at indicated times and plasma was collected. To 0.1 ml of plasma were added 50 μl of antiphosvitin; the immunoprecipitates were collected and washed and the absorbance and phosphorus were measured as described previously (9, 29). Triglycerides were analyzed by AutoAnalyzer methods (9).

Finally, the plasma levels of albumin were measured by the Laurell method (38) with an antiserum specific for hen albumin. As with apoA-I, the concentration of albumin was relatively unaltered with estrogen (Fig. 2).

Thus, a single injection of estrogen elicited a specific response: i.e., the selective augmentation of VLDL and vitellogenin levels without significant effects on the levels of HDL or albumin. Since the plasma concentration of a protein is a balance between the rate of its synthesis and that of its removal, we have studied the rate of synthesis of VLDL protein. To gain a better understanding of the significance of such studies, we have characterized the VLDL protein in terms of its primary amino acid sequence and lipid-binding properties.

CHARACTERIZATION AND PROPERTIES OF VLDL PROTEINS

Approximately 10% of hen VLDL is protein (9). After delipidation, the VLDL apoproteins have been fractionated (9) on Sephadex G-150 to yield a high-molecular-weight fraction that is similar to human apoVLDL (apoB) and a low-molecular-weight fraction that consists of one major protein designated apoVLDL-II (9). The primary amino acid sequence of apoVLDL-II has been determined (28) and is shown in Figure 4. The apolipoprotein consists of two polypeptides of identical sequence linked by a disulfide bond at cysteine-76. The same protein has also been isolated and sequenced from

Lys-Ser-Ile-Ile-Asp-Arg-Glu-Arg-Arg-Asp-Trp-Leu-Val-Ile-Pro-
5   10   15

Asp-Ala-Ala-Ala-Ala-Tyr-Ile-Tyr-Glu-Ala-Val-Asn-Lys-Val-Ser
20   25   30

Pro-Arg-Arg-Ala-Gly-Glu-Phe-Leu-Leu-Asp-Thr-Val-Ser-Gln-Thr-
35   40   45

Val-Val-Ser-Gly-Ile-Arg-Asn-Phe-Leu-Ile-Asn-Thr-Ala-Glu-Arg-
50   55   60

Leu-Thr-Lys-Leu-Ala-Glu-Gln-Leu-Met-Glu-Lys-Ile-Lys-Asp-Leu-
65   70   75

Cys-Tyr-Thr-Lys-Val-Leu-Gly
80

FIG. 4. Amino acid sequence of hen plasma apoVLDL-II described by Jackson et al. (28).

hen egg yolk (14). Goat antisera prepared against apoVLDL-II were specific for the apoprotein and did not react with the protein (apoB) that eluted at the void volume of Sephadex G-150, or with apoA-I, vitellogenin, or albumin.

Since all the plasma apolipoproteins studied to date (30) have been shown to bind phospholipid, it was of interest to determine the lipid-binding properties of apoVLDL-II. The lipid-binding experiments were performed with bilamellar vesicles of dimyristoyl phosphatidylcholine (DMPC). The addition of DMPC vesicles to the apoprotein resulted in a lipid-protein complex that was isolated by ultracentrifugation in KBr (Fig. 5); the complex was isolated between d 1.09 and 1.11 g/ml and contained 5.3 mg DMPC/mg apoprotein. As a result of binding, there was an increase in helical content of the apoprotein from 51% to 59%, as determined by circular dichroism (Fig. 6). The addition of phospholipid produced no change in the fluorescence (346 nm) of the single tryptophan at residue 11.

As noted previously in other apoproteins whose sequences are known (43), the plasma lipoprotein proteins have helical segments with unique features that may account for their lipid-associating properties. Each helical segment has one face that is apolar and contains hydrophobic amino acids,

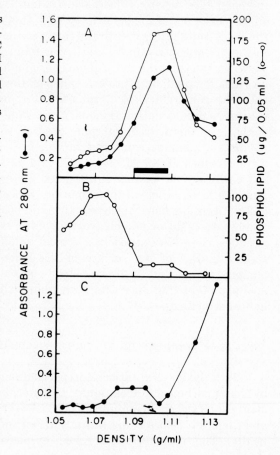

FIG. 5. Ultracentrifugal profiles of apoVLDL-II–dimyristoyl phosphatidylcholine (DMPC) complex (A); DMPC vesicles alone (B); and apoVLDL-II alone (C). ApoVLDL-II (1 mg) and DMPC vesicles (5 mg) were incubated in 2.0 ml of standard buffer at 28°C. After 12 h incubation, linear gradients (ranging from d = 1.02 g/ml to d = 1.12 g/ml) of salt were prepared in 5.0-ml polyallomer tubes with a Buchler Auto DensiFlo gradient maker. All solutions contained 0.01 M tris(hydroxymethyl)aminomethane (Tris)-HCl, 0.5 M NaCl, 0.001 M ethylenediaminetetraacetic acid (EDTA), pH 7.4, and KBr to provide the proper density; all solutions had a final volume of 2.4 ml. Each sample was placed in the d = 1.02 g/ml side of the gradient maker. In addition to the complex, apoVLDL-II (1 mg/4.8 ml) alone and DMPC (5 mg/4.8 ml) alone were subjected to gradient ultracentrifugation. Samples were centrifuged in a Beckman SW 50.1 rotor at 50,000 rpm (234,000 g) for 96 h. Contents of each tube were fractionated and analyzed for protein at 280 nm and total phosphorus; density of each fraction was obtained from its refractive index measured on a Bausch & Lomb refractometer.

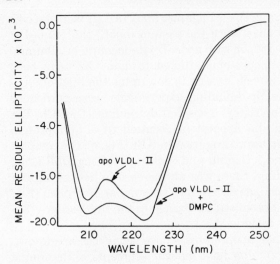

FIG. 6. Circular dichroic spectra of apoVLDL-II and of isolated apoprotein-DMPC complex. The spectrum analysis of the apoprotein was performed at a concentration of 0.5 mg/ml; the spectrum analysis of the complex was performed on the sample indicated in Figure 5.

whereas the other face is polar. The acidic residues appear at the center of the polar face, whereas the basic residues, lysine and arginine, are located on the periphery of the polar face. With this arrangement, the apolar face of the helix could interact with the fatty acyl groups of the phospholipid. Since in the present study apoVLDL-II was found to associate with phospholipid, we wished to examine the sequence for amphipathic helical segments. Based on rules for predicting protein conformation derived by Chou and Fasman (11), the conformational parameter $(P\alpha)$ for amino acids in helices was utilized to predict helical regions. Three helical segments accounting for 59% of the apoprotein were detected based on these rules; the isolated DMPC-apoprotein complex contained 59% helical structure. The helical regions were residues 16 $\rightarrow$ 26, 34 $\rightarrow$ 48, and 53 $\rightarrow$ 75. Corey-Pauling-Kendrew space-filling models were constructed for each helix and the polypeptides placed into an α-helical conformation. Since residues 16 $\rightarrow$ 26 and 34 $\rightarrow$ 48 did not contain basic residues, these helical segments were not typically amphipathic. However, construction of the helical segment corresponding to residues 53 $\rightarrow$ 75 resulted in a typical amphipathic helix with a polar face occupying 180° of the surface of the helix and a hydrophobic face that occupied the other 180° of the helical surface. Thus, apoVLDL-II is another apolipoprotein that interacts with phospholipid and contains amphipathic helical structures.

EFFECTS OF ESTROGEN ON APOPROTEIN VLDL-II SYNTHESIS

With the specific antisera prepared against apoVLDL-II, it was possible by immunochemical techniques to determine the effects of estrogen on synthesis of the apolipoprotein. Cockerels were first treated with the hormone and then, 3 h before being killed, [³H]leucine was administered intraperitoneally. The animals were killed by decapitation, and the amount of

[³H]leucine incorporated into apoVLDL-II in the plasma was determined by specific immunoprecipitation. As shown in Table 1, estrogen treatment resulted in a rapid increase of radioactivity incorporated into apoVLDL-II; there was a 10-fold increase at 30 h. Since trichloroacetic acid (TCA)-soluble counts were comparable, changes in pool size or permeability were unlikely to be the cause of the estrogen effects on these proteins. Hence, estrogen appears to stimulate the synthesis of apoVLDL-II.

Enhanced apoVLDL-II synthesis can also be shown in liver slices. In these experiments, cockerels were first treated with a single injection of DES (2.5 mg). The livers were removed at various times and liver slices were incubated in vitro with L-[³H]lysine. Maximum synthesis of VLDL occurred 24 h after DES administration (Fig. 7). At this time, there was a sixfold increase in VLDL synthesis over control animals. The effects of DES

TABLE 1. *Effects of estradiol on plasma apoVLDL-II synthesis*

	Time after Estradiol, h				
	0	3	6	18	48
Plasma apoVLDL-II, mg/ml	3	3	4	27	70

Plasma apoVLDL-II levels were determined by specific immunoprecipitation methods described previously (9) and in the text.

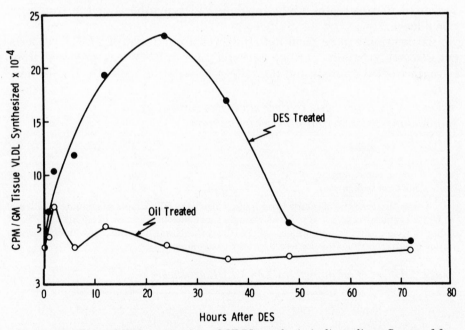

FIG. 7. Effects of DES on protein and VLDL synthesis in liver slices. Groups of four cockerels were treated with a single subcutaneous injection of either DES (2.5 mg) or sesame oil. At indicated times after injection, liver slices were incubated in vitro with [³H]lysine and the amount of VLDL synthesized was determined by immunoprecipitation as described previously (9).

on total protein synthesis were neither as consistent nor as dramatic. In general, DES-injected animals showed a twofold increase in the rate of total protein synthesis that lasted for about 36 h. To exclude the possibility that the observed stimulation of VLDL synthesis by DES might be part of a general phenomenon of the effect of the hormone on total protein synthesis in the liver, the immunoprecipitable counts in VLDL were divided by the TCA-precipitable count and this fraction was plotted against the time after DES treatment. From this plot, it could be shown that VLDL synthesis peaked at 24 h and returned to basal values by 48 h (9). At the peak of stimulation, VLDL constituted approximately 11% of the total soluble protein synthesized by the liver slices.

To further confirm that the labeled immunoprecipitable VLDL indeed represented newly synthesized VLDL, the VLDL synthesized in vitro were isolated by ultracentrifugation at d 1.006 g/ml. As shown in Table 2, the ratios of radioactivity present in the VLDL isolated by ultracentrifugation to counts obtained by immunoprecipitation were similar at 2, 24, and 48 h after estrogen treatment.

To determine the effects of an RNA synthesis inhibitor on the estrogen induction of VLDL, actinomycin D was given (5 mg/kg) by intramuscular injection to 3-wk-old cockerels simultaneously with 2.5 mg DES subcutaneously. Cockerels treated with DES alone served as the controls. As shown in Table 3, actinomycin D inhibited the increase in VLDL synthesis, which suggested that estrogen might regulate VLDL synthesis at the transcriptional level.

To determine more accurately the level of regulation of VLDL synthesis by estrogen, partially purified cockerel liver mRNA was prepared from estrogen-treated animals and the mRNA activity for apoVLDL-II was mea-

TABLE 2. *VLDL synthesis in liver slices determined by immunoprecipitation and ultracentrifugation*

Method	Time after DES, h		
	2	24	48
Immunoprecipitation	3.2	7.0	1.7
Ultracentrifugation	2.7	6.9	1.6

Values are the ratio of counts per minute VLDL after DES:counts per minute VLDL at 0 h. White Leghorn cockerels were given a single subcutaneous injection of 2.5 mg of DES. At indicated times, animals were killed, and VLDL synthesis was determined by immunoprecipitation or ultracentrifugation as described previously (9).

TABLE 3. *Effect of actinomycin D on VLDL synthesis*

Treatment	VLDL, counts/min $\times 10^{-6}$
None	3.6
DES	13.5
DES + actinomycin D	4.0

Values are for counts per minute of immunoprecipitable VLDL per gram of liver. The DES (2.5 mg) or DES (2.5 mg) + actinomycin D (5 mg/kg) were given, and 6 h later the livers were removed and VLDL synthesis was determined as described previously (9).

sured in a wheat-germ translation system (9). The apoVLDL-II mRNA was
found to increase from a low base-line value to a maximum 16–24 h after
estrogen treatment, returning toward base-line values at 30 h. At the peak
of induction, apoVLDL-II constituted 12% of the total protein synthesized.
The kinetics of induction of apoVLDL-II mRNA activity is very similar to
that found in liver slice experiments. This observation suggests that estrogen
stimulates VLDL synthesis, at least partially, by enhancing the accumulation of the mRNA for one of the major apoproteins (9).

EFFECTS OF PROGESTERONE ON VLDL SYNTHESIS

Since progesterone exerts a protective effect on the estrogen-induced
hypertriglyceridemia in women, it was of interest to study the effects of this
steroid on the accumulation of plasma VLDL, triglycerides, and apoVLDL-II
(8). In these experiments, the plasma levels of VLDL triglycerides and
proteins were measured after a single injection of estradiol-17β (1 mg) or
progesterone (2 mg). As shown in Figure 8, estradiol administration resulted
in an eightfold increase in plasma triglycerides and the simultaneous
administration of progesterone had no significant effect on the degree of
stimulation. Similar results were obtained when VLDL protein was analyzed
(Fig. 8). Both in the presence and absence of progesterone, after estrogen
treatment VLDL rose within 5 h, reached a peak at 48 h, and returned to
control levels at 68 h. We next studied the effect of progesterone on the rate
of estrogen-induced VLDL synthesis in liver slices (8). Animals were first
treated with a single injection of estradiol, progesterone and estradiol, or oil
alone. At various times after the injection, the animals were killed and their
livers removed. Treatment with either estradiol alone or estradiol plus
progesterone resulted in a fourfold stimulation of VLDL synthesis above
controls treated with oil alone (Table 4). This stimulation was first detected
12 h after hormone administration and was maximal at 17 h. Thus, the

FIG. 8. Effects of estradiol and estradiol
plus progesterone on plasma VLDL proteins and
triglycerides. Groups of four 3-wk-old cockerels
were given a single subcutaneous injection of
estradiol alone (1 mg) or estradiol (1 mg) plus
progesterone (2 mg). At various times after hormone treatment, the animals were sacrificed,
blood from each of the four animals was pooled,
VLDL were isolated, and VLDL proteins and
triglycerides were determined (8).

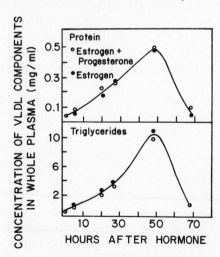

TABLE 4. *Effects of estradiol and estradiol + progesterone on VLDL synthesis*

| Treatment | VLDL Synthesis, counts/min $\times 10^{-4}$ | | | | | |
| | Time after treatment, h | | | | | |
	0	4	12	16	24	72
Control	1.7	1.7	1.7	1.7	1.6	2.2
Estradiol	1.7	3.0	4.1	6.5	3.4	2.8
Estradiol + progesterone	1.7	2.0	3.3	6.4	5.2	3.2

Groups of 4 cockerels were treated with a single subcutaneous injection of either estradiol (1 mg), estradiol (1 mg) + progesterone (2 mg), or sesame oil. At indicated times after injection, liver slices were incubated in vitro with [3H]lysine and VLDL were quantitated after 2 h by immunoprecipitation (8).

results shown in Figure 8 and Table 4 suggest that progesterone is without significant effect on the estrogen-induced hypertriglyceridemia in the cockerel. In this regard, the effects of progesterone are similar in man and the cockerel, viz., progesterone does not affect VLDL synthesis. In man, however, progesterone does increase the amount of lipoprotein lipase activity and probably accounts for the protective effect of the hormone. In the estrogen-treated cockerel (Fig. 8), VLDL levels returned to base-line values at about the same time whether estradiol alone or estradiol plus progesterone was given. This suggests that progesterone has no significant effect on VLDL catabolism in the chicken (8). Since it recently has been shown that phosvitin inhibits the activity of lipoprotein lipase (32), it may well be that the chicken has a compensatory mechanism to inhibit VLDL catabolism so as to produce more lipoprotein for egg production.

INTERACTION OF ESTROGEN WITH LIVER NUCLEI

Thus far, we have shown that estrogen administration to the cockerel produces a selective increase in hepatic VLDL synthesis. This increase is due to an accumulation of mRNAs coding for at least one major apolipoprotein. Estrogen thus appears to regulate VLDL synthesis at the transcriptional level. Since the site of gene transcription resides in the nucleus, we next examined the interaction of estrogen with liver nuclei in the cockerel (10).

Nuclei were isolated from cockerel liver at various times after DES administration. Specific high-affinity binding sites for estrogen in these isolated nuclei were assayed by the [3H]estradiol exchange method (2). Only a single class of binding sites was detected with an apparent K_d of 2×10^{-9} M that remained unaltered by estrogen treatment. In the absence of the hormone, liver nuclei bound about 0.08 fmol estradiol/μg DNA. Treatment of the cockerel with DES resulted in a marked stimulation in the number of these sites up to 0.6 fmol/μg DNA in the liver. Increases were first noted in 60 min; they reached a maximum by 4 h, when there was an eightfold stimulation. By 48 h, the number of sites had returned to control values.

The nuclear binding sites were estrogen specific, and 20% of the [³H]estradiol bound could be extracted by 0.4 M KCl. When the KCl-extractable complex was analyzed by sucrose-gradient centrifugation, the estrogen-receptor complex was found to sediment at the 5S region.

After its binding to specific receptors in the liver cell nucleus, estrogen appeared to stimulate RNA polymerase I and II activities, as measured in isolated nuclei, and to increase the number of RNA synthesis initiation sites assayed on isolated liver chromatin (L. D. Snow et al., manuscript in preparation). This was followed by an increased rate of synthesis of VLDL and, finally, by hypertriglyceridemia (Fig. 9).

DISCUSSION

Estrogen has been used as an experimental tool to induce hypertriglyceridemia in the cockerel. We have studied the mechanism by which estrogen "turns on" the transcription of the apoVLDL-II gene and found that the sequence of events is as follows: the hormone appears to first bind to specific receptors in the liver cell nuclei, resulting in *1)* enhanced RNA polymerase I

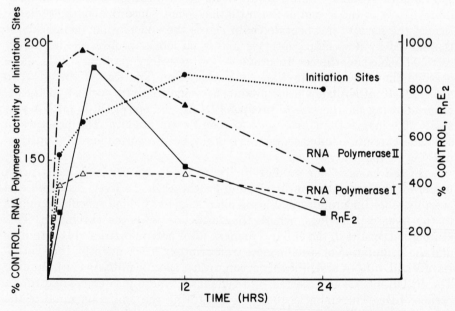

FIG. 9. Effects of DES treatment on nuclear estrogen-receptor levels, RNA polymerase I and II activities, and number of RNA synthesis initiation sites. Three-week-old cockerels were sacrificed at times indicated after treatment with 2.5 mg DES. Liver chromatin was isolated and RNA synthesis initiation sites were measured as described by Tsai et al. (48). Liver cell nuclei were prepared and endogenous RNA polymerase activities were measured as described by Hardin et al. (22). Nuclear estrogen receptors were quantitated by the method of Anderson et al. (2).

and II activities, *2)* increase in number of RNA synthesis initiation sites, and *3)* accumulation of apoVLDL-II mRNA. This is followed by an increased rate of VLDL synthesis and, finally, by hypertriglyceridemia.

To further understand the molecular mechanism of the estrogen stimulation of VLDL synthesis in the cockerel, we have purified the mRNA for a major apolipoprotein (apoVLDL-II) to apparent homogeneity (35, 49; L. Chan et al., manuscript in preparation). The purified RNA sedimented at 6–7S on sucrose gradients and had an electrophoretic mobility compatible with an apparent molecular weight of 130,000. When its in vitro translation product was analyzed by sodium dodecyl sulfate (SDS)-urea slab gel and fluorography, the product was found to have a molecular weight of 11,000, compared with 9400 for apoVLDL-II isolated from the cockerel plasma. It thus appears that apoVLDL-II is initially synthesized as a precursor molecule (preapoVLDL-II). This observation is consistent with Blobel's hypothetical model for secretory protein biosynthesis (5, 6, 13). On the basis of observations on a number of secretory proteins, Blobel and co-workers (5, 6, 13) postulated that there are intracellular precursors to most, if not all, of these proteins. According to their "signal" hypothesis, segregation of specific secretory proteins in the rough endoplasmic reticulum is accomplished by a metabolically short-lived "signal" sequence in the nascent polypeptide chain. This unique sequence would result from the translation of codons located immediately to the 3′ end of the initiation codon. Once the signal sequence "leads" the nascent polypeptide chain across the endoplasmic membrane, it is removed by a specific peptidase and is no longer present in the finally secreted molecule. Since lipoproteins are secretory proteins, it is quite possible that they contain the signal sequence. The size of the in vitro apoVLDL-II mRNA translation product is compatible with such a hypothesis. Even allowing for the size of preapoVLDL-II, the apoVLDL-II mRNA was about 30% longer than necessary to code for its product. The presence of stretches of nontranslated sequences has also been reported for other purified mRNAs (4, 15, 41).

On the basis of our studies in the cockerel, we can now construct a model for the regulation of lipoprotein synthesis in the liver. Estrogen and possibly other lipoprotein-regulating agents appear to bind specific receptors in the liver cell nucleus, where they associate with the chromatin. This association results in the enhancement of RNA polymerase I and II activities and the stimulation of specific gene transcription. Consequently, the synthesis of VLDL mRNA and probably of some other specific mRNAs is stimulated. The VLDL mRNA is exported into cytoplasm where it is translated into a preapoVLDL. The signal sequence, constituting the amino terminal of the nascent chain, is thought to be cleaved by a specific peptidase. On completion of translation of the mRNA, the apoVLDL is released and vectorially discharged. The apoVLDL then binds phospholipids and triglycerides that are synthesized mainly in the smooth endoplasmic reticulum (1, 46, 51). The VLDL are transported to the Golgi apparatus and are concentrated in secretory vesicles. They are finally secreted by fusion of the vesicular membrane with the plasma membrane of the hepatocyte.

We have presented an experimental model system for hormonal regulation of lipoprotein synthesis in the cockerel liver. Oral contraceptives containing estrogen most likely induce hypertriglyceridemia in women via a similar mechanism (10). We believe that our experimental approach to the regulation of lipoprotein metabolism can be applied to other lipid-modifying agents. Hopefully, with studies along similar lines, we will have a better understanding of hyperlipoproteinemia, a major pathogenetic factor in the development of atherosclerosis.

The authors' research is supported by National Institutes of Health Grant HL-16512. R. L. Jackson and L. Chan are Established Investigators of the American Heart Association. A. R. Means is an ACS Faculty Research Awardee.

REFERENCES

1. ALEXANDER, C. A., R. L. HAMILTON, AND R. J. HAVEL. Subcellular localization of B apoprotein of plasma lipoproteins in rat liver. *J. Cell Biol.* 69: 241–263, 1976.

2. ANDERSON, J., J. H. CLARK, AND E. J. PECK, JR. Oestrogen and nuclear binding sites. Determination of specific sites by [³H]oestradiol exchange. *Biochem. J.* 126: 561–567, 1972.

3. APPELBAUM, D. M., A. P. GOLDBERG, O. J. PYKALISTO, J. D. BRUNZELL, AND W. M. HAZZARD. Effect of estrogen on post-heparin lipolytic activity. Selective decline in hepatic triglyceride lipase. *J. Clin. Invest.* 59: 601–608, 1977.

4. BARALLE, F. E. Complete nucleotide sequence of the 5' noncoding region of rabbit β-globin mRNA. *Cell* 10: 549–558, 1977.

5. BLOBEL, G., AND B. DOBBERSTEIN. Transfer of proteins across membranes. I. Presence of proteolytically processed and unprocessed nascent immunoglobulin light chains on membrane-bound ribosomes of murine myeloma. *J. Cell Biol.* 67: 835–851, 1975.

6. BLOBEL, G., AND B. DOBBERSTEIN. Transfer of proteins across membranes. II. Reconstitution of functional rough microsomes from heterologous components. *J. Cell Biol.* 67: 852–862, 1975.

7. BRIGGS, M. H., AND M. BRIGGS. Molecular biology and oral contraception. *New Zealand Med. J.* 83: 257–261, 1976.

8. CHAN, L., R. L. JACKSON, AND A. R. MEANS. Female steroid hormones and lipoprotein synthesis in the cockerel: effects of progesterone and nafoxidine on the estrogenic stimulation of very low density lipoproteins (VLDL) synthesis. *Endocrinology* 100: 1636–1643, 1977.

9. CHAN, L., R. L. JACKSON, B. W. O'MALLEY, AND A. R. MEANS. Synthesis of very low density lipoproteins in the cockerel: effects of estrogen. *J. Clin. Invest.* 58: 368–379, 1976.

10. CHAN, L., AND B. W. O'MALLEY. Mechanism of action of the sex steroid hormones. *New Engl. J. Med.* 294: 1322–1328, 1976.

11. CHOU, P. Y., AND G. D. FASMAN. Conformational parameters for amino acids in helical, β-sheet and random coil regions calculated from proteins. *Biochemistry* 13: 211–245, 1974.

12. DEELEY, R. G., K. P. MULLINIX, W. WETEKAM, H. M. KRONENBERG, M. MEYERS, J. D. ELDRIDGE, AND R. F. GOLDBERGER. Vitellogenin synthesis in the avian liver: vitellogenin is the precursor of the egg yolk phosphoproteins. *J. Biol. Chem.* 250: 9060–9066, 1975.

13. DEVILLERS-THIERY, A., T. KINDT, G. SCHEELE, AND G. BLOBEL. Homology in amino-terminal sequence of precursors to pancreatic secretory proteins. *Proc. Natl. Acad. Sci. US* 72: 5016–5020, 1975.

14. DOLPHEIDE, T. A. A., AND A. S. INGLIS. Primary structure of apovitellogenin I from hen egg yolk and its comparison with emu apovitellogenin I. *Australian J. Biol. Sci.* 29: 175–180, 1976.

15. EFSTRATIADIS, A., F. C. KAFATOS, AND T. MANIATIS. The primary structure of rabbit β-globin mRNA as determined from cloned DNA. *Cell* 10: 571–585, 1977.

16. EHNHOLM, C., J. K. HUTTUNEN, P. J. KINNUNEN, T. A. MIETTINEN, AND E. A. NIKKILA. Effect of oxandrolone treatment on the activity of lipoprotein lipase, hepatic lipase and phospholipase A of human postheparin plasma. *New Engl. J. Med.* 292: 1314–1317, 1975.

17. EISENBERG, S., AND R. I. LEVY. Lipoprotein metabolism. *Advan. Lipid Res.* 13: 1–89, 1975.

18. GLUECK, C. J., R. W. FALLAT, AND D. SCHEEL. Effects of estrogenic compounds on triglyceride kinetics. *Metab. Clin. Exptl.* 24: 537–545, 1975.

19. GLUECK, C. J., P. GARTSIDE, R. W. FALLAT, AND S. MENDOZA. Effect of sex hormones on protamine inactivated and resistant postheparin plasma lipases. *Metab. Clin. Exptl.* 25: 625–632, 1976.

20. GOLDMAN, J. A., AND J. L. OVADIA. The effect of estrogen on intravenous glucose tolerance in women. *Am. J. Obstet. Gynecol.* 103: 172–178, 1969.

21. HAMOSH, M., AND P. HAMOSH. The effect of estrogen on the lipoprotein lipase activity of rat adipose tissue. *J. Clin. Invest.* 55: 1132–1135, 1975.

22. HARDIN, J. W., J. H. CLARK, S. R. GLASSER, AND E. J. PECK, JR. RNA polymerase activity and uterine growth: differential stimulation by estradiol, estriol and nafoxidine. *Biochemistry* 15: 1370–1374, 1976.

23. HAZZARD, W. R., J. D. BRUNZELL, D. T. NOTTER, M. J. SPIGER, AND E. L. BIERMAN. Estrogens and triglyceride transport: increased endogenous production as the mechanism for the hypertriglyceridemia of oral contraceptive therapy. *Excerpta Med. Intern. Congr. Ser.* 273: 1006–1012, 1973.

24. HAZZARD, W. R., D. T. NOTTER, M. J. SPIGER, AND E. L. BIERMAN. Oral contraceptives and triglyceride transport: acquired heparin resistance as the mechanism for impaired post-heparin lipolytic activity. *J. Clin. Endocrinol. Metab.* 35: 425–437, 1972.

25. HAZZARD, W. R., M. J. SPIGER, J. D. BAGDADE, AND E. L. BIERMAN. Studies on the mechanism of

increased plasma triglyceride levels induced by oral contraceptives. *New Engl. J. Med.* 280: 471–474, 1969.

26. HILLYARD, L. A., C. ENTENMAN, AND I. L. CHAIKOFF. Concentration and composition of serum lipoproteins of cholesterol-fed and stilbestrol-injected birds. *J. Biol. Chem.* 223: 359–368, 1950.

27. JACKSON, R. L., H.-Y. LIN, L. CHAN, AND A. R. MEANS. Isolation and characterization of the major apolipoproteins from chicken high density lipoproteins. *Biochim. Biophys. Acta* 420: 342–349, 1976.

28. JACKSON, R. L., H.-Y. LIN, L. CHAN, AND A. R. MEANS. The amino acid sequence of a major apoprotein from hen plasma very low density lipoproteins. *J. Biol. Chem.* 252: 250–253, 1977.

29. JACKSON, R. L., H.-Y. LIN, L. CHAN, AND A. R. MEANS. Estrogen induction of plasma vitellogenin in the cockerel: studies with a phosvitin antibody. *Endocrinology* 101: 849–857, 1977.

30. JACKSON, R. L., J. D. MORRISETT, AND A. M. GOTTO. Lipoprotein structure and metabolism. *Physiol. Rev.* 56: 259–316, 1976.

31. KEKKI, M., AND E. A. NIKKILA. Plasma triglyceride turnover during use of oral contraceptives. *Metab. Clin. Exptl.* 20: 878–889, 1971.

32. KELLEY, J. L., D. GANESAN, H. B. BASS, R. H. THAYER, AND P. ALAUPOVIC. Effect of estrogen on triacylglycerol metabolism: inhibition of post-heparin plasma lipoprotein lipase by phosvitin, an estrogen-induced protein. *Fed. European Biochem. Soc. Letters* 67: 28–31, 1976.

33. KIM, H. J., AND R. K. KALKHOFF. Sex steroid influence on triglyceride metabolism. *J. Clin. Invest.* 56: 888–896, 1975.

34. KISSEBAH, A. H., P. HARRIGAN, AND V. WYNN. Mechanism of hypertriglyceridemia associated with contraceptive steroids. *Hormone Metab. Res.* 5: 184–190, 1973.

35. KONECKI, D., J. M. CIMADEVILLA, G. KRAMER, AND B. HARDESTY. A simple method for the purification of reticulocyte globin messenger ribonucleic acid. *Mol. Biol. Rept.* 2: 335–341, 1975.

36. KUDZMA, D. J., P. M. HEGSTAD, AND R. E. STOLL. The chick as a laboratory model for the study of estrogen-induced hyperlipidemia. *Metab. Clin. Exptl.* 22: 423–424, 1973.

37. LARSSON-COHN, U., L. A. CARLSON, AND J. BOBERG. Effects of an oral contraceptive agent on plasma lipids, plasma lipoproteins, the intravenous fat tolerance and the post-heparin lipoprotein lipase activity. *Acta Med. Scand.* 190: 301–305, 1971.

38. LAURELL, C. B. Quantitative estimation of proteins by electrophoresis in agarose gel containing antibodies. *Anal. Biochem.* 15: 45–52, 1966.

39. LUSKEY, K. L., M. S. BROWN, AND J. L. GOLDSTEIN. Stimulation of the synthesis of very low density lipoproteins in rooster liver by estradiol. *J. Biol. Chem.* 249:

5939–5947, 1974.

40. OLIVER, M. R. Oral contraceptives and myocardial infarction. *Brit. Med. J.* 2: 210–213, 1970.

41. PROUDFOOT, N. J. Complete 3′ noncoding region sequence of rabbit and human β-globin messenger RNAs. *Cell* 10: 559–570, 1977.

42. ROSSNER, S., U. LARSSON-COHN, L. A. CARLSON, AND J. BOBERG. Effects of an oral contraceptive agent on plasma lipids, plasma lipoproteins, the intravenous fat tolerance and the post-heparin lipoprotein lipase activity. *Acta Med. Scand.* 190: 301–305, 1971.

43. SEGREST, J. P., R. L. JACKSON, J. D. MORRISETT, AND A. M. GOTTO. A molecular theory of lipid-protein interactions in the plasma lipoproteins. *Fed. European Biochem. Soc. Letters* 38: 247–253, 1974.

44. SPELLACY, W. N., R. P. BENDEL, W. C. BUHI, AND S. A. BIRK. Insulin and glucose determinations after two and three years of use of a combination type oral contraceptive. *Fertility Sterility* 20: 892–902, 1969.

45. SPELLACY, W. N., W. C. BUHI, C. H. SPELLACY, L. E. MOSES, AND J. W. GOLDZIEHER. Glucose, insulin and growth hormone studies in long-term users of oral contraceptives. *Am. J. Obstet. Gynecol.* 106: 173–182, 1970.

46. STEIN, Y., AND O. STEIN. Lipoprotein synthesis, intracellular transport and secretion in liver. In: *Artherosclerosis III*, edited by G. Schettler and A. Weizel. Berlin: Springer-Verlag, 1974, p. 652–657.

47. STOKES, T., AND V. WYNN. Serum lipids in women on oral contraceptives. *Lancet* 2: 677–680, 1971.

48. TSAI, M.-J., R. J. SCHWARTZ, S. Y. TSAI, AND B. W. O'MALLEY. Effects of estrogen on gene expression in the chick oviduct. IV. Initiation of RNA synthesis on DNA and chromatin. *J. Biol. Chem.* 250: 5165–5174, 1975.

49. WOO, S. L. C., S. E. HARRIS, J. M. ROSEN, L. CHAN, P. J. SPERRY, A. R. MEANS, AND B. W. O'MALLEY. Use of sepharose 4B for preparative scale fractionation of eukaryotic messenger RNAs. *Prep. Biochem.* 4: 555–572, 1974.

50. WYNN, V., J. W. H. DOAR, G. L. MILLS, AND T. STOKES. Fasting serum triglyceride, cholesterol and lipoprotein levels during oral contraceptive therapy. *Lancet* 2: 756–760, 1969.

51. VAN GOLDE, L. M. G., B. FLEISCHER, AND S. FLEISCHER. Some studies on the metabolism of phospholipids in Golgi complex from bovine and rat liver in comparison to other subcellular fractions. *Biochim. Biophys. Acta* 249: 318–330, 1971.

52. VESSEY, M. P., AND R. DOLL. Investigation of relation between use of oral contraceptives and thrombo-embolic disease. A further report. *Brit. Med. J.* 2: 651–657, 1969.

53. ZORRILLA, E., M. HULSE, A. HERNANDEZ, AND H. GERSHBERG. Severe endogenous hypertriglyceridemia during treatment with oestrogen and oral contraceptives. *J. Clin. Endocrinol. Metab.* 28: 1793–1796, 1968.

9

Hepatic Secretion and Metabolism of High-Density Lipoproteins

ROBERT L. HAMILTON

*Cardiovascular Research Institute and Department of Anatomy,
University of California, San Francisco, California*

THE MAJOR SOLUBLE LIPOPROTEINS found in normal blood and lymph plasmas share a common fundamental structure: an oily or nonpolar "core" of triglycerides and cholesteryl esters surrounded by a more polar monomolecular "surface" of phospholipids, unesterified cholesterol, and apoproteins (Zilversmit, chapt. 4). The term *pseudomicellar* has been proposed for this structure (21); the term *lamellar* has been proposed for two unusual lipoproteins (shown in Fig. 2) that are comprised principally of surface lipids and apoproteins and have the structure of a lipid bilayer (19, 22).

Two major lipoproteins characterized by a triglyceride-rich core, namely, chylomicrons from intestinal absorptive epithelium and very-low-density lipoproteins (VLDL) from hepatocytes, originate by intracellular processes generally similar to those of other secretory cells that elaborate specialized macromolecules for export (15). The two other major plasma lipoproteins characterized by cores enriched in cholesteryl esters, namely, low-density lipoproteins (LDL) and high-density lipoproteins (HDL), apparently originate by significantly different processes. Low-density lipoproteins are predominantly catabolic products of VLDL (35). The conversion of VLDL to LDL probably occurs extracellularly during a stepwise hydrolytic process at two different cell surfaces. The VLDL triglycerides are first hydrolyzed at the endothelial plasma surface in extrahepatic capillaries by lipoprotein lipases, giving rise to smaller remnant particles that are cleared rapidly by the liver (Fielding, chapt. 5). The specific mechanisms of the remnant remodeling process (the second step) that produces LDL are not established but may occur within the spaces of Disse in the liver among hepatocyte microvilli, the hypothetical site of action of hepatic triglyceride lipase (19).

One therefore might predict that plasma HDL also may originate either by direct secretion of mature pseudomicellar particles from liver and/or intestine or by some degradation process associated with catabolism of triglyceride-rich lipoproteins. Recent observations suggest that neither process alone adequately accounts for the origin of plasma HDL although both may play a significant role in the complicated evolution of the end product.

BACKGROUND

Two key observations led us to an initial hypothesis subsequently tested by simple experiments. The first was our repeated failure to obtain positive evidence for the presence of pseudomicellar plasma HDL within the Golgi apparatus of liver cells. Presumably other investigators also have not published their negative results. Lipid and protein material that floats in the HDL fraction can be recovered from Golgi fractions, but it contains insignificant amounts of cholesteryl esters, has neither the proper size nor staining characteristics of plasma HDL, and generally looks like membrane fragments in the electron microscope.

One group reported in abstract form that Golgi HDL ($d < 1.21$) migrated with alpha mobility on agarose gel electrophoresis and contained, by immunochemical analysis, the major apoprotein of plasma HDL (25). I reported that nascent HDL fractions from hepatocyte Golgi apparatus, isolated liver cells, and perfused liver contain disks with a lipid bilayer structure (15). The disks in Golgi fractions were seen by electron microscopy in negative stains after rupture of the membranes by the French pressure cell but have not been separated from microsomal fragments. In retrospect, the published half-life of 10–11 h for HDL apoprotein in the rat (31) suggests that the intracellular pool of nascent HDL may be too small to permit adequate recoveries by current separatory techniques. Lamellar particles, recovered from media in which isolated hepatocytes had been incubated, later were found to come from phospholipids already present as a major contaminant in the commercial preparations of bovine serum albumin added to the media. The discoidal HDL from liver perfusions, however, appear to represent a physiologic secretory product by hepatocytes (see below).

The second key observation, published in 1970 by Torsvik et al. (41) and in 1971 by Forte et al. (12), demonstrated by electron microscopy that HDL fractions of human subjects genetically lacking the enzyme lecithin:cholesterol acyltransferase (LCAT) contained predominantly discoidal particles. Because pseudomicellar HDL of blood plasma previously represented the best substrate for this enzyme (1, 9), and because the edge thickness of the disks was the same dimension as that known for membrane bilayers (43), we thought the disks might consist of phospholipid and unesterified or free cholesterol plus apoprotein. If the latter prediction proved correct, the discoidal HDL could represent the accumulation of the natural substrate for the absent LCAT in these patients and thereby a nascent or early form of HDL.

Glomset et al. (14) had predicted earlier that a different smaller molecular weight HDL particle, also found in these patients, together with the discoidal particles both may represent newly secreted precursors of HDL.

EXPERIMENTAL MODEL

Because of the technical problems associated with isolated hepatocytes and Golgi fractions described above, we reasoned that a recirculating liver-perfusion system might allow sufficient time to accumulate adequate material for analyses. Review of previous studies that had used this approach suggested that neither pseudomicellar nor discoidal HDL had been shown clearly to be secreted because of one or more aspects of the experimental technique [e.g., use of plasma already containing HDL, short or erythrocyte-free perfusions yielding insufficient material, inadequate characterization of HDL fractions, use of bovine serum albumin already containing phospholipid-rich substances of HDL density, or use of oxygenators that relied on gassing a thin film of perfusate, a procedure that might cause losses or structural changes of HDL (16)].

To reduce this latter risk, we first tested a simple Silastic lung to mimic in vivo gas exchange through a membrane (16). Much to our surprise, isolated livers survived well for prolonged periods (6–8 h) in the complete absence of added oncotically active proteins, provided that the perfusion media contained 25% washed rat erythrocytes. This finding simplified our experiments because it eliminated the tedious preparation of large quantities of lipoprotein-free serum, or toxin- and phospholipid-free bovine serum albumin. To really test our hypothesis, it seemed necessary to show, first, that in the presence of enzymatically active LCAT the perfused liver produced pseudomicellar HDL like plasma HDL and, second, the discoidal HDL were produced in this enzyme's absence. Because two independent groups showed that the perfused rat liver secreted this enzyme (30, 36), we needed a method of inhibiting LCAT during prolonged perfusions. A colleague (C. J. Fielding) directed us to a report showing that a sulfhydryl-blocking agent, 5,5′-dithionitrobenzoic acid (DTNB), fully inhibited human serum LCAT activity at low concentrations (39). Since no LCAT would be present in perfusates initially and would in fact probably never reach plasma levels found in vivo, in theory only trace quantities of DTNB would be required to block the small amount of LCAT secreted (30, 36). We found that in practice, by adding very small amounts of DTNB at 30-min intervals [the sum of which at the end of 6 h would have been 1.0–1.2 mM, which completely blocks LCAT (39) in human serum], the DTNB was mostly rendered inactive soon after being mixed in the perfusate. The DTNB caused no detectable liver damage. Analyses of perfused liver structure and function and of secretion rates of lipoprotein lipids (20) and apolipoproteins (8) were not significantly different in the presence and absence of DTNB.

The details of the technical aspects of the methods for these and other measurements used to obtain the results summarized in the next section have been published elsewhere (5–8, 20).

KEY OBSERVATIONS

Measurements of the capacity of control liver perfusates to esterify cholesterol are shown in Figure 1, representing LCAT secretion by the isolated perfused rat liver. The secretion rate of LCAT increased with time of perfusion, as did the secretion rate of lipoprotein lipids (20) and apolipoproteins (8). Inhibition of LCAT activity in the perfusates by DTNB averaged 86, 90, and 85% at 2, 4, and 6 h, respectively. The percent inhibition of LCAT in a single experiment is presented in Figure 1 to show that in individual perfusions there is some variability in the completeness of the enzyme inhibition by this method. The significance of this variability is brought out by studies of the chemical compositions of HDL fractions (1.075 > d > 1.175) from these perfusions (Table 1). Whereas the mean content of cholesteryl esters in HDL from DTNB perfusions was about 4%, individual values ranged from less than 1% to about 9%. Likewise, the cholesteryl ester content of HDL from control perfusions varied significantly from about 14 to 20%, sometimes approaching that found in HDL fractions isolated from rat plasma to which DTNB was immediately added (Table 1). We also observed that if precautions were not taken to inhibit LCAT in HDL fractions from plasma the weight percent of cholesteryl esters was increased from about 24% to as much as 30% (20). In general, apart from the content of triglyceride in HDL fractions from DTNB perfusions (discussed below), the chemical composition suggested that nascent discoidal particles were comprised predominantly of nonpolar surface lipids (phospholipids and cholesterol) together with specific apoproteins.

Electron-microscopic images of discoidal HDL fractions from liver perfusions with DTNB are consistent with the chemical composition data that,

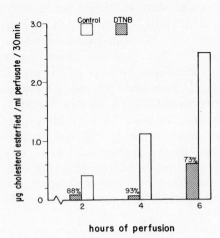

FIG. 1. Rate of cholesterol esterification in perfusates in the presence and absence of DTNB. Samples of perfusates were obtained from 2 livers perfused simultaneously. The DTNB was added at 30-min intervals to the perfusate of 1 liver. Samples were taken from the perfusate reservoir just before DTNB was added at each interval shown. [From Hamilton et al. (20).]

TABLE 1. *Chemical composition of high-density lipoproteins*

Source	Components, % by wt				
	Triglycerides	Cholesteryl esters	Free cholesterol	Phospho-lipids	Proteins
Plasma (DTNB added)*					
Mean (*n* = 5)	1.18	23.6	5.06	25.9	44.3
SD	0.88	1.20	0.30	1.68	0.94
Control perfusate (no DTNB)					
Mean (*n* = 5)	3.62†	16.8‡	6.30†	31.8†	41.5
SD	0.49	2.33	1.02	1.44	2.66
Perfusate (DTNB added)					
Mean (*n* = 5)	5.44§	4.28§	12.0§	39.9§	38.4
SD	0.90	3.42	2.12	3.10	2.35

* DTNB was added to freshly drawn plasma to give a final concentration of 1 mM. † Significantly different from values for plasma HDL (*P* < 0.01). ‡ Significantly different from value for plasma HDL (*P* < 0.05). § Significantly different from value for control perfusate HDL (*P* < 0.01). [From Hamilton et al. (20).]

taken together, strongly suggest the structure of a lipid bilayer. The electron-microscopic images in Figure 2 provide morphologic evidence that discoidal HDL (top) are essentially bilayer structures. For comparison, another lipid bilayer lipoprotein that occurs in cholestasis (called Lp-X) is shown in the bottom half of Figure 2. They are illustrated here together for two different reasons. First, it is important to emphasize the differences in size, shape, and structure as well as the similarities between these two quite different lipoproteins because they have been mistakenly described as the same or as similar particles in several recent papers. Second, the lipid bilayer structure of Lp-X has been firmly established (17–19) and is used here as a standard for comparison with the discoidal HDL. Each of these different lipoproteins may appear in stacks (Fig. 2, left side), called rouleaux, as described for erythrocytes, but this is an artifact of the drying process in the presence of phosphotungstate on the grid surface. In each case, they may also lie flat on the grid, appearing spherical, and thereby not be distinguishable from other pseudomicellar lipoproteins. Thus, although an artifact, the rouleau forms of these particles not only reveal their presence but also provide additional information about their structure. Because of this rouleau phenomenon, the edge thickness of nascent HDL disks from DTNB liver perfusions can be measured precisely from electron-microscopic images: 44–47 Å (SD 5–6 Å). This measurement is virtually the same as that published by Torsvik et al. (41) for the discoidal HDL of humans suffering from LCAT deficiency and is the appropriate measure of the thickness of a membrane bilayer containing cholesterol and protein (43). The diameter of the disks averaged 188–194 Å (SD 23–25 Å) in our rat liver perfusion studies (20), in contrast to 162 ± 56 Å in LCAT-deficient humans reported by Torsvik et al. (41). Note that the diameters of normal human pseudomicellar HDL are about 85 Å (41), whereas those of normal rat plasma are also proportionately larger, 114 ± 13 Å (20). Although not shown here, HDL fractions of control liver perfusions

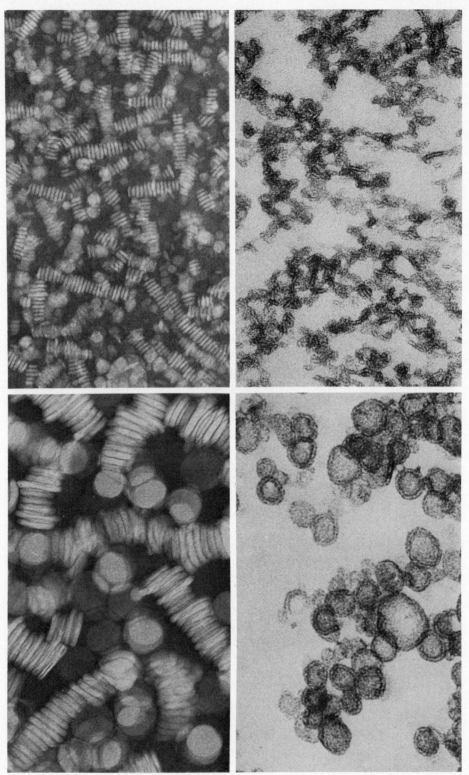

appeared to contain predominantly pseudomicellar particles (~75%) with a mean diameter slightly smaller than plasma HDL, together with some larger particles equal in diameter to that of disks. Equally significant is the observation that some disks in short stacks of rouleaux were also seen in control perfusate HDL and the occasional particle of disk diameter appeared in all fractions of rat plasma HDL (20). These observations of particle size (and structure) become important subsequently, when HDL fractions from these three different in vivo sources are compared in content of apoproteins and as substrates for LCAT in vitro (see Figs. 3 and 4).

The bottom images in Figure 2 are of Lp-X. The negative stain shows coin-shaped images but these differ from nascent HDL (top) because they are twice the thickness (>100 Å at edges) and more than twice the diameter (400–600 Å). Previous studies showed that this abnormal lipoprotein (Lp-X) was a lipid-bilayer liposome (17–19). During drying on the grid surface the liposomes collapse (due to evaporation of water from the trapped volume) into flattened vesicles in rouleaux. The individual edges of each consist of two bilayer thicknesses. The image at the bottom right of Figure 2 is the same lipoprotein fraction (Lp-X) after fixation in osmium tetroxide, staining in warm uranyl salts, followed by dehydration, embedding in plastic, and thin sectioning. This image shows the probable shape (spherical vesicle) of this particle as it exists in vivo but, more important, it shows the characteristic trilaminar staining of phospholipids as they occur in bilayers of biological membranes or lamellar aqueous suspensions. The three layers are seen because of the deposition of heavy metals in the region of the head groups separated by a space of 20–25 Å representing the unstained acyl chains in the center of the bilayer (38). These electron-microscopic images are consistent with the chemical composition (64% phospholipids, 33% cholesterol, and 3% protein) and X-ray diffraction data showing that Lp-X is a spherical liposome about 400–600 Å in diameter (17–19).

The thin-section images of discoidal HDL from DTNB liver perfusions show the same trilaminar staining pattern (Fig. 2, top right). The difference is that they appear as linear, open-ended bilayer pieces of membrane of much smaller size. Because these small particles are only about one-third to one-fourth in greatest dimension as the section thickness (600–800 Å), and because they are randomly oriented within the section, only those few particles that are oriented perpendicular to the plane and are free of superimposition of aggregates form clear images. Thus, the chemical compo-

---

FIG. 2. *Top left:* nascent HDL from rat livers perfused with DTNB (20). Image was obtained by negative staining, which causes rouleau formations of disks. Most individual particles are ~45 Å in thickness and ~190 Å in diameter. *Top right:* same lipoprotein as top left, but prepared by thin-sectioning techniques to show trilaminar staining (20). *Bottom left:* Lp-X, an abnormal plasma lipoprotein from a human with cholestasis, was isolated as previously described (17). Negative staining also causes these vesicular particles to collapse, forming rouleaux. This sometimes breaks the bilayer (note end particle of rouleaux). *Bottom right:* same lipoprotein as bottom left but again prepared by thin-sectioning techniques to show trilaminar staining of bilayer shell of spherical liposome containing an internal trapped volume (18). [×200,000.]

sition, edge thickness, and staining characteristics indicate that the predominant structure of the discoidal HDL is that of a bilayer membrane containing substantial amounts of protein (about one-third by weight, Table 1).

The apoproteins of HDL fractions from control and DTNB liver perfusions were compared with plasma HDL. The predominant apoprotein of plasma HDL was apoA-I, whereas the predominant apoprotein of discoidal particles was slightly slower in electrophoretic mobility, corresponding to the arginine-rich protein (ARP). The HDL fractions from control perfusions appeared to contain about equal amounts of apoA-I and ARP, as judged from the staining of tetramethylurea-soluble apoproteins in alkaline polyacrylamide gels (20). These differences are more clearly shown in sodium dodecyl sulfate (SDS)-polyacrylamide gel electropherograms as illustrated in Figure 3. There appears to be a progressive shift in proportions of ARP to apoA-I corresponding to the structural and lipid composition differences, which in turn correlate with the extent of LCAT activity. To quantitate the apoprotein differences, radioimmunoassays were developed for rat apoA-I and ARP (6, 7) and applied to these HDL fractions (8). The apoprotein content (ARP:apoA-I ratio), cholesteryl ester content, and structure (lamellar vs. pseudomicellar) appeared to represent a progression. The discoidal HDL contained the highest ratio of ARP:apoA-I (10:1) and lowest amount of cholesteryl esters (2%); control perfusate HDL (mixtures of pseudomicellar particles with some disks) contained intermediate ARP:apoA-I (2:1) and cholesteryl ester content (18%); however, the predominately pseudomicellar particles from plasma

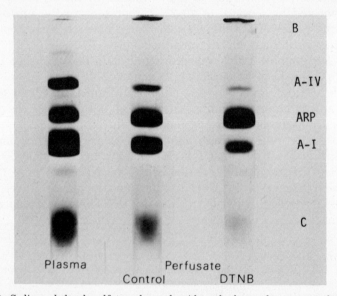

FIG. 3. Sodium dodecyl sulfate-polyacrylamide gel electropherograms showing major staining apoproteins of rat HDL fractions obtained from 3 different sources. These HDL fractions are also compared in Fig. 4 and Table 1. For details of methods or results of quantitative measurements of the apoprotein content of these HDL fractions, see Felker et al. (8).

contained 1:7 ARP:apoA-I and 24% cholesteryl esters (8). Measurements of the hepatic secretion rates of these apolipoproteins showed that ARP was a major secretory product that increased in concentration in perfusates in a linear or increasing rate over 6 h in amounts comparable to that of apoB, whereas apoA-I secretion by the liver was about one-seventh that of ARP, most of which was released during the first 2–4 h of perfusion (8). By contrast, the intestine produces most of the apoA-I and apparently little ARP (22). The SDS-gel electrophoresis patterns of Figure 3 show the presence of protein near the top of the gels of perfusate HDL fractions, which appeared more evident in the DTNB liver perfusions. Subsequently, a separate particle containing B apoprotein was found as a contaminant in perfusate HDL fractions, but it could be removed by concanavalin A-Sepharose chromatography with the discoidal particles otherwise left preserved (5). This contaminating particle apparently accounted for much of the perfusate HDL triglyceride (Table 1) and all of the apoB and corresponds to like findings reported for discoidal HDL fractions from humans with LCAT deficiency (29).

All the data summarized thus far suggest that discoidal HDL represent a nascent or precursor form of pseudomicellar HDL and therefore would be a preferred substrate for LCAT. The results presented in Figure 4 confirm this prediction. Purified LCAT from human plasma synthesized cholesteryl esters at a substantially faster rate from substrate lipids of perfusate HDL fractions, compared with plasma HDL, and the highest rate invariably was obtained with the discoidal HDL from DTNB liver perfusions (20). The differences in synthetic rates shown in Figure 4 were found whether the initial substrates were matched for unesterified cholesterol or protein content or when increasing amounts of unesterified cholesterol in HDL fractions were compared. The results of the enzyme studies (Fig. 4), taken together with the morphologic, chemical composition, and apoprotein data, support the hypothesis

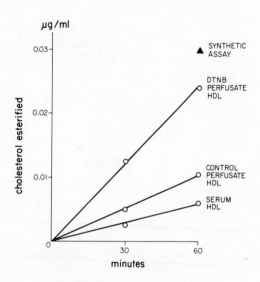

FIG. 4. Activity of purified human LCAT on rat HDL from different sources. Results are representative of 4 experiments. Rate against a synthetic substrate containing an optimal molar ratio of cholesterol:lecithin (1:4) and saturating concentration of apoprotein cofactor is shown (synthetic assay). [From Hamilton et al. (20).]

that the disk HDL become transformed into pseudomicellar HDL primarily because of the action of LCAT. The data also suggest the probability that a small fraction of discoidal particles in the HDL fractions from plasma may account for a substantial fraction of the observed activity of LCAT on this lipoprotein class in vitro. Furthermore, it has been proposed recently that the nascent discoidal particle may represent a small fraction of the total plasma HDL pool in vivo in humans that rapidly turns over newly formed cholesteryl esters produced by LCAT (2).

DISCUSSION OF HYPOTHESES

Schematic diagrams depicting the central ideas of our present hypotheses on the possible origins of pseudomicellar HDL of plasma are presented in Figures 5 and 6. I will discuss a few of the major aspects in an attempt to *1*) assess potential artifacts of the experimental system, *2*) explain the rationale for including the major concepts presented, and *3*) identify some key questions requiring future work.

A major criticism of this work is the use of the chemical reagent DTNB to selectively block one specific enzyme (LCAT) in a living tissue containing many proteins with sensitive sulfhydryl groups. Although it was reasoned that the amounts of the reagent used were small, that most of the DTNB was inactivated in the perfusate, and that certain measurements indicated

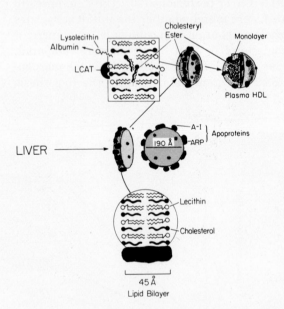

FIG. 5. Schematic diagram depicting the central ideas of our hypothesis of the hepatic origins of pseudomicellar HDL of plasma. It suggests that the liver secretes disk-shaped HDL into the blood plasma. One disk appears tilted on edge and the other one is flat to show apoproteins and diameter of 190 Å. Enlarged cutaway of 1 particle indicates a basic structure of a phospholipid bilayer containing cholesterol, as in cell membranes. Hydrocarbon edge of the disks of necessity would be protected from aqueous plasma by proteins, mainly arginine-rich apoprotein. Upper part of diagram illustrates the proposed molecular events that result from the LCAT reaction. Binding of LCAT to the surface (or edge) of the disk is followed by formation of cholesteryl esters, which, by virtue of their insolubility in water, move into the hydrocarbon domain of the bilayer. Polar lysolecithin transfers from the surface to serum albumin. The enzymatic transformation consumes surface molecules and generates an oily core that pushes apart the bilayer until a spherical pseudomicellar HDL of smaller size is formed. [From Hamilton et al. (20).]

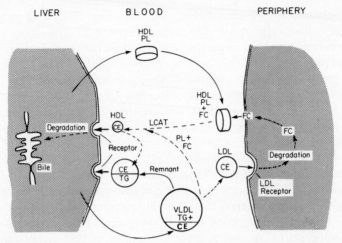

FIG. 6. Diagram depicting some speculation on possible role of discoidal HDL in cholesterol transport. Liver is shown secreting nascent VLDL containing predominantly triglycerides (TG) with only small amounts of cholesteryl esters (CE), whereas the disk contains mostly phospholipids (PL). In the blood or at the periphery, the disk picks up free cholesterol (FC) from cell membranes and from excess surface of triglyceride-rich particles shown here as VLDL conversion to remnants occurs. The LCAT would generate cholesteryl esters in the disk from these lipids that either transform the disk into a sphere (Fig. 5) or become transferred rapidly to the remnant during lipolysis of the triglycerides. Each of these cholesteryl ester-enriched particles, HDL and remnants, may then be recognized by hepatocyte receptors leading to uptake, to degradation, and finally to biliary excretion of cholesterol and bile salts. Alternatively either particle may be modified by the hepatocyte and returned to the plasma. Remnants in humans are mostly converted to LDL (35), whereas in rats most are catabolized by liver (21). The HDL may unload their CE contents at the hepatocyte membrane and recycle many times to periphery prior to degradation (4). The LDL derived from VLDL presumably transport their CE contents (synthesized largely by the HDL-LCAT system but transferred to remnants) to peripheral cells by way of the LDL-receptor mechanism, thereby providing cholesterol for membrane turnover (Brown and Goldstein, chapt. 10). This flux of LDL cholesterol into the peripheral tissues must be returned to the liver, suggesting a potentially fundamental role for the nascent disk in the HDL-LCAT system and cholesterol homeostasis.

viability apparently was not altered, other reactions within the hepatocyte could have been affected by DTNB, leading to the presence of the discoidal HDL. It seems unlikely that DTNB impaired cholesterol esterification within the liver because fatty acyl:CoA cholesterol transferase, a microsomal cholesterol-esterifying enzyme of liver, was not affected by DTNB since the amounts of cholesteryl esters in perfusate VLDL were the same in control and DTNB perfusions. The likelihood that DTNB causes disks through mechanisms other than the specific inhibition of LCAT appears remote because discoidal HDL are secreted by normal rat livers in the absence of DTNB (20). Discoidal HDL also occur in vivo in the absence of DTNB in several circumstances other than the genetic disease of LCAT deficiency. They occur in plasmas of cholestatic humans (18, 19) and rats (unpublished observations) and in other instances of liver damage associated with reduced levels of plasma LCAT activity (32, 33). Discoidal HDL also accumulate in plasma of guinea pigs fed a diet containing excess cholesterol (34) and in liver perfusates of these experimental animals (unpublished observations).

It is proposed that the liver secretes discoidal HDL (Figs. 5 and 6). Control perfusions in the absence of the liver have shown that neither red cells nor other pseudomicellar lipoproteins give rise to disks (20). Single-pass perfusion experiments show the presence of both VLDL and discoidal HDL in perfusates rapidly chilled to eliminate enzymic activities that might otherwise have occurred during prolonged recirculation at 37°C (26, 27; unpublished observations). Disks of HDL size are present in whole-liver perfusates (unpublished observations) and in whole plasma of human patients with LCAT deficiency (unpublished observations) and cholestasis (19), reducing the likelihood that they are ultracentrifugal by-products of VLDL or LDL. Other investigators have shown that HDL are recovered from either recirculating or single-pass perfusions of rat livers that are not secreting VLDL due to orotic acid poisoning (26, 45). This appears to eliminate VLDL as a potential source. Three major mechanisms of origin remain plausible. 1) The liver synthesizes disks intracellularly and secretes them as such into the plasma (Figs. 5 and 6). 2) The liver secretes ARP, free of lipid, which either in the space of Disse or in association with endothelial cells or erythrocytes combines with cell membrane lipids, resulting in extracellular self-assembly of disks. This seems unlikely, although not impossible, because disks are present in single-pass perfusions with erythrocyte-free media and because nascent VLDL isolated from Golgi fractions already contain considerable amounts of ARP (28; unpublished observations). 3) Arginine-rich protein, in association with surface lipids, may dissociate spontaneously from VLDL on release from the hepatocyte. Future studies clearly are needed to attempt to resolve this key question.

Arguments presented above favor a lipid bilayer arrangement as the predominant molecular structure of newly secreted discoidal HDL from perfused rat liver. However, this structure would demand the presence of detergentlike molecules around the edges of the disk to serve as a covering for the otherwise water-exposed hydrocarbons. The liver secretes another bimolecular disk of phospholipid in which bile salts protect the hydrophobic edges of a mixed micelle that solubilizes cholesterol in bile (37). Presumably, the HDL disk also is an efficient solubilizer of cholesterol sent to the peripheral tissues by the liver for this function (Fig. 6; see SPECULATIONS ON CHOLESTEROL TRANSPORT). However, in place of bile salts, which would be lost to plasma albumin and excreted by the kidney, the hydrophobic edges of disks secreted into blood are sealed instead by specific apoproteins, most probably ARP (Fig. 5). Many apoproteins have lipid-binding properties that may be dependent on numerous regions of amphipathic helices characterized by polar and nonpolar surfaces on opposite faces of the apoprotein (24). Such a conformation of apoprotein would provide the optimal topographical requirements to fit its nonpolar face alongside the acyl chains of phospholipids while presenting its polar amino acid residues toward the water. Both apoA-

I and ARP can bind spontaneously to phospholipids suspended in water, causing the formation of lipid-protein complexes with properties of bilayer disks (unpublished observations). Perhaps more compelling are reports that in several species in vivo the predominant apoprotein of discoidal HDL is ARP (see 20). In discoidal HDL from perfused livers of cholesterol-fed guinea pigs, ARP is the exclusive apoprotein (unpublished observations). Thus, ARP is shown to be the major structural apoprotein of the nascent HDL disk of perfused livers, with smaller amounts of apoA-I present perhaps also along the edge (Fig. 5). The alignment of the active site of LCAT with the substrate lipids of the disk somehow may be brought about by the unique spatial relationships afforded by this hydrocarbon edge (which is absent from all other plasma lipoproteins) interacting with the apoA-I apoprotein that activates this enzyme (10).

The hypothesis (Fig. 5) suggests a molecular model whereby a disk-shaped particle of known dimensions, comprised of surface lipids (phospholipids and unesterfied cholesterol) and sealed on its hydrocarbon edge by specific apoproteins (ARP and apoA-I), may be converted into a typical psuedomicellar (liquid lipid-core) plasma lipoprotein by a single enzyme reaction. The LCAT, bound to the disk particle, becomes activated by apoA-I to hydrolyze the β-fatty acid ester of phospholipid releasing water-soluble lysolecithin to a nearby molecule of plasma albumin. The LCAT transfers this fatty acid to the 3-hydroxyl of an adjacent cholesterol, forming a nonpolar cholesteryl ester, which, due to its complete insolubility in both surface water and polar lipids, pushes into the hydrocarbon domains within the center of the bilayer. As the LCAT reaction continues, a separate oil phase of cholesteryl esters pushes apart the leaflets of the bilayers of the disk from within, generating an oily core until a pseudomicellar HDL of smaller diameter is created, still covered by a surface monomolecular film of polar lipids and apoproteins (Fig. 5).

The LCAT esterification rate would be rapid initially because these disks contain optimal proportions (11) of phospholipid and unesterified cholesterol (Table 1) whereas discoidal HDL of LCAT-deficient subjects (29) and cholesterol-fed guinea pigs (34) theoretically would be poor substrates because they contain an equimolar (or more) ratio of cholesterol to phospholipid. In vitro measurements have shown that a high ratio of free cholesterol to phospholipid greatly inhibits LCAT activity (11). The catalytic rate of LCAT presumably would become slower as the disk accumulated cholesteryl esters, which also effectively inhibit the reaction (11). In vivo, transfers of surface lipids from plasma membranes of cells and from surfaces of partially catabolized triglyceride-rich lipoproteins presumably would replenish substrate lipids for the continued reaction (Fig. 6). Presented with an excess of dietary cholesterol, these processes might generate an abnormally swollen core of cholesteryl esters, leading to enlarged species of HDL such as HDL_c (Mahley, chapt. 11).

The model shown in Figure 5 is oversimplified because it includes only the proposed hepatic contributions to the formation of pseudomicellar HDL of plasma. The rat intestine has been shown to synthesize HDL apoproteins (44) and appears to be the major source of apoA-I (22). There is no firm evidence that the intestine secretes either a nascent or precursor HDL[1] particle or LCAT. However, the small-molecular-weight HDL of LCAT-deficient patients contain predominantly apoA-I and therefore may be of intestinal origin (13, 29). It is worth noting that the perfused rat liver did not appear to synthesize measurable amounts of comparable small-molecular-weight HDL (20). Glomset et al. (14) predicted that the small-molecular-weight HDL and the discoidal particles in LCAT-deficient humans both were precursor forms of plasma HDL. It is not yet known how apoA-I becomes the major component and ARP a minor component of plasma HDL. It may involve transfers or exchanges between HDL and triglyceride-rich particles from the intestine because the latter particles originally carry apoA-I in intestinal lymph that apparently is replaced by ARP in the process of remnant formation. Although specific details of this process are unclear, it may be coupled with the mechanism by which cholesteryl esters generated by the LCAT-HDL system become incorporated into remnants (Fig. 6; 13, 21).

SPECULATIONS ON CHOLESTEROL TRANSPORT

What is the major function of HDL and how do discoidal particles participate in the physiology of lipid transport? A greatly oversimplified scheme is shown in Figure 6 in an attempt to speculate on the possible role of discoidal HDL in cholesterol homeostasis. The major function of the HDL-LCAT system is probably to scavenge cholesterol from cell membranes from peripheral tissues and from excess surfaces of triglyceride-rich lipoproteins (13). A unique vehicle to specifically transport cholesterol from the periphery (nonliver tissues) presumably would be necessary to recruit and carry cholesterol back to the liver for excretion. This transport system is predicted first because peripheral cells turn over cholesterol but lack enzymes to catabolize it and second because recent discoveries indicate that peripheral tissues synthesize little of their own cholesterol in vivo but obtain it instead by taking up and catabolizing cholesteryl ester-enriched LDL (see Brown and Goldstein, chapt. 10). If cholesterol synthesis in peripheral tissues normally is suppressed by the LDL receptor mechanism as proposed, calculations indicate a substantial (1–2 g/day) flux of cholesterol by this pathway (42). Except for the amount used by those cells of the endocrines converting cholesterol into steroid hormones (Brown and Goldstein, chapt. 10), the bulk of LDL cholesterol must subsequently be returned to the liver for excretion. The discoidal HDL may play an important role in this process. Phospholipids and especially phospholipid plus HDL-apoprotein complexes appear to be effective removers of cholesterol from cell membranes (23). Apoprotein A-I

---

[1] *Note added in proof.* An abstract published in October 1977 describes discoidal HDL from rat mesenteric lymph. (P. GREEN, A. TALL, AND R. GLICKMAN. Rat intestine secretes discoidal nascent HDL. *Circulation* 56: III-56, 1977.).

solubilizes phospholipids (23, 40) and ARP interacts with receptors on cells from peripheral tissues like LDL (3; Mahley, chapt. 11). Of considerable interest is the consistent finding that ARP is greatly increased in plasma lipoproteins in response to the demands for increased cholesterol transport (Mahley, chapt. 11). Therefore, in addition to being a preferred substrate for LCAT, the discoidal HDL have many properties that appear to facilitate the scavenging of cholesterol from cell surfaces (Fig. 6).

Arginine-rich protein may serve a broader fundamental role in the transport of cholesterol away from peripheral tissues to the liver (Fig. 6). If it is correct that the liver secretes apoB (contained initially in nascent VLDL) with the ultimate function of delivering cholesterol to peripheral cells, it may be predicted that the liver also secretes a different apoprotein the function of which is to return equal amounts of cholesterol from those same peripheral cells to the liver for excretion. The ARP may serve this general function because of the following: *a)* ARP is synthesized largely by the liver in amounts comparable to apoB (8, 22); *b)* cholesterol excess apparently stimulates ARP synthesis, presumably by the liver, because it is greatly increased in plasma lipoproteins in hypercholesterolemias caused by cholesterol feeding in many species (34; Mahley, chapt. 11); *c)* ARP appears to be an affector apoprotein on remnants, resulting in their recognition and rapid removal by the liver, a major pathway of returning cholesteryl esters to the liver for excretion (Fig. 6; Sherrill, chapt. 6); *d)* ARP is the major apoprotein of nascent discoidal HDL whose properties would appear to facilitate uptake of unesterified cholesterol from plasma membranes of peripheral cells (see DISCUSSION OF HYPOTHESES); and *e)* ARP apparently is recognized by the same peripheral cells that contain receptors for LDL (3; Mahley, chapt. 11). Thus, nascent discoidal HDL initially may be comprised predominantly of phospholipids and ARP and may be recognized by the plasma membranes of peripheral cells that release unesterified cholesterol to the disks. In the thoracic duct lymph and in the blood the disks may pick up additional apoA-I, synthesized by the intestine, that binds to and activates LCAT on the discoidal particles when they reach the bloodstream. The LCAT reaction produces cholesteryl esters within the disks (Fig. 5), a reaction further stimulated by transfer of substrate lipids from surfaces of triglyceride-rich lipoproteins (Fig. 6). Both normal pseudomicellar HDL of plasma and the abnormal pseudomicellar HDL_c therefore may represent largely end products of this process, carrying their cargo of cholesteryl esters back to the liver for excretion.

Although a number of studies have indicated that liver can take up HDL, the quantities found were always disappointingly small. In a recent experiment with isolated hepatocytes, the uptake of cholesteryl esters from HDL suggested a calculated in vivo half-life of only 30 min (4) in sharp contrast to the in vivo half-life measurement for HDL apoprotein of about 10 h (31). Drevon et al. (4) proposed that an HDL particle may recirculate between the periphery and liver, selectively giving up cholesteryl esters many times to the liver, prior to complete degradation. Alternatively, the bulk of the cholesteryl esters generated by LCAT may be transferred, in association with ARP, to remnants during their formation from triglyceride-rich particles and be taken up rapidly by the liver for removal and degradation (Fig. 6) or returned to plasma in LDL (2, 13, 21, 29). Direct in vivo quantitative measurements of these several different possible pathways of cholesterol return to liver for biliary excretion now appear to be promising objectives of current and future research.

CONCLUSIONS

Evidence that the liver secretes a nascent precursor of plasma HDL that differs greatly from the final product is discussed. The nascent particle is discoidal with many physical and chemical properties best described as phospholipid bilayer like a cell membrane. This structure requires the presence of detergentlike molecules to seal the edge from water. Arginine-rich apoprotein appears to have this structural role. The discoidal HDL occur because of the absence or reduced activity of the enzyme lecithin:cholesterol acyltransferase. Discoidal HDL are the best substrates for LCAT in vitro compared with all other plasma lipoproteins. The data suggest a molecular model whereby discoidal particles comprised of bilayer lipids become transformed into typical pseudomicellar HDL of plasma by the synthesis of core cholesteryl esters produced by the LCAT reaction. It is proposed that the structural properties of the nascent HDL may facilitate the scavenging of excess cholesterol from the membranes of extrahepatic tissues, providing a return transport system to liver for cholesterol deposited in the periphery through the LDL-receptor pathway.

The author's personal research was supported by the Public Health Service (SCOR Grant HL-14237). The following coinvestigators contributed much to the personal research described: M. N. Berry, M. Fainaru, T. E. Felker, C. J. Fielding, P. E. Fielding, R. J. Havel, and in particular M. C. Williams, whose helpful criticism of this manuscript is greatly appreciated.

REFERENCES

1. AKANUMA, Y., AND J. GLOMSET. In vitro incorporation of cholesterol-^{14}C into very low density lipoprotein cholesteryl esters. J. Lipid Res. 9: 620–626, 1968.
2. BARTER, P. J., AND W. E. CONNER. The transport of esterified cholesterol in plasma high density lipoproteins of human subjects: a mathematical model. J. Lab. Clin. Med. 88: 627–639, 1976.
3. BERSOT, T. P., AND R. W. MAHLEY. Interaction of swine lipoproteins with the low density lipoprotein receptor in human fibroblasts. J. Biol. Chem. 251: 2395–2398, 1976.
4. DREVON, C. A., T. BERG, AND K. R. NORUM. Uptake and degradation of cholesterol ester-labelled rat plasma lipoproteins in purified rat hepatocytes and nonparenchymal liver cells. Biochim. Biophys. Acta 487: 122–316, 1977.
5. FAINARU, M., T. E. FELKER, R. L. HAMILTON, AND R. J. HAVEL. Evidence that a separate particle containing β-apoprotein is present in high density lipoproteins

from perfused rat liver. Metabolism 26: 999–1004, 1977.
6. FAINARU, M., R. J. HAVEL, AND T. E. FELKER. Radioimmunoassay of lipoprotein apoprotein A-I of rat serum. Biochim. Biophys. Acta 446: 56–58, 1976.
7. FAINARU, M., R. J. HAVEL, AND K. IMAIZUMI. Radioimmunoassay of arginine-rich apolipoprotein of rat serum. Biochim. Biophys. Acta 490: 144–155, 1977.
8. FELKER, T., M. FAINARU, R. L. HAMILTON, AND R. J. HAVEL. Secretion of the arginine-rich and A-I apolipoproteins by the isolated perfused rat liver. J. Lipid Res. 18: 465–473, 1977.
9. FIELDING, C. J., AND P. E. FIELDING. Purification and substrate specificity of lecithin-cholesterol acyltransferase from human plasma. Fed. European Biochem. Soc. Letters 15: 355–358, 1971.
10. FIELDING, C. J., V. G. SHORE, AND P. E. FIELDING. A protein cofactor of lecithin:cholesterol acyltransferase. Biochem. Biophys. Res. Commun. 46: 1493–1498, 1972.
11. FIELDING, C. J., V. G. SHORE, AND P. E. FIELDING.

Lecithin:cholesterol acyltransferase: effects of substrate composition upon enzyme activity. *Biochim. Biophys. Acta* 270: 513-518, 1972.

12. FORTE, T., K. R. NORUM, J. A. GLOMSET, AND A. V. NICHOLS. Plasma lipoproteins in familial lecithin:cholesterol acyltransferase deficiency: structure of low and high density lipoproteins as revealed by electron microscopy. *J. Clin. Invest.* 50: 1141-1148, 1971.

13. GLOMSET, J. A., AND K. R. NORUM. The metabolic role of lecithin:cholesterol acyltransferase: perspectives from pathology. *Advan. Lipid Res.* 11: 1-65, 1973.

14. GLOMSET, J. A., K. R. NORUM, AND W. KING. Plasma lipoproteins in familial lecithin:cholesterol acyltransferase deficiency: lipid composition and reactivity in vitro. *J. Clin. Invest.* 49: 1827-1837, 1970.

15. HAMILTON, R. L. Synthesis and secretion of plasma lipoproteins. Pharmacological control of lipid metabolism. *Advan. Exptl. Med. Biol.* 26: 7-24, 1972.

16. HAMILTON, R. L., M. N. BERRY, M. C. WILLIAMS, AND E. M. SEVERINGHAUS. A simple and inexpensive membrane "lung" for small organ perfusion. *J. Lipid Res.* 15: 182-186, 1974.

17. HAMILTON, R. L., R. J. HAVEL, J. P. KANE, A. E. BLAUROCK, AND T. SATA. Cholestasis: lamellar structure of the abnormal human serum lipoprotein. *Science* 172: 475-478, 1971.

18. HAMILTON, R. L., R. J. HAVEL, AND M. C. WILLIAMS. Lipid bilayer structure of plasma lipoproteins in cholestasis (abstr.). *Federation Proc.* 33: 351, 1974.

19. HAMILTON, R. L., AND H. J. KAYDEN. The liver and the formation of normal and abnormal plasma lipoproteins. In: *The Liver: Normal and Abnormal Functions,* edited by F. F. Becker. New York: Dekker, 1974, part A, p. 531-572.

20. HAMILTON, R. L., M. C. WILLIAMS, C. J. FIELDING, AND R. J. HAVEL. Discoidal bilayer structure of nascent high density lipoproteins from perfused rat liver. *J. Clin. Invest.* 58: 667-680, 1976.

21. HAVEL, R. J. Lipoproteins and lipid transport. In: *Lipids, Lipoproteins and Drugs,* edited by D. Kritchevsky, R. Paoletti, and W. L. Holmes. New York: Plenum, 1975, p. 37-59.

22. HAVEL, R. J., AND R. L. HAMILTON. Synthesis and secretion of plasma lipoproteins and apolipoproteins. In: *Fourth International Atherosclerosis Symposium.* New York: Springer-Verlag, in press.

23. JACKSON, R. L., A. M. GOTTO, O. STEIN, AND Y. STEIN. A comparative study on the removal of cellular lipids from Landschütz ascites cells by human plasma apolipoproteins. *J. Biol. Chem.* 250: 7204-7209, 1975.

24. JACKSON, R. L., J. D. MORRISETT, AND A. M. GOTTO. Lipoprotein structure and metabolism. *Physiol. Rev.* 56: 259-316, 1976.

25. MAHLEY, R. W., T. P. BERSOT, R. I. LEVY, H. G. WINDMUELLER, AND V. S. LE QUIRE. Identity of lipoprotein apoproteins of plasma and liver Golgi apparatus in the rat (abstr.). *Federation Proc.* 29: 629, 1970.

26. MARSH, J. B. Apoproteins of the lipoproteins in a nonrecirculating perfusate of rat liver. *J. Lipid Res.* 17: 85-90, 1976.

27. MARSH, J. B. Lipoproteins in a nonrecirculating perfusate of rat liver. *J. Lipid Res.* 15: 544-550, 1974.

28. NESTRUCK, C. A., AND D. RUBINSTEIN. The synthesis of apoproteins of very low density lipoproteins isolated from the Golgi apparatus of rat liver. *Can. J. Biochem.* 54: 617-628, 1976.

29. NORUM, K. R., J. A. GLOMSET, A. V. NICHOLS, T. FORTE, J. J. ALBERS, W. C. KING, C. D. MITCHELL, K. R. APPLEGATE, E. L. GONG, V. CABANA, AND E. GJONE. Plasma lipoproteins in familial lecithin:cholesterol acyltransferase deficiency: effects of incubation with lecithin:cholesterol acyltransferase in vitro. *Scand. J. Clin. Lab. Invest. Suppl.* 142: 31-55, 1975.

30. OSUGA, T., AND O. W. PORTMAN. Origin and disappearance of plasma lecithin:cholesterol acyltransferase. *Am. J. Physiol.* 220: 735-741, 1971.

31. ROHEIM, P. S., D. RACHMILEWITZ, O. STEIN, AND Y. STEIN. Metabolism of iodinated high density lipoproteins in the rat. I. Half-life with circulation and uptake by organs. *Biochim. Biophys. Acta* 248: 315-329, 1971.

32. SABESIN, S. M., H. L. HAWKINS, L. KUIKEN, AND J. B. RAGLAND. Abnormal plasma lipoproteins and lecithin-cholesterol acyltransferase deficiency in alcoholic liver disease. *Gastroenterology* 72: 510-518, 1977.

33. SABESIN, S. M., L. B. KUIKEN, AND J. B. RAGLAND. Lipoprotein and lecithin:cholesterol acyltransferase changes in galactosamine-induced rat liver injury. *Science* 190: 1302-1304, 1975.

34. SARDET, C., H. HANSMA, AND R. OSTWALD. Characterization of guinea pig plasma lipoproteins: the appearance of new lipoproteins in response to dietary cholesterol. *J. Lipid Res.* 13: 624-639, 1972.

35. SIGGURDSSON, G., A. NICOLL, AND B. LEWIS. Conversion of very low density lipoprotein to low density lipoprotein. A metabolic study of apolipoprotein B kinetics in human subjects. *J. Clin. Invest.* 56: 1481-1490, 1975.

36. SIMON, J. B., AND J. L. BOYER. Production of lecithin:cholesterol acyltransferase by the isolated perfused rat liver. *Biochim. Biophys. Acta* 218: 549-551, 1971.

37. SMALL, D. M. In: *The Bile Acids—Chemistry, Physiology and Metabolism,* edited by P. P. Nair and D. Kritchevsky. New York: Plenum, 1971, vol. I, chapt. 8, p. 247-354.

38. STOECKENIUS, W., AND D. M. ENGELMAN. Current models for the structure of biological membranes. *J. Cell Biol.* 42: 613-646, 1969.

39. STOKKE, K. T., AND K. R. NORUM. Determination of lecithin:cholesterol acyltransferase in human blood plasma. *Scand. J. Clin. Lab. Invest.* 27: 21-27, 1971.

40. TALL, A. R., AND D. M. SMALL. Solubilization of phospholipid membranes by human plasma high density lipoproteins. *Nature* 265: 163-164, 1977.

41. TORSVIK, H., M. H. SOLAAS, AND E. GJONE. Serum lipoproteins in plasma lecithin:cholesterol acyltransferase deficiency, studied by electron microscopy. *Clin. Genet.* 1: 139-150, 1970.

42. WEINSTEIN, D. B., T. E. CAREW, AND D. STEINBERG. Uptake and degradation of low density lipoprotein by swine arterial smooth muscle cells with inhibition of cholesterol biosynthesis. *Biochim. Biophys. Acta* 424: 404-421, 1976.

43. WILKINS, M. H. F., A. E. BLAUROCK, AND D. M. ENGELMAN. Bilayer structure in membranes. *Nature New Biol.* 230: 72-76, 1971.

44. WINDMUELLER, H. G., P. N. HERBERT, AND R. I. LEVY. Biosynthesis of lymph and plasma lipoprotein apoproteins by isolated perfused rat liver and intestine. *J. Lipid Res.* 14: 215-223, 1973.

45. WINDMUELLER, H. G., AND R. I. LEVY. Total inhibition of hepatic β-lipoprotein production in the rat by orotic acid. *J. Biol. Chem.* 242: 2246-2254, 1967.

10

General Scheme for Regulation of Cholesterol Metabolism in Mammalian Cells

MICHAEL S. BROWN AND JOSEPH L. GOLDSTEIN

*Department of Internal Medicine, University of Texas
Health Science Center, Dallas, Texas*

A MAJOR ACHIEVEMENT OF BIOCHEMICAL RESEARCH over the past 30 years was the elucidation of the complex pathway by which animal cells synthesize cholesterol from acetyl coenzyme A, a metabolic intermediate that can be derived from the catabolism of carbohydrate, fat, and protein (Fig. 1). Virtually all nucleated mammalian cells have the capacity to convert acetyl-CoA into cholesterol (9), and in every cell with this capacity the rate of such cholesterol synthesis appears to be tightly regulated (1, 2, 6, 7).

The specific factors that regulate the quantitative flux of cholesterol in specific cells are diverse (discussed below), but the final mechanism for the regulation of cholesterol synthesis seems to be similar in every cell. That is, when intracellular cholesterol (or perhaps some metabolite derived from cholesterol) accumulates within the cell, the activity of the enzyme 3-hydroxy-3-methylglutaryl coenzyme A reductase (HMG-CoA reductase) is reduced. This enzyme catalyzes the reduction of the six-carbon intermediate HMG-CoA to mevalonate, a reaction that is regarded as the first step committed solely to cholesterol biosynthesis because HMG-CoA, but not mevalonate, can be used for other purposes in some tissues (28, 29). Under some conditions, other enzymes of the cholesterol biosynthetic pathway in addition to HMG-CoA reductase can be suppressed by cholesterol. For example, in the liver of rats that have been fed cholesterol, the activity of cytosolic HMG-CoA synthase rapidly becomes reduced (16), and eventually the activities of several of the later enzymes in the cholesterol biosynthetic pathway, such as those involved in the conversion of squalene to cholesterol, become suppressed. However, the changes in HMG-CoA reductase occur more quickly and are of greater amplitude than those of the other enzymes; hence, HMG-CoA reductase is still believed to be the primary rate-controlling enzyme for cholesterol biosynthesis in all tissues studied so far (28, 29).

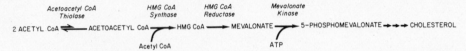

FIG. 1. Cholesterol biosynthetic pathway. HMG-CoA reductase is the major rate-controlling enzyme in the overall conversion of acetyl-CoA to cholesterol.

CHOLESTEROL HOMEOSTASIS AT THE CELLULAR LEVEL

Although the liver and intestine had long been thought to be the only tissues in which cholesterol synthesis is subject to regulation, more recent studies of a variety of cultured cells, as well as studies of excised tissues from a variety of animals, have disclosed that the above scheme for the regulation of HMG-CoA reductase appears to operate in nearly all mammalian cells (1, 2, 13, 19). In each cell, the regulatory mechanism senses the adequacy of the intracellular pool of cholesterol that is available for metabolic utilization by the cell and adjusts HMG-CoA reductase activity accordingly. For each cell the size of the metabolically active sterol pool is governed by a balance between cholesterol input and output (Fig. 2; 5, 8, 12, 13). In general, *cholesterol input* can be derived from two sources: *1*) uptake of cholesterol from circulating plasma lipoproteins or *2*) synthesis of cholesterol from acetyl-CoA within the cell. *Cholesterol output* from the metabolically active pool can also occur by two general mechanisms: *1*) utilization of cholesterol for plasma membrane synthesis during periods of cell growth and division and *2*) loss of cholesterol from the cell. The loss of cholesterol can occur in several ways: *1*) surface membrane cholesterol appears to be continuously lost by all cells through passive transfer to plasma lipoproteins (3); *2*) cholesterol is actively secreted in the form of lipoproteins by certain cells such as those of the liver and intestine; and *3*) cholesterol is converted to metabolic products such as bile acids in the liver or steroid hormones in endocrine glands.

Figure 2 summarizes the general features of cellular cholesterol balance and lists the specific input and output components for certain specialized body cells. In the steady state in each cell, the total input (i.e., the sum of *A* + *B*) must equal the total output of cholesterol (i.e., the sum of *C* + *D*). In general, if the sterol output of a cell is constant, then *A* and *B* (i.e., the rate of cholesterol input from lipoproteins and the rate of cholesterol synthesis in the cell) are related inversely. Thus, when the rate of cholesterol input from exogenous lipoproteins is high, all normal cells so far studied will suppress their cholesterol synthesis at the level of HMG-CoA reductase (13, 19). The differences among different cell types are attributable largely to two factors: *1*) the nature of the plasma lipoproteins recognized by the cell, i.e., a liver cell recognizes chylomicron remnants whereas a kidney cell recognizes low-density lipoproteins (LDL) (2); and *2*) the rate of utilization of cholesterol, i.e., the sum of processes *C* + *D* in Figure 2. For example, rapidly growing cells, such as dividing fibroblasts and lymphoblasts in tissue culture, have a larger requirement for cholesterol to support their net membrane synthesis

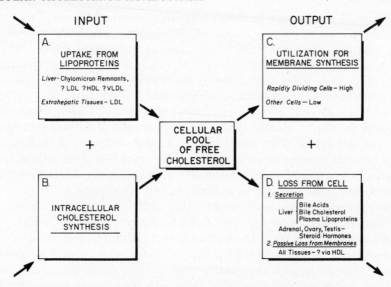

FIG. 2. Diagrammatic representation of major factors determining the content of free cholesterol in individual mammalian cells. In the steady state, the total input of cholesterol into the cellular free-cholesterol pool $(A + B)$ equals the total output of cholesterol from this pool $(C + D)$.

than do nondividing cells, such as lymphocytes circulating in the bloodstream (24). Moreover, in cells that excrete large amounts of cholesterol or steroid hormones, such as liver cells or adrenal cells, the requirement for cholesterol is dictated by the rate of such secretion. For example, hepatic cholesterol synthesis is enhanced when bile acid secretion is stimulated by the administration of the bile acid-binding resin cholestyramine (17); similarly, adrenal cholesterol synthesis is enhanced when steroid secretion is stimulated by ACTH (18, 26).

In many cells an increase in the rate of cholesterol output concomitantly evokes both an increase in the rate of cholesterol synthesis and an increase in the rate at which the cell takes up cholesterol from lipoproteins (13, 19). Thus, in cultured mouse adrenal cells (discussed below in more detail), stimulation of steroid synthesis with ACTH leads both to an enhanced rate of cholesterol synthesis and to an increase in the number of LDL receptors that transport LDL cholesterol into the cell (18). In these mouse adrenal cells, as well as in cultured human fibroblasts, lymphoblasts, and smooth muscle cells, the cells prefer to use exogenous cholesterol contained in plasma LDL rather than to synthesize their own cholesterol. Hence, when LDL are present in the culture medium, a stimulation of sterol efflux in these cells is balanced by an increase in the uptake of LDL, which in turn keeps sterol synthesis suppressed (13, 18, 19).

In addition to their content of free cholesterol, mammalian cells contain varying amounts of cholesteryl esters. These sterol esters serve to dampen transient changes in free-cholesterol content that might otherwise occur during sudden alterations in sterol flux. In general, cholesteryl esters are formed by a cell when the input of cholesterol transiently exceeds the output, and they are hydrolyzed when sterol output exceeds input. Whereas the content of cholesteryl esters in most cells is much lower than the content of free cholesterol, three specialized types of cells tend to accumulate much larger amounts of cholesteryl esters. These are: *1*) steroid hormone-secreting cells, such as adrenal cortical cells, that may have sudden demands for cholesterol to support steroid synthesis; *2*) liver cells of animal species such as the rat and rabbit after consumption of large amounts of cholesterol in the diet; and *3*) phagocytic cells and vascular smooth muscle cells of tissues that have been exposed to an abnormally high influx of plasma lipoproteins such as occurs pathologically in xanthomas and atheromas.

Cholesteryl esters are formed within cells through the action of a microsomal enzyme, fatty acyl-CoA:cholesterol acyltransferase, which transfers an activated fatty acid to the 3-hydroxyl group of cholesterol (21). On the other hand, cholesteryl esters can be hydrolyzed by several different enzymes. One of these, a nonspecific acid lipase located within lysosomes, hydrolyzes the cholesteryl esters that enter cells bound to plasma lipoproteins (20). Whether this acid lipase also functions to hydrolyze endogenously synthesized cholesteryl esters stored within the cell is not yet established. It seems likely that in certain tissues the stored cholesteryl esters may be hydrolyzed by nonlysosomal cholesterol esterases with more neutral pH optima, such as those found in both cytosolic and membrane fractions of liver (21, 27) and in the cytosolic fraction of the adrenal gland (10).

LDL-RECEPTOR PATHWAY IN MAMMALIAN CELLS

Extensive studies of cultured cells have revealed a major mechanism by which a variety of different cell types obtain cholesterol from plasma LDL (13, 19). As shown in Figure 3, the critical component of this mechanism, which has been called the LDL-receptor pathway, consists of a high-affinity receptor localized on the plasma membrane of these cells. This receptor specifically binds LDL and thereby initiates a sequence of events by which the cells take up the lipoprotein through adsorptive endocytosis, hydrolyze its protein and cholesteryl ester components within lysosomes, and release free cholesterol for use by the cell.

In the presence of a fixed output of cellular cholesterol (Fig. 2, *panels C + D*), the uptake of LDL cholesterol through the receptor pathway (Fig. 2, *panel A*) acts to suppress intracellular cholesterol synthesis (Fig. 2, *panel B*). As mentioned above, this is achieved through a suppression of the activity of HMG-CoA reductase.

Table 1 lists the different mammalian cell types in which the role of LDL receptors in the regulation of cellular cholesterol synthesis has been studied. In each cell type, the presence of LDL receptors is associated with a suppression of HMG-CoA reductase activity when the cells are grown in whole serum containing LDL and an increase in HMG-CoA reductase

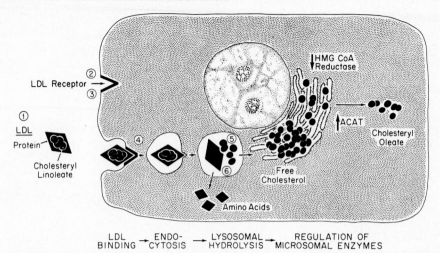

FIG. 3. Sequential steps in the LDL-receptor pathway. Numbers indicate the sites at which mutations have been identified in human cells: 1) abetalipoproteinemia; 2) familial hypercholesterolemia, receptor-negative; 3) familial hypercholesterolemia, receptor-defective; 4) familial hypercholesterolemia, internalization defect; 5) Wolman's disease; and 6) cholesteryl ester-storage disease. HMG-CoA reductase denotes 3-hydroxy-3-methylglutaryl coenzyme A reductase; ACAT denotes acyl-CoA:cholesterol acyltransferase. [Modified from Brown and Goldstein (13).]

activity when the cells are exposed to lipoprotein-deficient serum (i.e., serum from which the LDL have been removed).

The critical role of the LDL receptor in this regulatory process has been established through analysis of human cells bearing mutations in the gene encoding the LDL receptor (11, 14). Cells from subjects who exhibit the genetic disorder homozygous familial hypercholesterolemia are unable to bind LDL and hence are unable to utilize the lipoprotein to supply their cholesterol needs. As a result, when these mutant cells are in need of cholesterol for metabolic purposes, they must synthesize the sterol within the cell. Thus, when fibroblasts, lymphoblasts, and aortic smooth muscle cells from these familial hypercholesterolemia homozygotes are grown in tissue culture in the presence of whole serum containing LDL, these mutant cells, in contrast to normal cells, must maintain a high level of HMG-CoA reductase activity and a high rate of cholesterol synthesis (11, 14). In addition, when lymphocytes are freshly isolated from the bloodstream of subjects with homozygous familial hypercholesterolemia and incubated in the absence of lipoproteins, the subsequent addition of LDL fails to cause a suppression of HMG-CoA reductase activity (24).

A situation similar to that of the homozygous familial hypercholesterolemia cells has been observed in the V-79 clone of Chinese hamster cells. These V-79 cells appear to have undergone an alteration (mutation?) in cell culture that prevents the expression of the LDL receptor. As a result, these V-79 cells, like the homozygous familial hypercholesterolemia cells, must synthesize all their own cholesterol for growth and are unable to use the cholesterol contained in plasma lipoproteins (unpublished observations).

TABLE 1. *Relation between presence of LDL receptors and level of HMG-CoA reductase activity in various mammalian cell types cultured in whole serum and in lipoprotein-deficient serum*

Cell Type	Presence of LDL Receptors	HMG-CoA Reductase Activity		Ref
		Whole serum	Lipopotein-deficient serum	
Human				
Fibroblasts*	Yes	Low	High	19
Lymphoblasts*	Yes	Low	High	23, 25
Aortic smooth muscle cells*	Yes	Low	High	11
Circulating lymphocytes*	Yes	Low	High	22, 24
HeLa cells	Yes	Low	High	†
Endothelial cells	Yes	Low	High	30
Mouse				
Y-1 adrenal cells	Yes	Low	High	18
L cells	Yes	Low	High	†
Chinese hamster				
Lung fibroblasts	Yes	Low	High	†
CHO cells (ovary)	Yes	Low	High	†
V-79 cells (lung)	No	High	High	†
Swine				
Aortic smooth muscle cells	Yes	Low	High	4, 31

* Cell types in which genetic absence of LDL receptors results in a high level of HMG-CoA reductase activity when cells are cultured in whole serum.   † Unpublished observations.

REGULATION OF STEROL METABOLISM IN CULTURED ADRENAL CELLS

Recent insight into the interrelationships among sterol uptake, synthesis, and output in mammalian cells has come from studies of a line of steroid-secreting cultured mouse adrenal cells. These cells were derived from the Y-1 clone of functional mouse adrenal tumor cells that was adapted to culture by Buonassisi et al. (15). The Y-1 adrenal cells secrete large amounts of steroid hormones when exposed to ACTH (18), and this property allows the investigator to vary sterol output from the cells at will.

When these Y-1 cells are exposed to ACTH they obtain the large amounts of cholesterol needed for hormone synthesis both from an enhanced synthesis of cholesterol mediated by an increase in HMG-CoA reductase activity and from an increased uptake of plasma LDL through the LDL receptor (18). Under these conditions, the cholesterol liberated from LDL by the receptor pathway supplies more than 75% of the sterol that is converted to steroid hormones. The intracellular event that triggers these adaptive responses is a depletion of the cellular pool of free cholesterol that occurs when ACTH stimulates the cleavage of the cholesterol side chain to form steroid hormones. In the presence of aminoglutethimide, the side-chain cleavage enzymes are blocked, intracellular cholesterol is not depleted by ACTH, and cholesterol synthesis and LDL receptor activity are not enhanced (18).

SUMMARY

The understanding of cellular cholesterol homeostasis that has emerged from studies of cultured mammalian cells points the way to further studies designed to reveal the precise mechanisms by which these control mechanisms are exerted both in isolated cells and in the whole body. In addition, the elucidation of these pathways should provide further insights into the derangements that lead to clinical disorders of cholesterol metabolism in man.

REFERENCES

1. ANDERSEN, J. M., AND J. M. DIETSCHY. Regulation of sterol synthesis in 16 tissues of rat. I. Effect of diurnal light cycling, fasting, stress, manipulation of enterohepatic circulation, and administration of chylomicrons and Triton. J. Biol. Chem. 252: 3646–3651, 1977.

2. ANDERSEN, J. M., AND J. M. DIETSCHY. Regulation of sterol synthesis in 15 tissues of rat. II. Role of rat and human high and low density plasma lipoproteins and of rat chylomicron remnants. J. Biol. Chem. 252: 3652–3659, 1977.

3. ARBOGAST, L. Y., G. H. ROTHBLAT, M. H. LESLIE, AND R. A. COOPER. Cellular cholesterol ester accumulation induced by free cholesterol-rich lipid dispersions. Proc. Natl. Acad. Sci. US 73: 3680–3684, 1976.

4. ASSMANN, G., B. G. BROWN, AND R. W. MAHLEY. Regulation of 3-hydroxy-3-methylglutaryl coenzyme A reductase activity in cultured swine aortic smooth muscle cells by plasma lipoproteins. Biochemistry 14: 3996–4002, 1975.

5. BAILEY, J. M. Regulation of cell cholesterol content. In: Ciba Found. Symp. Atherogenesis: Initiating Factors. Amsterdam: Elsevier, 1973, vol. 12 (new series), p. 63–92.

6. BALASUBRAMANIAM, S., J. L. GOLDSTEIN, J. R. FAUST, AND M. S. BROWN. Evidence for regulation of 3-hydroxy-3-methylglutaryl coenzyme A reductase activity and cholesterol synthesis in nonhepatic tissues of rat. Proc. Natl. Acad. Sci. US 73: 2564–2568, 1976.

7. BALASUBRAMANIAM, S., J. L. GOLDSTEIN, J. R. FAUST, G. Y. BRUNSCHEDE, AND M. S. BROWN. Lipoprotein-mediated regulation of 3-hydroxy-3-methylglutaryl coenzyme A reductase activity and cholesteryl ester metabolism in the adrenal gland of the rat. J. Biol. Chem. 252: 1771–1779, 1977.

8. BATES, S. R., AND G. H. ROTHBLAT. Regulation of cellular sterol flux and synthesis by human serum lipoproteins. Biochim. Biophys. Acta 360: 38–55, 1974.

9. BLOCH, K. The biological synthesis of cholesterol. Science 150: 19–28, 1965.

10. BOYD, G. S., AND W. H. TRZECIAK. Cholesterol metabolism in the adrenal cortex: studies on the mode of action of ACTH. Ann. N.Y. Acad. Sci. 212: 361–377, 1973.

11. BROWN, M. S., R. G. W. ANDERSON, AND J. L.

GOLDSTEIN. Mutations affecting the binding, internalization, and lysosomal hydrolysis of low density lipoprotein in cultured human fibroblasts, lymphocytes, and aortic smooth muscle cells. J. Supramol. Struct. 6: 85–94, 1977.

12. BROWN, M. S., J. R. FAUST, AND J. L. GOLDSTEIN. Role of the low density lipoprotein receptor in regulating the content of free and esterified cholesterol in human fibroblasts. J. Clin. Invest. 55: 783–793, 1975.

13. BROWN, M. S., AND J. L. GOLDSTEIN. Receptor-mediated control of cholesterol metabolism. Science 191: 150–154, 1976.

14. BROWN, M. S., AND J. L. GOLDSTEIN. Familial hypercholesterolemia: a genetic defect in the low-density lipoprotein receptor. New Engl. J. Med. 294: 1386–1390, 1976.

15. BUONASSISI, V., G. SATO, AND A. I. COHEN. Hormone-producing cultures of adrenal and pituitary tumor origin. Proc. Natl. Acad. Sci. US 48: 1184–1190, 1962.

16. CLINKENBEARD, K. D., T. SUGIYAMA, W. D. REED, AND M. D. LANE. Cytoplasmic 3-hydroxy-3-methylglutaryl coenzyme A synthase from liver. J. Biol. Chem. 250: 3124–3135, 1975.

17. DANIELSSON, H., AND J. SJÖVALL. Bile acid metabolism. Ann. Rev. Biochem. 44: 233–253, 1975.

18. FAUST, J. R., J. L. GOLDSTEIN, AND M. S. BROWN. Receptor-mediated uptake of low density lipoprotein and utilization of its cholesterol for steroid synthesis in cultured mouse adrenal cells. J. Biol. Chem. 252: 4861–4871, 1977.

19. GOLDSTEIN, J. L., AND M. S. BROWN. The LDL pathway in human fibroblasts: a receptor-mediated mechanism for the regulation of cholesterol metabolism. Current Topics Cellular Regulation 11: 147–181, 1976.

20. GOLDSTEIN, J. L., S. E. DANA, J. R. FAUST, A. L. BEAUDET, AND M. S. BROWN. Role of lysosomal acid lipase in the metabolism of plasma low density lipoprotein: observations in cultured fibroblasts from a patient with cholesteryl ester storage disease. J. Biol. Chem. 250: 8487–8495, 1975.

21. GOODMAN, DeW. S. Cholesterol ester metabolism. Physiol. Rev. 45: 747–839, 1965.

22. HO, Y. K., M. S. BROWN, D. W. BILHEIMER, AND J. L. GOLDSTEIN. Regulation of low density lipoprotein

receptor activity in freshly isolated human lymphocytes. *J. Clin. Invest.* 58: 1465–1474, 1976.

23. HO, Y. K., M. S. BROWN, H. J. KAYDEN, AND J. L. GOLDSTEIN. Binding, internalization, and hydrolysis of low density lipoprotein in long-term lymphoid cell lines from a normal subject and a patient with homozygous familial hypercholesterolemia. *J. Exptl. Med.* 144: 444–455, 1976.

24. HO, Y. K., J. R. FAUST, D. W. BILHEIMER, M. S. BROWN, AND J. L. GOLDSTEIN. Regulation of cholesterol synthesis by low density lipoprotein in isolated human lymphocytes. *J. Exptl. Med.* 5: 1531–1549, 1977.

25. KAYDEN, H. J., L. HATAM, AND N. G. BERATIS. Regulation of 3-hydroxy-3-methylglutaryl coenzyme A reductase activity and the esterification of cholesterol in human long term lymphoid cell lines. *Biochemistry* 15: 521–528, 1976.

26. KOWAL, J. ACTH and the metabolism of adrenal cell cultures. *Recent Progr. Hormone Res.* 26: 623–676, 1970.

27. RIDDLE, M. C., E. D. SMUCKLER, AND J. A. GLOMSET. Cholesteryl ester hydrolytic activity of rat liver plasma membrane. *Biochim. Biophys. Acta* 388: 339–348, 1975.

28. RODWELL, V. W., J. L. NORDSTROM, AND J. J. MITSCHELEN. Regulation of HMG CoA reductase. *Advan. Lipid Res.* 14: 1–74, 1976.

29. SIPERSTEIN, M. D. Regulation of cholesterol biosynthesis in normal and malignant tissues. *Current Topics Cellular Regulation* 2: 65–100, 1970.

30. STEIN, O., AND Y. STEIN. High density lipoproteins reduce the uptake of low density lipoproteins by human endothelial cells in culture. *Biochim. Biophys. Acta* 431: 363–368, 1976.

31. WEINSTEIN, D. B., T. E. CAREW, AND D. STEINBERG. Uptake and degradation of low density lipoprotein by swine arterial smooth muscle cells with inhibition of cholesterol biosynthesis. *Biochim. Biophys. Acta* 424: 404–421, 1976.

11

Alterations in Plasma Lipoproteins Induced by Cholesterol Feeding in Animals Including Man

ROBERT W. MAHLEY

*Comparative Atherosclerosis and Arterial Metabolism Section, Laboratory
of Experimental Atherosclerosis, National Heart, Lung, and
Blood Institute, Bethesda, Maryland*

Canine and Rat Plasma Lipoproteins
Swine and Patas Monkey Plasma Lipoproteins
Characteristics of Cholesterol-Induced Hyperlipoproteinemia
Cholesterol Feeding in Man
Conclusions

THE ALARMINGLY HIGH INCIDENCE of coronary artery disease and atherosclerosis in the Western World has been directly correlated with plasma cholesterol levels. Among other facets of our style of living, our diet, particularly rich in calories and high in fat, has been strongly implicated as a causative factor [for review see Keys (10)]. The observation that plasma cholesterol levels in man can be changed by manipulation of polyunsaturated and saturated fats, as well as cholesterol, in the diet prompted us to embark on an investigation into the comparative responses of several animal species to high-fat, high-cholesterol diets. Included in these studies were dog, miniature swine, rat, *Erythrocebus patas* monkey, and man.

For the lower species, the design was to feed diets high in fat and cholesterol to determine the dietary and metabolic conditions necessary to induce a hypercholesterolemia sufficient to produce accelerated atherosclerosis in a reasonable period of time (6 mo to 2 yr). The plasma lipoproteins of each species were characterized, and the changes in the lipoproteins produced by the diets were correlated with the extent of atherosclerosis. Two factors that may influence susceptibility to atherosclerosis are the types of lipoproteins produced in response to an atherogenic diet and inherent differences in arterial wall metabolism. The latter has been implicated (17, 33) but not extensively studied in the different species. This chapter is intended to demonstrate that, although the plasma cholesterol level that produces accelerated atherosclerosis varies among species, there are certain consistent, diet-induced alterations in the plasma lipoproteins in both atherosclerosis-susceptible (pig and monkey) and atherosclerosis-resistant (dog and rat) species. In addition, recent studies indicate that similar changes occur in the lipoproteins of man on high-cholesterol diets.

181

CANINE AND RAT PLASMA LIPOPROTEINS

The major plasma lipoproteins of the atherosclerosis-resistant dog and rat are the high-density lipoproteins (HDL; $d > 1.06$), which normally carry approximately 75% of the plasma cholesterol. In the dog and rat the plasma cholesterol level is ~80 mg/100 ml. The main HDL of dog and rat (referred to as HDL_2) have α_1-mobility on paper electrophoresis (Fig. 1) and are similar to the typical HDL of man with respect to chemical composition, size (Table 1), and apoprotein content (Fig. 2). One difference is that rat

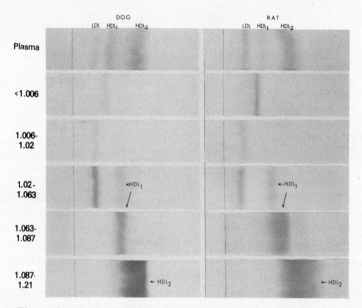

FIG. 1. Electrophoretograms of lipoproteins in ultracentrifugal density fractions from a dog and rat on commercial control chow.

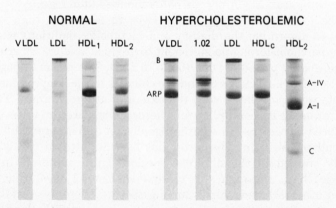

FIG. 2. Sodium dodecyl sulfate-polyacrylamide (10%) gel electrophoresis of apolipoproteins of control and cholesterol-fed rats. Apoprotein nomenclature is based on the characterization of the apoproteins previously reported (14, 30, 34).

TABLE 1. *Percent composition and size of canine and rat lipoproteins*

	Control Diet							
	Dog*				Rat†			
	VLDL	LDL	HDL$_1$	HDL$_2$	VLDL	LDL	HDL$_1$	HDL$_2$
Triglyceride	58.8	29.4	2.2	0.6	70.5	15.0	4.0	0.2
Total cholesterol	15.0	22.1	34.6	20.4	11.0	37.7	39.9	23.9
Phospholipid	16.3	24.8	40.6	36.4	12.5	21.8	26.0	32.0
Protein	9.8	23.6	22.6	42.6	6.1	25.5	30.1	43.9
Size, Å	260–900	160–250	120–350	60–90	300–700	180–250	140–250	80–120
	Cholesterol Fed							
	Dog				Rat			
	B-VLDL	LDL	HDL$_c$	HDL$_2$	B-VLDL	LDL	HDL$_c$	HDL$_2$
Triglyceride	40.1	8.3	0.9	1.2	14.3	0.8	1.0	0.1
Total cholesterol	35.0	43.8	51.5	21.0	58.0	57.8	42.8	28.1
Phospholipid	18.2	26.3	32.0	36.3	22.2	25.3	41.4	28.2
Protein	6.7	21.6	15.6	41.5	5.2	16.1	15.1	43.7
Size, Å	220–600	160–300	120–340	70–90	350–700	180–350	125–325	80–120

* Lipoproteins were obtained from the following ultracentrifugal fractions: VLDL or B-VLDL ($d < 1.006$), LDL, HDL$_1$ or HDL$_c$ (1.02–1.063), and HDL$_2$ (1.10–1.21). Cholesterol-fed dogs were surgically thyroidectomized and fed a diet containing 16% beef tallow, 1–3% cholesterol, and 0.75% taurocholate. In addition, they received 500 mg of propylthiouracil/day by capsule. The plasma cholesterol of the cholesterol-fed dog was 1120 mg/100 ml.   † Lipoproteins were obtained from the following ultracentrifugal fractions: VLDL or B-VLDL ($d < 1.006$), LDL, HDL$_1$ or HDL$_c$ (1.02–1.08), and HDL$_2$ (1.08–1.21). Cholesterol-fed rats were maintained on control chow plus 5% lard, 1% cholesterol, 0.3% taurocholate, and 0.1% propylthiouracil. The plasma cholesterol was 600 mg/100 ml.

HDL$_2$ normally contain the arginine-rich apoprotein (ARP), whereas the HDL of the other species studied, including man, contain very little (<2%) ARP.

In addition to the α_1-migrating HDL$_2$, the dog and rat have another HDL-like lipoprotein (referred to as HDL$_1$), which has a slower electrophoretic mobility (α_2) and extends to lower densities ($d = 1.03$–1.08) (Fig. 1). Both HDL$_1$ and HDL$_2$ have been classed as high-density lipoproteins because they lack the B apoprotein and contain the A-I apoprotein (20). The HDL$_1$ also contain the ARP; in the rat the ARP is the major protein constituent of HDL$_1$ (Fig. 2; 13, 34). In addition to HDL$_1$ and HDL$_2$, the dog and rat have lipoproteins equivalent to the very-low density lipoproteins (VLDL) and low-density lipoproteins (LDL) (14, 20, 34).

Neither the dog nor rat develops atherosclerosis naturally, and both species are resistant even to hypercholesterolemia. In the dog, for instance, a plasma cholesterol level in excess of 750 mg/100 ml must be maintained for more than 6 mo before significant atherosclerosis is observed (21). To accomplish this, the dog must be rendered hypothyroid and fed a diet containing 1–3% cholesterol, 15–20% fat, and 0.75% taurocholic acid (5, 18, 21). Alternatively, hypercholesterolemia can be induced in euthyroid dogs by feeding a semisynthetic diet containing 16% hydrogenated coconut oil as the only fat and 5% cholesterol (17, 25). The main characteristics of the hyperlipoproteinemia induced by both of these dietary protocols are essentially identical (17, 21). The rat, in response to a diet containing 5% lard, 1% cholesterol, 0.35% taurocholic acid, and 0.1% propylthiouracil, attains plasma cholesterol levels of 400–600 mg/100 ml (14). Plasma lipoprotein changes similar to those seen in dogs can then be observed. Cholesterol feeding alone in either the dog or rat results in only a minimal increase in the plasma cholesterol.

The alterations in canine plasma lipoproteins after cholesterol feeding (with either dietary protocol) can be seen by a comparison of electrophoretograms of the plasma lipoproteins (Fig. 3). The electrophoretic pattern of control dog plasma lipoproteins is contrasted with patterns obtained for plasma of four different hypercholesterolemic dogs with increasing plasma cholesterol levels. In control animals the lipoproteins seen are LDL, HDL_1, and HDL_2 (VLDL are in too low a concentration to be seen). Initially, as the plasma cholesterol increases, the cholesterol is carried principally by α_2-lipoproteins similar to HDL_1. We have called these cholesterol-rich lipoproteins HDL_c to indicate by the subscript c that they are cholesterol induced and to distinguish them from control HDL_1 (17, 21). Presumably, HDL_c represent an increased concentration of HDL_1. The HDL_c concentration increases with further increases in plasma cholesterol. Moreover, as the plasma cholesterol increases, there is an elevation of the LDL. For the plasma of dogs that develop significant atherosclerosis (those with cholesterol levels greater than 750 mg/100 ml; bottom two patterns in Fig. 3) the electrophoresis pattern is more complicated in that there is a broad β, pre-β band that corresponds to the presence of B-VLDL and LDL. There is also a prominent HDL_c band and a markedly reduced HDL_2 band. Similar changes in the lipoprotein pattern occur in the rat (12, 14).

As suggested by electrophoresis of the whole plasma, there are marked

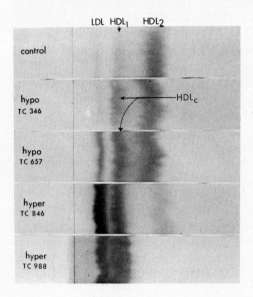

FIG. 3. Electrophoretograms of plasma lipoproteins from a dog on commercial control chow compared with dogs on the atherogenic diet (lard, cholesterol, taurocholate). Level of plasma cholesterol is indicated on each strip. [From Mahley et al. (21).]

changes in the distribution of the various lipoprotein classes after cholesterol feeding. To study these changes the lipoprotein classes were isolated by preparative ultracentrifugation (Fig. 4) and subjected to Geon-Pevikon block electrophoresis when a fraction contained more than one lipoprotein class (19). The preparative electrophoretic procedure has been particularly helpful in separating β-migrating LDL and α_2-migrating HDL$_c$, which overlap in particle size and cannot be separated by chromatographic techniques (21, 24).

In the $d < 1.006$ fraction of control dogs only pre-β-migrating VLDL occur. However, after cholesterol feeding, there is the appearance of β-migrating lipoproteins referred to as B-VLDL (Fig. 4). The B-VLDL of cholesterol-fed dogs are similar to the B-VLDL described in patients with type 3 hyperlipoproteinemia (8) and are composed of 40% triglyceride and 35% cholesterol (Table 1). However, the cholesterol content of the B-VLDL increases with increasing concentrations of plasma cholesterol. In addition to the appearance of B-VLDL, the $d = 1.006$–1.02 intermediate lipoproteins are increased (Fig. 4) and are also rich in cholesterol (Table 1). Other changes that can be appreciated in Figure 4 include an increase in the LDL and the occurrence of HDL$_c$. The LDL and HDL$_c$ are both rich in cholesterol (~70% of the cholesterol is esterified; Table 1) and yet they are quite different lipoproteins with respect to their apoprotein contents (see below).

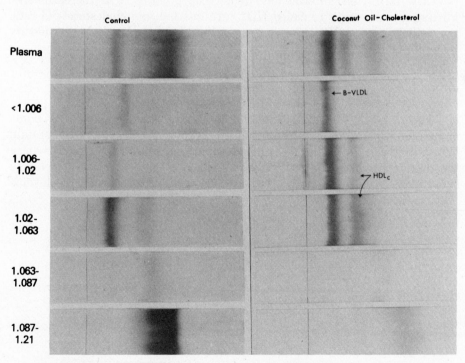

FIG. 4. Electrophoretograms of lipoproteins in ultracentrifugal density fractions from a control dog and a coconut oil-cholesterol-fed dog. [From Mahley et al. (17).]

Despite the relative and absolute decrease in HDL_2, the percent composition of the HDL_2 of control and cholesterol-fed animals is essentially unchanged. The particle sizes of the control and cholesterol-induced lipoproteins as determined by negative-staining electron microscopy are compared in Table 1.

A study of the apoprotein contents of the cholesterol-induced lipoproteins of the dog reveals that the B-VLDL contain primarily the B and arginine-rich apoproteins (Fig. 5). The presence of the ARP as a major constituent of the B-VLDL is similar to the apoprotein pattern obtained from B-VLDL of patients with type 3 hyperlipoproteinemia (8) and B-VLDL from cholesterol-fed rabbits (29). The HDL_c isolated from the various ultracentrifugal fractions lack the B apoprotein and contain the ARP as the major protein. In the cholesterol-fed dog, the HDL_c isolated from the $d = 1.006–1.02$ fraction contain the ARP as the exclusive protein constituent (17). At higher densities, the HDL_c contain both the ARP and A-I apoproteins. The presence of the ARP as a major apoprotein is a consistent feature of the various cholesterol-induced lipoproteins (17, 21).

Similar apoprotein changes have been observed in rats (Fig. 2). The total plasma arginine-rich apoprotein content increases twofold after cholesterol feeding in rats as determined by two-dimensional quantitative immunoelectrophoresis. The ARP content of the HDL_2 decreases and that of the B-VLDL, HDL_c, and intermediate-density lipoproteins (IDL) increases (14). Furthermore, when ^{125}I-labeled HDL_2 are injected into cholesterol-fed rats, the radiolabeled ARP redistributes to the cholesterol-rich lower density lipoproteins (34).

SWINE AND PATAS MONKEY PLASMA LIPOPROTEINS

The atherosclerosis-susceptible miniature swine and *Erythrocebus patas* monkey develop atherosclerosis naturally with age and have a lipoprotein distribution similar to that of man, with LDL being more prominent than in the dog or rat carrying 50–60% of the total plasma cholesterol (plasma cholesterol ~100 mg/100 ml). Both the swine and patas monkeys develop

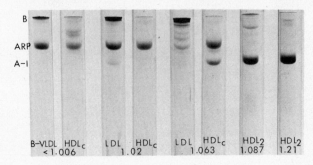

FIG. 5. Sodium dodecyl sulfate-polyacrylamide gel electrophoresis of apolipoproteins of a coconut oil-cholesterol-fed dog. [From Mahley et al. (17).]

hypercholesterolemia at a cholesterol level of 300–500 mg/100 ml by consuming a cholesterol-rich diet, and both develop significantly accelerated atherosclerosis within 8 mo to 2 yr.

Control swine have lipoproteins equivalent to human VLDL, LDL, and HDL (Fig. 6). Use of the control diet plus 15% lard and 1% cholesterol causes hypercholesterolemia and marked alterations in the plasma lipoproteins similar to the changes described in the dog and rat (24); B-VLDL appear along with VLDL in the $d < 1.006$ fraction (Fig. 6), IDL and LDL increase, and HDL$_c$ appear. The concentration of HDL$_c$ increases progressively with an increased plasma cholesterol level. As in the dog, the B-VLDL, LDL, and HDL$_c$ are rich in cholesterol esters and the arginine-rich apoprotein becomes a major protein constituent (24).

Erythrocebus patas is an Old World monkey that appears to represent a very useful nonhuman primate model for the study of lipoprotein metabolism and atherosclerosis (22, 23). The lipoproteins of this monkey on a control diet include VLDL, LDL, and HDL. In addition, patas monkeys have α_2-migrating lipoproteins that appear to be equivalent to human Lp(a) (23). The addition of 0.5% cholesterol to the control diet causes hypercholesterolemia and altered lipoprotein distribution. The B-VLDL are seen, and there is an increase in the IDL and LDL. The α_2-lipoproteins are altered in that they become richer in cholesterol and the ARP becomes a major protein constituent (22). However, unlike HDL$_c$ of the lower species, this lipoprotein does contain the B apoprotein. Because of the occurrence of Lp(a) in the monkey, it may be difficult to separate the B-containing lipoproteins from the HDL$_c$ equivalent, and clarification of this point must await better separation techniques.

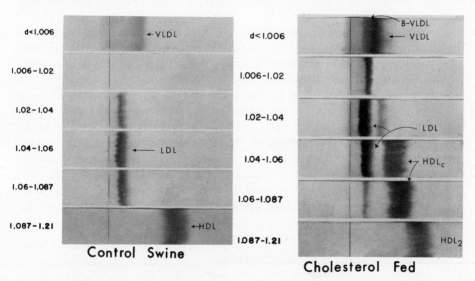

FIG. 6. Electrophoretograms of lipoproteins of miniature swine on a control diet and a high-fat, high-cholesterol diet. [From Mahley et al. (24).]

CHARACTERISTICS OF CHOLESTEROL-INDUCED HYPERLIPOPROTEINEMIA

The five major changes in the lipoproteins consistently observed after cholesterol feeding are listed in Table 2. The apoproteins of the cholesterol-rich B-VLDL induced by cholesterol feeding are compared with those of the B-VLDL of a patient with type 3 hyperlipoproteinemia in Figure 7. The B-VLDL are defined as β-migrating lipoproteins that float at $d < 1.006$ by preparative ultracentrifugation. Recently, data have been presented indicating that inclusion of 750–1500 mg of cholesterol/day in the diet of man resulted in the appearance of B-VLDL in 7 of 10 patients in which the plasma cholesterol increased (26).

Several possible origins for cholesterol-induced B-VLDL can be postulated. They may be synthesized directly by the intestine in response to cholesterol feeding. However, when we examine thoracic duct lymph from cholesterol-fed dogs, only large, triglyceride-rich particles are present at $d < 1.006$. Synthesis by the liver is a second possible origin for B-VLDL, and liver has been suggested as the source of the B-VLDL of the cholesterol-fed rabbit (27, 29). A third alternative, that B-VLDL and IDL are remnants of cholesterol-induced intestinal or liver lipoproteins, is strongly supported by the work of Ross and Zilversmit (28). Their data clearly substantiate the chylomicron-remnant hypothesis and furthermore indicate that nearly two-thirds of the esterified cholesterol in the rabbit $d < 1.006$ fraction is of dietary origin. Moreover, there appears to be a defect in the removal of chylomicron remnants from the plasma of cholesterol-fed rabbit (28). Therefore, the B-VLDL and IDL of cholesterol-fed animals may represent products of catabolism formed by the action of triglyceride lipases on lipoproteins of intestinal origin. To delve further into this hypothesis, we have attempted to determine whether changes in triglyceride lipase activity accompany cholesterol feeding.

After intravenous heparin injection, it is possible to measure in plasma the activities of two different triglyceride lipases: lipoprotein lipase, released from peripheral tissues, and hepatic lipase. Their activities can be measured separately with protamine sulfate used to inhibit selectively the peripheral enzyme activity as described by Krauss et al. (11). Postheparin lipolytic activities of euthyroid dogs on control diet, surgically thyroidectomized (hypothyroid) dogs on control diet, and hypothyroid dogs on the atherogenic (cholesterol-rich) diet are compared in Table 3. Hypothyroidism causes a significant increase in the peripheral lipase activity; after cholesterol feeding this activity remains elevated compared with that of control dogs. The hepatic lipase activity is unaffected by hypothyroidism but is decreased significantly after cholesterol feeding. Moreover, when the hepatic triglycer-

TABLE 2. *Characteristics of cholesterol-induced hyperlipoproteinemia*

1) Occurrence of B-VLDL
2) Increase in IDL ($d = 1.006–1.02$)
3) Increase in LDL
4) Occurrence of HDL$_c$
5) Decrease in typical HDL (HDL$_2$)

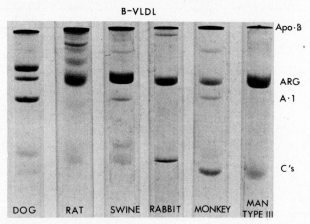

FIG. 7. Sodium dodecyl sulfate-polyacrylamide gel electrophoresis of β-migrating B-VLDL isolated from the $d < 1.006$ fraction of cholesterol-fed animals and a patient with type 3 hyperlipoproteinemia. [From Mahley et al. (22).]

TABLE 3. *Postheparin triglyceride lipase activities in dogs*

	No. of Dogs	Free Fatty Acids, μmol/ml plasma per h		
		Total	Hepatic	Peripheral
Control diet	24	24.1 ± 6	18.2 ± 5	6.0 ± 3
Hypothyroid controls	10	33.2 ± 8	19.5 ± 5	13.8 ± 5
Atherogenic diet	23	21.0 ± 5	9.9 ± 4	11.1 ± 4

Values are means ± SD. The dogs (NIH foxhounds) had been on the control or atherogenic diet (18) for 2 yr at the time the lipase assay was performed. Heparin (100 U/kg body wt) was injected intravenously and postheparin samples were obtained 10 min later.

ide lipase activity is plotted against the plasma cholesterol levels of the individual dogs at the time of the assay, there is a correlation between the decrease in enzyme activity and an increase in plasma cholesterol (Fig. 8).

The results of a short-term dietary study typify the response observed (Fig. 9). The peripheral and hepatic lipase activities were measured while the dog was on the control diet, 4 wk after thyroidectomy, and twice during the course of cholesterol feeding. The most significant change in lipolytic activity accompanying the cholesterol-induced hyperlipoproteinemia is the reduction in the hepatic lipase activity. In the dog hepatic lipase may play a role in determining the characteristics of the cholesterol-induced hyperlipoproteinemia, but this, along with clarification of the role of human hepatic lipase, awaits further studies.

In addition to the occurrence of B-VLDL and IDL, another major alteration in the lipoprotein pattern induced by cholesterol feeding is the appearance of HDL_c, which have characteristics in common with both LDL and the typical HDL (referred to as HDL_2 in the animals; Table 4) and overlap with LDL and HDL ultracentrifugal densities ($\sim d = 1.03$–1.10). As the plasma cholesterol level increases, HDL_c become richer in cholesterol esters and float at lower densities. The upper limit of $d = 1.10$ is arbitrary, and apparently HDL_c and the typical HDL form a continuum of particles.

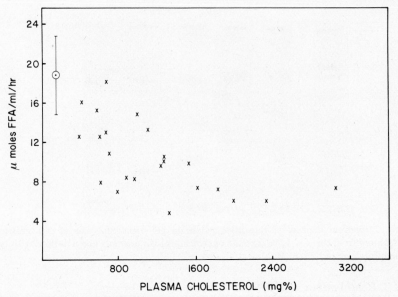

FIG. 8. Hepatic lipase activity in postheparin plasma of dogs on an atherogenic diet (described in Table 3) vs. level of plasma cholesterol. Bar (Φ) represents mean ±SD of hepatic lipase obtained for control dogs.

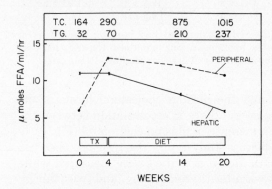

FIG. 9. Peripheral and hepatic lipase activity of a dog on control chow, 4 wk after thyroidectomy, and at 2 time points during cholesterol feeding. Plasma triglyceride and cholesterol levels (in mg/100 ml) are shown at each time point.

The HDL$_c$ particles are similar to LDL with respect to composition and size, but are strikingly dissimilar with respect to apoprotein content, since HDL$_c$ lack the B apoprotein (the major apoprotein of LDL) and contain ARP and apoA-I as major constituents. In fact, in canine HDL$_c$ ARP may be the exclusive apoprotein present (17). A comparison of the HDL$_c$ from various species is shown in Figure 10.

The HDL$_c$ can be precipitated by heparin/manganese at a concentration that precipitates LDL (15). The degree of HDL$_c$ precipitability appears to correlate with the presence of the arginine-rich apoprotein, the most readily precipitable HDL$_c$ containing the most ARP (15). Other common properties of HDL$_c$ and LDL include the ability to regulate HMG-CoA reductase activity and the ability to be bound, internalized, and degraded by fibroblasts and smooth muscle cells (Table 4; 2, 3, 15–17).

The origin of HDL$_c$ is uncertain. As suggested for B-VLDL, HDL$_c$ may represent remnants of intestinal lipoproteins. However, preliminary turn-over studies with iodinated lipoproteins have failed to support this hypothesis (unpublished observations). A second alternative is that HDL$_c$ are formed by an overloading of typical HDL (HDL$_2$) with cholesterol. This could occur by a transfer of cholesterol from cells or from other cholesterol-rich lipoproteins to the HDL, a process that may involve lecithin:cholesterol acyltransferase (LCAT) in the loading and esterification. The increased size of the HDL$_c$ compared with the 100-Å HDL could result from a fusion of HDL particles, a phenomenon observed when the apoA-I content is reduced by heat treatment of the HDL (32). It is postulated that this destabilizes the particles and they fuse. Such destabilization and fusion may occur by an overloading of the HDL with cholesterol. On the other hand, the increased size of HDL$_c$ (150–200 Å) compared with HDL may reflect the addition of cholesterol to the HDL, forming a cholesterol ester-rich core that expands the particle size. X-ray diffraction and differential scanning calorimetry indicate that swine HDL$_c$ have a layered cholesterol ester core similar to LDL (31).

TABLE 4. *Characteristics of HDL$_c$*

	HDL$_c$	LDL	HDL$_2$
Electrophoretic mobility	α_2	β	α_1
Density	1.03–1.10	1.02–1.06	1.06–1.21
Composition	CE rich	CE rich	Protein, PL
Size, Å	130–250	160–240	80–110
Apoproteins	ARP, A-I	B	A
Heparin precipitable	+	+	−
HMG-CoA regulation	+	+	−
LDL receptor binding	+	+	−

Generalizations were made in preparing this table. For precise characteristics of HDL$_c$ for each animal species, see references cited in text. CE, cholesteryl ester; PL, phospholipid.

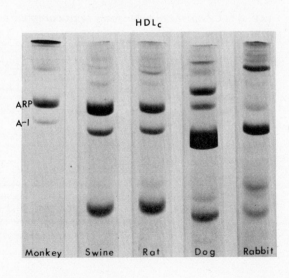

FIG. 10. Sodium dodecyl sulfate-polyacrylamide gel electrophoresis of HDL$_c$ of cholesterol-fed animals.

There are two lines of evidence suggesting that HDL (HDL$_2$) are involved in the formation of cholesterol-rich HDL$_c$. When 100-Å HDL are incubated with erythrocytes from a cholesterol-fed dog plus LCAT and lipoprotein-deficient serum, the HDL increase in size (150–300 Å) and exhibit a decreased electrophoretic (α_2) mobility (Fig. 11; unpublished observations). The second observation that supports the HDL-HDL$_c$ hypothesis is derived from a comparison of the cholesterol ester fatty acid composition of the lipoproteins from cholesterol-fed swine (Table 5). The fatty acid compositions of the cholesterol esters are very similar for HDL$_c$ and HDL$_2$ and are different from those of VLDL, IDL, and LDL. The fatty acid contents of VLDL, IDL, and LDL are similar. The high linoleate content of HDL$_c$ and HDL$_2$ may reflect a common origin from nascent HDL secondary to LCAT activity [for review see Glomset and Norum (6)]. The high oleate content of VLDL and LDL may reflect intestinal or hepatic cholesterol ester synthetic activity, since the principal fatty acid ester of cholesterol synthesized by the intestine and liver of the lower species has been demonstrated to be oleic acid [for review see Goodman (7)].

An important common characteristic of HDL$_c$ and LDL is the ability to

$$\text{HDL}\frac{\text{LCAT}}{\text{Cholesterol}} > \text{HDL}_c$$

HDL + RBCs + LCAT + Lp-deficient sera ($d > 1.21$)
Increased particle size
Decreased mobility

FIG. 11. High-density lipoproteins ($d = 1.10$–1.21; 1 ml) at a concentration of 20 mg/ml were incubated with 5 ml packed red blood cells (RBCs) plus 2.5 ml of lipoprotein-deficient sera for 14 h at 35°C. The RBCs were from a hypothyroid dog fed the fat and cholesterol diet (plasma cholesterol ~ 1000 mg/100 ml). The LCAT was isolated from normal dog plasma by the technique of Ho and Nichols (9). Activity was concentrated approximately 100-fold compared with the original plasma activity. After incubation, HDL were reisolated by ultracentrifugation.

TABLE 5. *Cholesterol ester fatty acid composition of lipoproteins from cholesterol-fed swine*

	Percent of Total Fatty Acids				
	$d < 1.006$	IDL	LDL	HDL$_c$	HDL$_2$
16:0	8.4	8.1	9.7	15.9	15.2
18:0	7.3	5.5	5.0	1.3	1.1
18:1	59.7	56.0	44.0	25.8	25.0
18:2	17.0	22.5	29.5	48.9	51.1

Percent composition of total fatty acids was determined by gas chromatography (only major fatty acids are listed). The LDL and HDL$_c$ were isolated by preparative electrophoresis from the ultracentrifugal fraction $d = 1.02$–1.063; HDL$_2$ were obtained by ultracentrifugation at $d = 1.10$–1.21. Diet consisted of commercial chow supplemented with 15% lard and 1% cholesterol and had been fed ~6 mo at the time of analysis.

be bound, internalized, and degraded by fibroblasts and smooth muscle cells (3, 15–17). As described by Goldstein, Brown, and co-workers (for review see 4), LDL are bound to cell surfaces through high-affinity receptor sites on fibroblasts. Originally, it appeared that the receptor might be specific for apoB. Subsequently, however, it has been shown that both canine and swine HDL_c are bound to the same cell surface receptors and yet lack the B apoprotein and contain the arginine-rich apoprotein (3, 15, 16). It has now been established that the protein is the important determinant for cell surface receptor binding and that either apoB or ARP can react with the receptor (16).

As a consequence of the binding, internalization, and degradation of LDL or HDL_c, there is an accumulation of cholesterol and cholesteryl esters in fibroblasts and smooth muscle cells in culture (17). As shown in Figure 12, B-VLDL ($d < 1.006$), LDL, two HDL_c fractions, and typical HDL from a cholesterol-fed dog were incubated with canine smooth muscle cells at a lipoprotein cholesterol concentration of 200 μg/ml, and the cellular sterol content was determined after 24 h. The apoprotein contents of the lipoproteins used in this experiment are shown in the upper panel of Figure 12. The

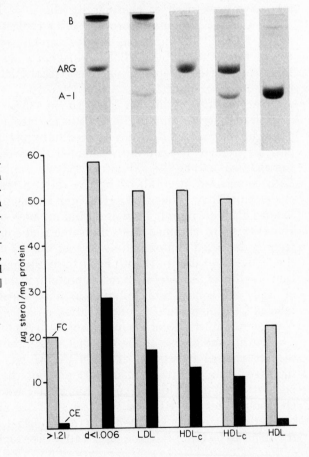

FIG. 12. Sterol accumulation by canine aortic smooth muscle cells in culture in response to 24-h incubation with lipoproteins (200 μg/ml cholesterol) from a cholesterol-fed dog. Apoprotein patterns of lipoproteins used are shown at top. FC, free cholesterol; CE, cholesteryl ester. [From Mahley et al. (17).]

basal or control contents of free and ester cholesterol in the cells were determined by incubation of the cells in lipoprotein-deficient serum ($d >$ 1.21). Use of LDL and HDL_c resulted in a similar marked increase in the cellular sterol content. However, typical HDL, which contain primarily apoA-I and neither apoB nor ARP, do not cause an increase in cellular cholesterol level.

CHOLESTEROL FEEDING IN MAN

An understanding of the types of changes induced by cholesterol feeding in both resistant and susceptible species provides a background on which to attempt to determine whether similar changes occur with cholesterol feeding in man. Recently, in collaboration with T. P. Bersot and T. L. Innerarity (manuscript in preparation), the plasma lipoproteins of young, healthy men and women were analyzed after their diets were supplemented with 4–6 eggs/day for 4 wk. Attention was focused on the high-density lipoproteins in an attempt to determine if there is an HDL_c equivalent in man. Two properties of HDL_c – cell surface receptor binding and heparin precipitability – have been used to characterize the $d = 1.095–1.21$ ultracentrifugal fraction of the patients before and after cholesterol feeding. As discussed above, HDL_c are precipitated by heparin/manganese at concentrations that do not precipitate typical HDL and compete with LDL for binding to the same cell surface receptors, whereas typical HDL are much less effectively bound to the receptor (15).

The abilities of human HDL ($d = 1.095–1.21$) to compete with ^{125}I-labeled LDL for binding to the cell surface receptor of fibroblasts before and after cholesterol feeding are compared in Figure 13 for two (A and B) of six patients studied. The concentration of HDL added to the media is plotted on the abscissa, and on the ordinate 100% represents the amount of ^{125}I-labeled LDL bound and internalized by the cells in the absence of HDL. Before cholesterol feeding (control), HDL did not significantly displace the ^{125}I-labeled LDL (5 µg/ml) from the binding sites on the fibroblasts (<10%). However, HDL obtained from the same individuals 4 wk after cholesterol feeding displaced approximately 25% of the ^{125}I-labeled LDL. Treatment of the HDL ($d = 1.095–1.21$) with heparin/manganese resulted in the precipitation of ~15% of the total lipoprotein protein, and the precipitable subfraction of HDL had considerable binding activity, displacing 45–60% of the ^{125}I-labeled LDL at a protein concentration of 200 µg/ml. The nonprecipitable fraction has much less or, as in *subject B*, no binding activity.

During the course of the egg diet, the plasma cholesterol of *subject A* did not change (remained at ~190 mg/100 ml), while that of *subject B* increased from 200 to ~250 mg/100 ml, but the HDL from both subjects behaved similarly. This suggests that after 4 wk of consumption of a high-cholesterol diet the HDL ($d = 1.095–1.21$) are altered whether or not the plasma cholesterol is elevated. The $d = 1.095–1.21$ lipoproteins have been fractionated by Geon-Pevikon preparative electrophoresis (19), and a subfraction of HDL with many of the characteristics of the HDL$_c$ of the lower species has been identified. This subfraction contains the arginine-rich apoprotein, lacks the B apoprotein (Fig. 14), and appears to account for the high-affinity binding of the HDL to the cell surface receptors. Alterations in human HDL after a high cholesterol intake have been previously noted by Mistry et al. (26), but others (1) have observed no effect.

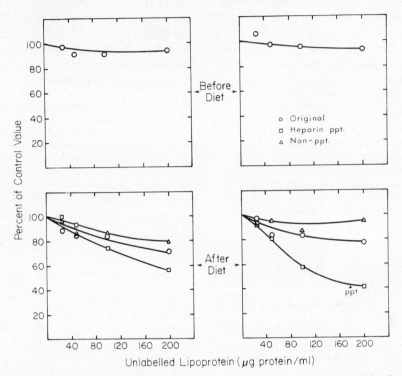

FIG. 13. Ability of an increasing concentration of HDL (d = 1.095–1.21) to displace ^{125}I-labeled LDL (5 μg/ml) from high-affinity binding sites of human fibroblasts in culture.

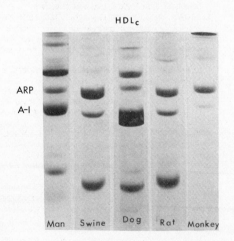

FIG. 14. Apoprotein content of HDL$_c$ isolated from the HDL fraction of a normal patient fed the high-cholesterol diet for 4 weeks compared with cholesterol-induced HDL$_c$ of the lower species.

CONCLUSIONS

Cholesterol feeding results in marked changes in the plasma lipoproteins and in alterations in lipoprotein metabolism. The B-VLDL, IDL, and LDL increased by cholesterol feeding may reflect a saturation of clearance mechanisms induced by the high cholesterol content of the diet. The HDL_c that occur with cholesterol feeding may represent HDL that are overloaded with cholesterol. The decrease in typical HDL may reflect in part this altered HDL metabolism. The cholesterol-induced HDL_c are bound to the LDL cell receptor and cause an increase in the sterol content of fibroblasts and arterial smooth muscle cells in culture. In the animal models such alterations in plasma lipoproteins are associated with accelerated atherosclerosis.

The author gratefully acknowledges the collaboration of the following co-workers who have contributed to this review: T. P. Bersot, D. L. Fry, K. S. Holcombe, T. L. Innerarity, S. Oh, R. E. Pitas, and K. H. Weisgraber. Animal colony studies were performed with members of other groups; collaborative studies were carried out 1) in dogs and miniature swine with Dr. Joseph E. Pierce, National Heart, Lung, and Blood Institute, and with Dr. Jere M. Philips, National Institute of Mental Health, and 2) in monkeys and swine with Dr. David K. Johnson, National Institutes of Health Division of Research Services, Veterinary Resources Branch. The assistance of Dr. R. M. Krauss in setting up the lipase assay and Miss C. Groff in typing the manuscript is appreciated.

REFERENCES

1. APPLEBAUM, D., J. CAIN, W. HAZZARD, J. ALBERS, M. CHEUNG, AND R. KUSHWAHA. Short-term cholesterol feeding in humans: failure to induce β-migrating very low density lipoproteins (β-VLDL). Clin. Res. 25: 158A, 1977.

2. ASSMANN, G., B. G. BROWN, AND R. W. MAHLEY. Regulation of 3-hydroxy-3-methylglutaryl coenzyme A reductase activity in cultured swine aortic smooth muscle cells by plasma lipoproteins. Biochemistry 14: 3996–4002, 1975.

3. BERSOT, T. P., R. W. MAHLEY, M. S. BROWN, AND J. L. GOLDSTEIN. Interaction of swine lipoproteins with the low density lipoprotein receptor in human fibroblasts. J. Biol. Chem. 251: 2395–2398, 1976.

4. BROWN, M. S., Y. HO, AND J. L. GOLDSTEIN. The low density lipoprotein pathway in human fibroblasts: relation between cell surface receptor binding and endocytosis of low density lipoprotein. Ann. N.Y. Acad. Sci. 275: 244–257, 1976.

5. FLAHERTY, J. T., V. J. FERRANS, J. E. PIERCE, T. E. CAREW, AND D. L. FRY. Localizing factors in experimental atherosclerosis. In: Atherosclerosis and Coronary Heart Disease, edited by W. Likoff, B. L. Segal, W. Insull, Jr., and J. H. Moyer. New York: Grune & Stratton, 1972, p. 40–83.

6. GLOMSET, J. A., AND K. R. NORUM. The metabolic role of lecithin:cholesterol acyl-transferase: perspectives from pathology. Advan. Lipid Res. 11: 1–61, 1973.

7. GOODMAN, D. S. Cholesterol ester metabolism. Physiol. Rev. 45: 747–839, 1965.

8. HAVEL, R. J., AND J. P. KANE. Primary dysbetalipoproteinemia; predominance of a specific apoprotein species in triglyceride-rich lipoproteins. Proc. Natl. Acad. Sci. US 70: 2015–2019, 1973.

9. HO, W. K. K., AND A. V. NICHOLS. Interaction of lecithin:cholesterol acyltransferase with sonicated dis-

persions of lecithin. Biochim. Biophys. Acta 231: 185–193, 1971.

10. KEYS, A. Coronary heart disease—the global picture. Atherosclerosis 22: 149–192, 1975.

11. KRAUSS, R. M., H. G. WINDMUELLER, R. I. LEVY, AND D. S. FREDRICKSON. Selective measurement of two different triglyceride lipase activities in rat posthep-arin plasma. J. Lipid Res. 14: 286–295, 1973.

12. LASSER, N. L., P. S. ROHEIM, D. EDELSTEIN, AND H. A. EDER. Serum lipoproteins of normal and cholesterol-fed rats. J. Lipid Res. 14: 1–18, 1973.

13. LUSK, L. T., L. F. WALTER, L. H. DuBIEN, AND G. S. GETZ. Characterization of a major rat lipoprotein containing predominantly arginine-rich peptide. Federation Proc. 36: 1142, 1977.

14. MAHLEY, R. W., AND K. S. HOLCOMBE. Alterations of plasma lipoproteins and apoproteins following cholesterol feeding in the rat. J. Lipid Res. 18: 314–324, 1977.

15. MAHLEY, R. W., AND T. L. INNERARITY. Interaction of canine and swine lipoproteins with the low density lipoprotein receptor of fibroblasts as correlated with heparin/manganese precipitability. J. Biol. Chem 252: 3980–3986, 1977.

16. MAHLEY, R. W., T. L. INNERARITY, R. E. PITAS, K. H. WEISGRABER, J. H. BROWN, AND E. GROSS. Inhibition of lipoprotein binding to cell surface receptors of fibroblasts following selective modification of arginyl residues in arginine-rich and B apoproteins. J. Biol. Chem. 252: 7279–7287, 1977.

17. MAHLEY, R. W., T. L. INNERARITY, K. H. WEISGRABER, AND D. L. FRY. Canine hyperlipoproteinemia and atherosclerosis: accumulation of lipid by aortic medial cells in vivo and in vitro. Am. J. Pathol. 87: 205–225, 1977.

18. MAHLEY, R. W., A. W. NELSON, V. J. FERRANS, AND D. L. FRY. Thrombosis in association with athero-

sclerosis induced by dietary perturbations in dogs. *Science* 192: 1139–1141, 1976.

19. MAHLEY, R. W., AND K. H. WEISGRABER. An electrophoretic method for the quantitative isolation of human and swine plasma lipoproteins. *Biochemistry* 13: 1964–1969, 1974.

20. MAHLEY, R. W., AND K. H. WEISGRABER. Canine lipoproteins and atherosclerosis. I. Isolation and characterization of plasma lipoproteins from control dogs. *Circulation Res.* 35: 713–721, 1974.

21. MAHLEY, R. W., K. H. WEISGRABER, AND T. L. INNERARITY. Canine lipoproteins and atherosclerosis. II. Characterization of the plasma lipoproteins associated with atherogenic and non-atherogenic hyperlipidemia. *Circulation Res.* 35: 722–733, 1974.

22. MAHLEY, R. W., K. H. WEISGRABER, AND T. L. INNERARITY. Atherogenic hyperlipoproteinemia induced by cholesterol feeding in the patas monkey. *Biochemistry* 15: 2979–2985, 1976.

23. MAHLEY, R. W., K. H. WEISGRABER, T. L. INNERARITY, AND H. B. BREWER, JR. Characterization of the plasma lipoproteins and apoproteins of the *Erythrocebus patas* monkey. *Biochemistry* 15: 1928–1933, 1976.

24. MAHLEY, R. W., K. H. WEISGRABER, T. L. INNERARITY, H. B. BREWER, JR., AND G. ASSMANN. Swine lipoproteins and atherosclerosis. Changes in the plasma lipoproteins and apoproteins induced by cholesterol feeding. *Biochemistry* 14: 2817–2823, 1975.

25. McCULLAGH, K. G., A. EHRHART, AND A. BUTKUS. Experimental canine atherosclerosis and its prevention: the dietary induction of severe coronary, cerebral, aortic, and iliac atherosclerosis and its prevention by safflower oil. *Lab. Invest.* 34: 394–405, 1976.

26. MISTRY, P., A. NICOLL, C. NIEHAUS, I. CHRISTIE, E. JANUS, AND B. LEWIS. Cholesterol feeding revisited. *Circulation* 54: II–178, 1976.

27. RODRIGUEZ, J. L., G. C. GHISELLI, D. TORREGGIANI, AND C. R. SIRTORI. Very low density lipoproteins in normal and cholesterol-fed rabbits: lipid and protein composition and metabolism. Part I. Chemical composition of very low density lipoproteins in rabbits. *Atherosclerosis* 23: 73–83, 1976.

28. ROSS, A. C., AND D. B. ZILVERSMIT. Chylomicron remnant cholesteryl esters as the major constituent of very low density lipoproteins in plasma of cholesterol-fed rabbits. *J. Lipid Res.* 18: 169–181, 1977.

29. SHORE, V. G., B. SHORE, AND R. G. HART. Changes in apolipoproteins and properties of rabbit very low density lipoproteins in induction of cholesterolemia. *Biochemistry* 13: 1579–1585, 1974.

30. SWANEY, J. B., F. BRAITHWAITE, AND H. A. EDER. Characterization of the apolipoproteins of rat plasma lipoproteins. *Biochemistry* 16: 271–278, 1977.

31. TALL, A. R., D. ATKINSON, D. M. SMALL, AND R. W. MAHLEY. Characterization of the lipoproteins of atherosclerotic swine. *J. Biol. Chem.* 252: 7288–7293, 1977.

32. TALL, A. R., AND D. M. SMALL. Solubilisation of phospholipid membranes by human plasma high density lipoproteins. *Nature* 265: 163–164, 1977.

33. WAGNER, W. D., AND T. B. CLARKSON. Genetic susceptibility to atherosclerosis at the artery level. *Federation Proc.* 38: 876, 1975.

34. WEISGRABER, K. H., R. W. MAHLEY, AND G. ASSMANN. Identification of the rat arginine-rich apoprotein and its redistribution following injection of iodinated lipoproteins into normal and hypercholesterolemic rats. *Atherosclerosis* 28: 121–140, 1977.

12

Genetic Dyslipoproteinemias

DONALD S. FREDRICKSON AND PETER N. HERBERT

National Institutes of Health, Bethesda, Maryland

Genetic Disorders Producing Hyperchylomicronemia
Genetic Disorders Elevating Plasma Very-Low-Density Lipoproteins
Genetic Disorders Producing Hyperbetalipoproteinemia
Familial Combined Hyperlipidemia
Genetic Deficiency States of the Chylomicron-VLDL-LDL System
Genetic HDL-Deficiency States
Familial Lecithin:Cholesterol Acyltransferase Deficiency
Tangier Disease
Comparison of Familial LCAT Deficiency and Tangier Disease
  High-density lipoproteins
  Chylomicron-VLDL-LDL system
  Tissue changes
Conclusion

GENETIC DISORDERS OF LIPOPROTEIN METABOLISM are first detected by changes in concentrations of cholesterol and triglycerides and are then sometimes classified more specifically according to the lipoproteins affected. The number of abnormalities at different genetic loci, however, greatly exceed the possible abnormal lipoprotein patterns; taxonomy or diagnosis is increasingly dependent on other clinical and biochemical features.

Dyslipoproteinemia (Fig. 1) can be secondary to other well-characterized diseases that only partially or quite incidentally affect plasma lipid metabolism. When such diseases are excluded, one is left with primary hyper- or hypolipoproteinemia to unravel further. The instances of primary dyslipoproteinemia that are clearly genetically determined are in the minority. For example, compared with most Asiatic Indians, most North Americans have hypercholesterolemia that is cultural – specifically dietary – in origin. Nevertheless, cultural influences must interact with constitutive, mainly genetic, factors for their expression. A considerable number of genes participate in the modulation of plasma lipid levels and their identification and modes of action present an enormous challenge to the biomedical researcher.

Genetic dyslipoproteinemia is due either to single gene defects or to polygenic determinants operating in concert with environmental influences. The single gene defects, most of them relatively rare, have been the most instructive to both physicians and biologists. Much of the information presented in this book concerning metabolic pathways, enzymes, or apolipoproteins was first suggested or confirmed through study of such human mutations. Since 1960, the number of single gene defects resulting in dyslipoproteinemia has grown from two well-established ones to 18 or more (Table 1). Among these a few common and several rare disorders of considerable heuristic value receive special attention in this chapter.

GENETIC DISORDERS PRODUCING HYPERCHYLOMICRONEMIA

Chylomicrons bear triglycerides of exogenous or dietary origin from the intestine, through the lymph to the bloodstream. A diet containing 100 g of

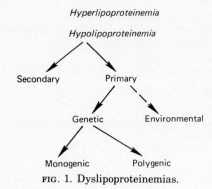

FIG. 1. Dyslipoproteinemias.

TABLE 1. *Genetic dyslipoproteinemias*

Familial hypercholesterolemia
   LDL receptor negative
   LDL receptor deficient

Familial lipoprotein lipase deficiency

Type 1 hyperlipoproteinemia without lipase deficiency

Apoprotein C-II deficiency

Familial type 3 hyperlipoproteinemia

Familial combined hyperlipidemia

Familial hypertriglyceridemia

Familial type 5 hyperlipoproteinemia

Abetalipoproteinemia
   Classical ABL
   Familial hypobetalipoproteinemia

Familial absence of HDL (Tangier disease)

Lecithin:cholesterol acyltransferase deficiency

Acid cholesteryl ester hydrolase deficiency
   Cholesteryl ester storage disease
   Wolman's disease

β-Sitosterolemia and xanthomatosis

Cerebrotendinous xanthomatosis (cholestanolosis)

fat could raise the blood triglyceride concentration several thousand milligrams per deciliter each day if chylomicron clearance were completely blocked. Normal individuals catabolize chylomicrons with great facility, however, and the biological half-life of these lipoproteins is a matter of minutes. The lipolytic dissolution of chylomicrons is catalyzed by lipoprotein lipase in the capillary walls.

Something like 100 people are known today who have no effective lipoprotein lipase activity in their capillaries due to mutation of one or more autosomal genes. This familial lipoprotein lipase deficiency (13) results in startling increases in plasma glycerides of 100-fold above normal, and the serum has the appearance of cream. The most important consequences of this are bouts of abdominal pain. Sometimes these are due to pancreatitis, which can be fatal.

Phenocopies of familial lipoprotein lipase deficiency have recently been recognized. We have studied two siblings with splenomegaly, chylomicronemia, and occasional pancreatitis since childhood. Both patients have low but detectable levels of lipoprotein lipase in their postheparin plasma. An individual has also been described (3) with fasting chylomicronemia secondary to a deficiency of apolipoprotein C-II (apoC-II), a protein required for maximal activity of lipoprotein lipase. Additional mutants with relatively pure hyperchylomicronemia probably will be recorded in the future.

Severe chylomicronemia in children usually is caused by genetic disease when obvious secondary causes such as paraproteinemia or diabetic ketoacidosis are excluded. Adult-onset hyperchylomicronemia, however, usually has its origin in disorders that elevate very-low-density lipoproteins (VLDL) first and chylomicrons only secondarily.

GENETIC DISORDERS ELEVATING PLASMA VERY-LOW-DENSITY LIPOPROTEINS

There are numerous ways in which VLDL metabolism could be affected to increase the plasma concentration of these lipoproteins, especially if one accepts evidence that in man the catabolism of VLDL is through mechanisms that normally run close to saturation. Lipoprotein lipase appears involved in the clearance of VLDL as well as chylomicrons, though the latter is the preferred substrate. When augmented synthesis or diminished catabolism leads to high plasma VLDL concentrations, VLDL may saturate clearance sites and chylomicron accumulation also ensues (7). Simple elevations of plasma VLDL therefore are expected only at triglyceride concentrations less than 400 mg/dl.

Increased VLDL levels, designated type 4 hyperlipoproteinemia in the generic classification of abnormal lipoprotein patterns (15), are a common accompaniment of many diseases. There are primary forms too, several of them due to single gene defects, and they occur in relatively high frequency in the American population. These include familial (endogenous) hypertriglyceridemia and a rarer, more severe form that seems to be a separate defect and is called familial type 5 hyperlipoproteinemia, because VLDL and chylomicrons accumulate abnormally in plasma. It can be argued that these two disorders represent varied expression of the same mutation, but we have been impressed by the concentration of severe hypertriglyceridemia in certain affected families. In both disorders, half the adult first-degree relatives have hypertriglyceridemia. An intriguing feature is the typical delay of expression of these abnormalities into late childhood or adulthood. Not clearly explained also is their common association with diabetes and hyperuricemia and the great sensitivity of triglyceride levels in those affected to the total caloric intake and alcohol.

One of the more obscure and yet quite interesting disorders in VLDL metabolism is that termed familial type 3 hyperlipoproteinemia. It represents one of few instances when chemically abnormal lipoproteins appear in the circulation. The unusual lipoprotein pattern is not always due to genetic disease. It has been seen in some diabetics during periods of severe insulin deficiency and also occasionally accompanies hypothyroidism. The majority of patients in whom it has been found, however, have a mutant genome that causes the abnormality to appear in adulthood.

In any adult who has elevated concentrations of both plasma cholesterol and triglycerides, the chance is not greater than 1 in 100 that the cause is attributable to this mutation. Type 3 is characterized by the presence in plasma of detectable quantities of what is called β-VLDL or intermediate-density lipoproteins (IDL). Such IDL may be lipoprotein particles that normally arise during the conversion of VLDL to low-density lipoproteins (LDL) and that appear only fleetingly in plasma. When these lipoproteins accumulate in plasma in any significant concentration, they are accompanied by a distressing proclivity to coronary and peripheral vascular disease. The hazard of premature vascular disease in type 3 hyperlipoproteinemia is greater than that seen in all but one or two other lipoprotein disorders.

Many important questions about type 3 hyperlipoproteinemia are still unanswered. Even the diagnosis depends on criteria that are not specific. We initially favored a test based on the identification of lipoproteins of β-mobility among the VLDL or plasma (15). Based on evidence that the test is nonspecific, we have abandoned it in favor of a chemical measurement that depends on the presence of cholesterol-enriched VLDL in the plasma (16). However, earlier proponents of a chemical test now favor the electrophoresis test for "floating-beta" lipoproteins (28). Both criteria are useful; neither is adequate.

Recently, the apoprotein content of type 3 VLDL has become of interest in relation to diagnosis, mechanism, and genetics. There is a deficiency of C apoproteins in type 3 VLDL and at least a relative increase in the content of apoB and the arginine-rich apoprotein, also called apoE (27). The latter protein can be resolved into several components by isoelectric focusing, and one group has reported that a component of apoE is missing in patients with type 3 hyperlipoproteinemia (45).

Although a seemingly unique subpopulation of hyperlipidemic subjects is fairly well segregated by the several diagnostic tests for type 3 hyperlipoproteinemia, the genetic mode is unsettled. Expression of abnormality takes years, longer in women than in men (36). There are only five known cases in children (18, 20, 33, 35). Eventually, half of first-degree relatives are hyperlipidemic. About half of these have β-VLDL or IDL; the other half have simple endogenous hypertriglyceridemia. Hyperlipidemia is thus "dominant"; β-VLDL is "recessive." Recently, it has been suggested that the component of apoE missing in homozygotes is diminished in heterozygotes, suggesting a protein deficiency that is recessive in terms of clinical expression (44). An important piece of the puzzle, the function of apoE, is still missing.

GENETIC DISORDERS PRODUCING HYPERBETALIPOPROTEINEMIA

An excessive concentration of LDL in plasma is known as type 2 hyperlipoproteinemia in the convenient shorthand designation. The plasma cholesterol concentration is increased; the triglyceride concentration is normal unless VLDL levels are also increased. Both the number of causes and the number of patients having excess LDL (hyperbetalipoproteinemia) depend in part on where the line representing normality is drawn.

The most extreme and serious form of hyperbetalipoproteinemia occurs in familial hypercholesterolemia (FH), which is numerically a minor cause of type 2 hyperlipoproteinemia. An estimated 1 of 20 patients with this lipoprotein pattern have FH. This form of "hereditary xanthomatosis" was first segregated by Thannhauser and Magendantz in the late 1930's (42). Heterozygotes commonly have a plasma cholesterol concentration greater than 300 mg/dl. As adults, they tend to develop tendon xanthomas. Such lesions are fairly well restricted to patients with FH and thus they are helpful in diagnosis.

It is fitting that on this oldest of the genetic dyslipoproteinemias has been bestowed an important role in the single most dramatic extension in knowledge of lipoprotein metabolism in the past few years. This is the demonstration of the presence on cell surfaces of a receptor that binds LDL and thereby regulates both LDL degradation and cholesterol synthesis (21). Details and references to this seminal work by Brown and Goldstein are provided elsewhere in this book and are not repeated here. There appear to be several allelic forms of the disease. In one mutant, homozygotes have no apparent functioning receptors and heterozygotes have about 50% of the normal binding capacity (6). A second group of "homozygotes" (which may represent a genetic compound state — two different mutant alleles at the FH locus) are "receptor defective" and appear to possess kinetically abnormal LDL receptors capable of binding small amounts of LDL (1, 4, 24). The FH cell surface defect has now been detected in circulating leukocytes (10) and when the tests become standardized the use of such cells may greatly facilitate in vitro subclassification of patients with type 2 hyperlipoproteinemia.

One of the by-products of the research of Goldstein, Brown, and their colleagues is an assortment of useful tests for FH developed in cultured fibroblasts. The best test thus far appears to be the degree of cholesteryl ester synthesis stimulated by exposure of the cells to LDL. The esterification rate depends directly on the number of functioning LDL receptors and on a fully intact chain of events from the binding of LDL to the hydrolysis of its cholesteryl esters.

In addition to FH cells, fibroblasts from another rare set of patients receive low marks in this test. These are patients with acid cholesteryl ester hydrolase deficiency (24). There are some 35 reported instances of severe deficiency of the lysosomal acid cholesteryl esterase (14). The majority of patients are infants who survive briefly and succumb to what is better known as Wolman's disease. The minority are older and have a more benign course; they are labeled as having cholesteryl ester storage disease. These diseases, thought for some time to be quite independent, now appear to be allelic series, i.e., different phenotypes for the same defect caused by slightly different mutations at a genetic locus determining the activity of the esterase.

The tissues of all such patients contain prodigious quantities of cholesteryl esters and also excessive amounts of triglycerides. The "acid lipase" that is defective has a broad substrate specificity. The infants have severe malabsorption, adrenal calcification, and low lipoprotein concentrations. The adults, in contrast, usually have hyperbetalipoproteinemia. It is tempting to speculate that this latter is explicable on the basis of in vitro studies showing that high intracellular cholesterol concentrations lead to diminished surface receptors and reduced catabolism of cholesterol-rich lipoproteins (24).

The rationale for treatment of the dyslipoproteinemias is not the object of this brief chapter, but a word of caution against undue pessimism in the treatment of familial hypercholesterolemia is appropriate. The specter has been raised that successful attempts to lower the plasma LDL concentration may increase cholesterol synthesis in local tissues such as the arterial wall and obviate the apparent benefits of treatment (13, 22). It can be argued, however, that the augmented cholesterol synthesis in FH cells may be a compensatory mechanism to generate sterol to meet cellular requirements. Fibroblasts of subjects with homozygous FH grown in fetal calf serum contain normal quantities of cholesterol (5). Abetalipoproteinemia (see below) is an extreme example of removal of the feedback control initiated by LDL uptake, and yet there is no evidence of intracellular storage of cholesterol in this disease. It seems likely that the cholesteryl esters accumulating in atheromas in FH are derived from the plasma, not from in situ synthesis. Reduction of the gradient between plasma and cellular cholesterol therefore still appears to be a justifiable objective of therapy.

FAMILIAL COMBINED HYPERLIPIDEMIA

One of the most common causes of primary hypercholesterolemia and/or hypertriglyceridemia has been named familial combined hyperlipidemia

(CHL) by Goldstein and associates (25). It appears to be the most common form of single gene defects resulting in primary hyperlipoproteinemia. Affected subjects, or even the same patient on different occasions, may have one of several abnormal lipoprotein patterns. The diagnosis is reached only after family screening (25). Relatives with the disorder have high cholesterol, high triglycerides, or both. Like familial hypertriglyceridemia, but in contrast to familial hypercholesterolemia, lipid elevations are rarely expressed before 20 yr of age. The appellation CHL should not be indiscriminately applied to everyone with elevations of both VLDL and LDL. If family screening is not feasible, the noncommittal designation "mixed hyperlipidemia" is more appropriate.

The variation in lipoprotein patterns in CHL reflects the sensitive balance between rates of production of VLDL and of catabolism of these lipoproteins and their products, the LDL. In different subjects, and at different times in the same subject, the concentrations of VLDL may be moderately increased, or both VLDL and LDL or LDL alone may be increased. The lipoprotein elevations are generally moderate and do not reach a level at which lipid becomes deposited in the skin or tendons. Nevertheless, there appears to be a proclivity toward premature atherosclerosis in this disorder (25) that demands attention to both the mechanisms and the management of the hyperlipidemia. Tests more specific than simple lipid and lipoprotein measurements are sorely needed to better define CHL.

GENETIC DEFICIENCY STATES OF THE CHYLOMICRON-VLDL-LDL SYSTEM

No other genetic form of dyslipoproteinemia carries so stark a message about the importance of an apolipoprotein as does abetalipoproteinemia (ABL), discovered by Salt and co-workers in 1960 (39). Abetalipoproteinemia is still only presumptively due to a defect in apoB synthesis, but this mutation provides powerful evidence of the precursive relationship of the triglyceride-bearing lipoproteins to LDL. Abetalipoproteinemia wipes out from the plasma of its victims all chylomicrons, VLDL, and LDL and therefore all but a trace of triglycerides. Even the most severe malnutrition cannot produce such extreme deficiency. On only one occasion have we seen it secondary to any disease and that was associated with apparent antibodies to LDL arising in a peculiar form of autoimmune disease.

The fat malabsorption that attends ABL typically is associated with severe symptoms in the child, but only mild gastrointestinal complaints in the adult. Nevertheless, the retinal and neuromuscular degeneration usually progresses until most patients in the past were confined to a wheelchair by the end of their third decade (Fig. 2). We therefore were fortunate to have had the opportunity to study a woman with ABL who was functioning capably as a housewife in her fifth decade (2; Fig. 2). She had all the biochemical findings typical of ABL save one—there were low but detectable quantities of vitamin E in her plasma when no supplements were provided. Moreover, pedigree demonstrated that she represented a mutant in which

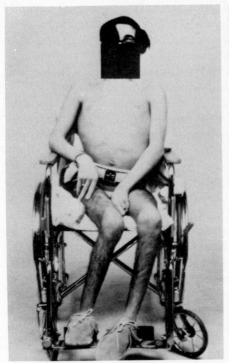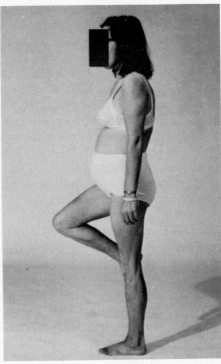

FIG. 2. A 17-yr-old boy with abetalipoproteinemia who cannot walk unassisted is contrasted with a woman of 42 with homozygous hypobetalipoproteinemia. [From Herbert et al. (29).]

hypobetalipoproteinemia is manifest in the heterozygous state and abetalipoproteinemia in homozygotes (2). This form of ABL has come to be called familial homozygous hypobetalipoproteinemia (8, 29). The outstanding difference between abetalipoproteinemia and familial hypobetalipoproteinemia is the inability of the bearers of a single allele for the latter disorder to maintain a normal concentration of LDL (29). Subjects heterozygous for both abnormalities are usually totally asymptomatic. The finding of detectable plasma vitamin E in the only known adult with homozygous FH may be noteworthy because there is an emerging consensus that vitamin E may play a critical role in preventing or arresting the retinal and neuromuscular degeneration in ABL (29, 37).

GENETIC HDL-DEFICIENCY STATES

Many of the genetic dyslipoproteinemias listed in Table 1 are associated with reduced plasma concentrations of HDL, and in several we are still uncertain whether the low plasma HDL are a primary or secondary abnormality. Familial lipoprotein lipase deficiency, whether absolute or relative, is accompanied by HDL concentrations that are about half normal. Dietary fat restriction and the achievement of low plasma triglyceride concentrations have little effect on the HDL concentration in this disorder. Other hypertriglyceridemic states including familial hypertriglyceridemia, familial type 5 hyperlipoproteinemia, familial type 3 hyperlipoproteinemia, and familial combined hyperlipoproteinemia regularly manifest low HDL levels when plasma triglyceride levels are uncontrolled. In some but not all instances therapy directed at the hypertriglyceridemia normalizes the HDL concentration. Patients with homozygous familial hypercholesterolemia have low apoA-I (31) and HDL levels that can be raised if the hypercholesterolemia is successfully treated.

The first recognized patient with cholesteryl ester storage disease was observed by us for over 15 yr (12). She had at all times a deficiency in plasma HDL and sometimes the concentrations were vanishingly small. Several other patients reported since have also had similar deficiencies in HDL (14). This deficiency in HDL brings us back for a moment to the observations on LDL catabolism. What maintains the balance of cholesterol in cells that are both synthesizing and receiving sterol from LDL uptake? One hypothesis is that the excess, perhaps in the substance of discarded cell membranes, must be excreted from the cell and retransported in plasma. For some time, HDL have been suspected to be the vehicle for such transport.

From comparisons of the distributions of lipids among LDL and HDL among species and of the neonatal changes in lipoprotein in man (19, 32), one may conclude that HDL represent a different and perhaps more primitive transport mechanism than LDL and their triglyceride-bearing precursors. The origin, fate, and functions of HDL are quarries that still remain at large, but the net is drawing tighter. As detailed by Hamilton in chapter 9, the precursors of HDL, flat disks of lipid and protein, appear to be secreted by the liver. They are expanded to particles resembling normal HDL by exposure to the cholesterol-esterifying activity of the enzyme lecithin:cholesterol acyltransferase (LCAT). Two genetic dyslipoproteinemias, familial LCAT deficiency and Tangier disease, deserve special mention because of the lessons they embody concerning the functions and fate of HDL.

FAMILIAL LECITHIN:CHOLESTEROL ACYLTRANSFERASE DEFICIENCY

The story of LCAT is exemplary of the sometimes irregular pace of the maturation of concepts in biology and of how discovery of a new disease may accelerate this process. A "cholesterol esterase" in plasma was discovered by Sperry in 1935 (40). For 25 years this activity was considered to be of little or no importance. Then it was reexamined by Glomset et al. (17), who renamed it and proposed that it could possibly account for nearly all the esterification of cholesterol in plasma. The normal substrate for LCAT appears to be HDL (17). A fatty acid is transferred from lecithin, a large pool of which is provided by HDL, to unesterified cholesterol. The resultant cholesteryl esters are transferred mainly to other lipoproteins. The core of most lipoproteins is believed to include the nonpolar cholesteryl esters, and the normal spherical shape of lipoproteins thus is dependent on an adequate supply of them. This appears to be particularly critical in maintaining stability of the "remnants" derived from chylomicrons and VLDL as they shed their triglyceride burden during intravascular lipolysis.

It was the discovery in 1966–67 of three Norwegian sisters with profound deficiency of LCAT activity in plasma (38) that proved the importance of the LCAT enzyme. In all known instances of familial LCAT deficiency, very low concentrations of plasma cholesteryl esters and abnormally high levels of unesterified cholesterol are found. The plasma lipoprotein and tissue derangements that accompany LCAT deficiency are of signal importance and they are considered after brief mention of the other major genetically determined disorders of HDL metabolism.

TANGIER DISEASE

In 1960 large orange tonsils were removed from a 5-yr-old boy who lived on an island called Tangier in the Chesapeake Bay. Histological examination suggested the presence of neutral lipid in the tissue. An exhaustive search of Tangier Island for similarly affected subjects uncovered a single additional case, the 6-yr-old sister of the index patient. Normal HDL were found to be virtually absent from the plasma of both siblings and in the last 17 years, 24 additional examples of Tangier disease have been discovered, the majority of them in either the United States or Germany (29). In all there is a reduction of the concentrations of the major HDL apolipoproteins, apoA-I and apoA-II, to extremely low levels. Plasma levels of HDL and the A apoproteins are approximately half-normal in obligate heterozygotes. In all homozygotes examined before puberty, the orange tonsils are a singular finding, and thus Tangier disease is the genetic dyslipoproteinemia most likely to be discovered, or inadvertently discarded, by otolaryngologists.

COMPARISON OF FAMILIAL LCAT DEFICIENCY AND TANGIER DISEASE

Biomedical research is often better, and certainly it is more gratifying, if one can simultaneously study both the normal and abnormal. It is a special advantage to compare separate mutants affecting contiguous elements in some biological system. Such an opportunity is presented by the deletion of LCAT activity in one disease, and, in another, of the HDL substrate of LCAT. The consequences in each disorder have interesting similarities and perhaps a critical difference.

High-Density Lipoproteins

In LCAT deficiency HDL are present in reduced quantities. Most HDL are disk-shaped lipoproteins about 40 Å thick and 150–200 Å in diameter and have a tendency to form rouleaux (11). These are rich in lecithin and unesterified cholesterol and bear striking resemblance to what has been termed "nascent" HDL (26). There are also smaller amounts of particles resembling normal HDL and still smaller spheres that contain lipid and apoA-I (43). Most of the apoA-I in LCAT-deficient plasma is in the lipoprotein-free fraction of plasma ($d > 1.21$ g/ml). The relationship of these abnormalities to the missing enzyme seems certain, for added LCAT converts the disks to spheres and enriches the HDL in apoA-I.

The trace amounts of HDL in Tangier plasma include a pleiomorphic collection of lipoprotein forms (29). Among these are discoidal lipoproteins that stack in rouleaux, large (>1000-Å) translucent particles, and tiny spherical lipoproteins. The origin of the disk-shaped lipoproteins is uncertain, but they may well represent a form of nascent HDL. The large bizarre particles seem to be chylomicron remnants, and their numbers can be greatly diminished by withdrawal of dietary fat. The small particles may be remnant HDL and contain primarily apoA-II. In Tangier disease, as in familial LCAT deficiency, most of the plasma apoA-I is recovered in the lipoprotein-free fraction of plasma.

Chylomicron-VLDL-LDL System

Both familial LCAT deficiency and Tangier disease are characterized by moderate hypertriglyceridemia, and in both the VLDL have less than normal mobility. The LDL in both diseases contain excessive triglyceride relative to cholesterol. In LCAT deficiency, in addition, large "membrane-like" bodies similar to those found in Tangier HDL are demonstrable in LDL (11). As in the case of Tangier disease, the numbers of these strange particles can be greatly diminished by removing fat from the diet. Thus, we can conclude that the hypothesis attributing an important function to both LCAT and HDL in assuring smooth intravascular degradation of chylomicrons and VLDL is probably correct.

Tissue Changes

In Tangier disease reticuloendothelial cells and cornea are burdened with cholesteryl esters. The Schwann cells of peripheral nerves also store cholesteryl esters. The latter is associated with peripheral neuropathy, to date the most serious known consequence of Tangier disease (29).

In LCAT deficiency, unesterified cholesterol and phospholipids accumulate in the kidney, liver, spleen, and the cornea. But there are more ominous consequences in LCAT deficiency. Vessels from major arteries to capillaries undergo destruction associated with lipid deposition (30). The most serious lesions occur in the glomerular tufts of the kidney, where membrane structures, similar to the plasma particles, are retained. The inevitable result is renal failure. Kidneys transplanted into LCAT-deficient recipients soon undergo similar changes (41).

The vascular changes in LCAT deficiency afford a sharp contrast with Tangier disease. The ultrastructure of kidneys in Tangier disease has never been examined, but there is no clinically apparent renal disease. Capillaries and other small vessels in extrarenal tissues show no significant accumulation of lipid (9).

Comparison of these two mutants leaves unsettled the question: What is the function of HDL? Do HDL accept excess cholesterol from cells for return to the liver or other sites and thus maintain the equilibrium affected by LDL reception and uptake of its cholesterol? The two mutants in which normal HDL are virtually absent do demonstrate intracellular accumulation of cholesterol. However, this might be explained by unstable metabolism of triglyceride-bearing lipoproteins and their uptake by macrophages. More evidence for primary storage of cholesterol in Tangier disease is needed. This unresolved question of HDL function is central to latter-day revival of the old hypothesis: that "deficiency" of HDL is a determinant of atherogenesis, especially in older subjects (34). Is it possible that the functional level of LCAT may prove to be more critical in this regard? Is it unreasonable to postulate that the HDL that clear tissues of effete membrane and lipoprotein cholesterol are not the predominant species in plasma replete with cholesteryl ester but rather the more nascent discoidal HDL found even in Tangier plasma? Perhaps this is the critical lesson residing in these genetic HDL-deficiency states.

CONCLUSION

The concept of plasma lipids as parts of lipoproteins has survived, and the properties and metabolism of the latter have proved to be predictable and important in the study of both health and disease. The study of derangements in plasma lipoproteins has become a subdiscipline of its own. Both genetic and extrinsic determinants are involved. A small universe of hereditary dyslipoproteinemias has been charted and is still expanding, although the greatest single pulse in its growth may be over.

We all have been preoccupied mainly with gross defects due to single gene mutants. It is only a small subset of the universe. Where plasma lipids and lipoproteins influence health and longevity in the great bulk of the population, the admixture of multiple genes and of culture poses a more difficult problem.

Within the broad span of normal distribution lie the major interactions that require understanding for better control. Why, for example, though we eat at the same table and have such similar lives, do I have a cholesterol concentration of 240 and you have one of 140, or I an HDL level of 50 and you one of 35? Such heterogeneity, we continue to learn, is most important. It is one of the principal challenges remaining. Perhaps our preoccupation with the concentrations of lipids in plasma, especially those in the morning before breakfast, and with the structure of lipoproteins, has limited our perceptions of both normal mechanisms and disease.

Present address of P. N. Herbert: The Miriam Hospital, Division of Clinical and Experimental Atherosclerosis, 164 Summit Avenue, Providence, RI 02906.

REFERENCES

1. AVIGAN, J., S. J. BHATHENA, AND M. E. SCHREI-NER. Control of sterol synthesis and of hydroxymethyl-glutaryl CoA reductase in skin fibroblasts grown from patients with homozygous type II hyperlipoproteinemia. *J. Lipid Res.* 16: 151–154, 1975.

2. BIEMER, J. J., AND R. E. McCAMMON. The genetic relationship of abetalipoproteinemia and hypobetalipo-proteinemia: a report of the occurrence of both diseases within the same family. *J. Lab. Clin. Med.* 85: 556–565, 1975.

3. BRECKENRIDGE, W. C., J. A. LITTLE, G. STEINER, A. CHOW, AND M. POAPST. Hyperlipoproteinemia associated with an absence of C-II apoprotein in plasma lipoproteins. *Circulation* 54: II–25, 1976.

4. BRESLOW, J. L., D. R. SPAULDING, S. E. LUX, R. I. LEVY, AND R. S. LEES. Homozygous familial hypercho-lesterolemia: a possible biochemical explanation of clini-cal heterogeneity. *New Engl. J. Med.* 293: 900–903, 1975.

5. BROWN, M. S., J. R. FAUST, AND J. L. GOLDSTEIN. Role of the low density lipoprotein receptor in regulating the content of free and esterified cholesterol in human fibroblasts. *J. Clin. Invest.* 55: 783–793, 1975.

6. BROWN, M. S., AND J. L. GOLDSTEIN. Familial hyper-cholesterolemia: defective binding of lipoproteins to cul-tured fibroblasts associated with impaired regulation of 3-hydroxy-3-methylglutaryl coenzyme A reductase activ-ity. *Proc. Natl. Acad. Sci. US* 71: 788–792, 1971.

7. BRUNZELL, J. D., W. R. HAZZARD, D. PORTE, JR., AND E. L. BIERMAN. Evidence for a common, saturable, triglyceride removal mechanism for chylomicrons and very low density lipoproteins in man. *J. Clin. Invest.* 52: 1578–1585, 1973.

8. COTTRILL, C., C. J. GLUECK, V. LEUBA, F. MIL-LETT, D. PUPPIONE, AND W. V. BROWN. Familial homozygous hypobetalipoproteinemia. *Metabolism* 23: 779–791, 1974.

9. FERRANS, V. J., AND D. S. FREDRICKSON. The pathology of Tangier disease. A light and electron micro-scopic study. *Am. J. Pathol.* 78: 101–136, 1975.

10. FOGELMAN, A. M., J. EDMOND, J. SEAGER, AND G. POPJAK. Abnormal induction of 3-hydroxy-3-methyl-glutaryl coenzyme A reductase in leukocytes from sub-jects with heterozygous familial hypercholesterolemia. *J. Biol. Chem.* 250: 2045–2055, 1975.

11. FORTE, T., A. NICHOLS, J. GLOMSET, AND K. NO-RUM. The ultrastructure of plasma lipoproteins in leci-thin:cholesterol acyltransferase deficiency. *Scand. J. Clin. Lab. Invest.* 33, Suppl. 137: 121–132, 1974.

12. SLOAN, H. R., AND D. S. FREDRICKSON. Rare famil-ial diseases with neutral lipid storage: Wolman's disease, cholesteryl ester storage disease, and cerebrotendinous xanthomatosis. In: *The Metabolic Basis of Inherited Disease* (3rd ed.), edited by J. B. Stanbury, J. B. Wyn-gaarden, and D. S. Fredrickson. New York: McGraw-Hill, 1972, p. 808–832.

13. FREDRICKSON, D. S., M. S. BROWN, AND J. L. GOLDSTEIN. Familial hyperlipoproteinemia. In: *The Metabolic Basis of Inherited Disease* (4th ed.), edited by J. B. Stanbury, J. B. Wyngaarden, and D. S. Fredrick-son. New York: McGraw-Hill, 1977, in press.

14. FREDRICKSON, D. S., AND V. J. FERRANS. Choles-teryl ester hydrolase deficiency: Wolman's disease and cholesteryl ester storage disease. In: *The Metabolic Basis of Inherited Disease* (4th ed.), edited by J. B. Stanbury, J. B. Wyngaarden, and D. S. Fredrickson. New York: McGraw-Hill, 1977, in press.

15. FREDRICKSON, D. S., R. S. LEES, AND R. I. LEVY. Fat transport in lipoproteins – an integrated approach to mechanisms and disorders. *New Engl. J. Med.* 276: 148–156, 215–226, 1967.

16. FREDRICKSON, D. S., J. MORGANROTH, AND R. I. LEVY. Type III hyperlipoproteinemia: an analysis of two contemporary definitions. *Ann. Internal Med.* 82: 150–157, 1975.

17. GLOMSET, J. A., E. J. JANSSEN, R. KENNEDY, AND J. DOBBINS. Role of plasma lecithin:cholesteryl acyl-transferase in the metabolism of high density lipopro-teins. *J. Lipid Res.* 7: 638–648, 1966.

18. GLUECK, C. J., R. W. FALLAT, M. J. MELLIES, AND P. M. STEINER. Pediatric familial type 3 hyperlipopro-teinemia. *Metabolism* 25: 1269–1274, 1976.

19. GLUECK, C. J., F. HECKMAN, M. SCHOENFELD, P. STEINER, AND W. PEARCE. Neonatal familial type II hyperlipoproteinemia: cord blood cholesterol in 1,800 births. *Metabolism* 20: 597–608, 1971.

20. GODOLPHIN, W. J., G. CONRADI, AND D. J. CAMP-BELL. Type III hyperlipoproteinemia in a child. *Lancet* 1: 209–210, 1972.

21. GOLDSTEIN, J. L., AND M. S. BROWN. Binding and degradation of low density lipoproteins by cultured hu-man fibroblasts. *J. Biol. Chem.* 249: 5153–5162, 1974.

22. GOLDSTEIN, J. L., AND M. S. BROWN. Familial hyper-cholesterolemia: a genetic regulatory defect in choles-terol metabolism. *Am. J. Med.* 15: 147–150, 1975.

23. GOLDSTEIN, J. L., S. E. DANA, G. Y. BRUNSCHEDE, AND M. S. BROWN. Genetic heterogeneity in familial hypercholesterolemia: evidence for two different muta-tions affecting functions of low density lipoprotein recep-tor. *Proc. Natl. Acad. Sci. US* 72: 1092–1096, 1975.

24. GOLDSTEIN, J. L., S. E. DANA, J. R. FAUST, A. L. BEAUDET, AND M. S. BROWN. Role of lysosomal acid lipase in the metabolism of plasma low density lipopro-tein. *J. Biol. Chem.* 250: 8487–8495, 1975.

25. GOLDSTEIN, J. L., H. G. SCHROTT, W. R. HAZZARD, E. L. BIERMAN, AND A. G. MOTULSKY. Hyperlipid-emia in coronary heart disease. II. Genetic analysis of lipid levels in 176 families and delineation of a new inherited disorder, combined hyperlipidemia. *J. Clin. Invest.* 52: 1544–1568, 1973.

26. HAMILTON, R. L., M. C. WILLIAMS, C. J. FIELDING, AND R. J. HAVEL. Discoidal bilayer structure of nascent high density lipoproteins from perfused rat liver. *J. Clin. Invest.* 58: 667–680, 1976.

27. HAVEL, R. J., AND J. P. KANE. Primary dysbetalipo-proteinemia: predominance of a specific apoprotein spe-cies in triglyceride-rich lipoproteins. *Proc. Natl. Acad. Sci. US* 70: 2015–2019, 1973.

28. HAZZARD, W. R., T. F. O'DONNELL, AND Y. L. LEE. Broad-β disease (type III hyperlipoproteinemia) in a large kindred. Evidence for a monogenic mechanism. *Ann. Internal Med.* 82: 141–149, 1975.

29. HERBERT, P. N., A. M. GOTTO, AND D. S. FREDRICK-SON. Familial lipoprotein deficiency (abetalipopro-teinemia, hypobetalipoproteinemia and Tangier dis-ease). In: *The Metabolic Basis of Inherited Disease* (4th ed.), edited by J. B. Stanbury, J. B. Wyngaarden, and D. S. Fredrickson. New York: McGraw-Hill, 1977, in press.

30. HOVIG, T., AND E. GJONE. Familial lecithin:cholesterol acyltransferase deficiency. Ultrastructural studies on lipid deposition and tissue reactions. *Scand. J. Clin. Lab. Invest.* 33, Suppl. 137: 135–146, 1974.

31. KARLIN, J. B., D. J. JUHN, J. I. STARR, A. M. SCANU, AND A. H. RUBENSTEIN. Measurement of human high density lipoprotein apolipoprotein A-I in serum by radioimmunoassay. *J. Lipid Res.* 17: 30–37, 1976.

32. KWITEROVICH, P. O., JR., R. I. LEVY, AND D. S. FREDRICKSON. Neonatal diagnosis of familial type II hyperlipoproteinemia. *Lancet* 1: 118–121, 1973.

33. KWITEROVICH, P. O., C. NEILL, S. MARGOLIS, M. THAMER, AND P. BACHORIK. Allelism, non-allelism and genetic compounds in familial hyperlipoproteinemia. *Clin. Res.* 23: 262A, 1975.

34. MILLER, G. J., AND N. E. MILLER. Plasma high-density-lipoprotein concentration and development of ischaemic heart-disease. *Lancet* 1: 16–19, 1975.

35. MISHKEL, M. A., D. J. NAZIR, AND S. CROWTHER. A longitudinal assessment of lipid ratios in the diagnosis of type III hyperlipoproteinemia. *Clin. Chim. Acta* 58: 121–136, 1975.

36. MORGANROTH, J., R. I. LEVY, AND D. S. FREDRICKSON. The biochemical, clinical, and genetic features of type III hyperlipoproteinemia. *Ann. Internal Med.* 82: 158–174, 1975.

37. MULLER, D. P. R., J. K. LLOYD, AND A. C. BIRD. Long-term management of abetalipoproteinemia: possible role for vitamin E. *Arch. Disease Childhood* 52: 202–214, 1977.

38. NORUM, K. R., AND E. GJONE. Familial plasma lecithin:cholesterol acyltransferase deficiency. Biochemical study of a new inborn error of metabolism. *Scand. J. Clin. Lab. Invest.* 20: 231–243, 1967.

39. SALT, H. B., O. H. WOLFF, J. K. LLOYD, A. S. FOSBROOKE, AND D. V. HUBBLE. On having no beta-lipoprotein. A syndrome comprising a-beta-lipoproteinemia, acanthocytosis, and steatorrhea. *Lancet* 2: 325–329, 1960.

40. SPERRY, W. M. Cholesterol esterase in blood. *J. Biol. Chem.* 111: 467–478, 1935. 1935.

41. STOKKE, K. T., K. S. BJERVE, J. P. BLOMHOFF, B. ÖYSTESE, A. FLOTMORK, K. R. NORUM, AND E. GJONE. Familial lecithin:cholesterol acyltransferase deficiency. Studies on lipid composition and morphology of tissues. *Scand. J. Clin. Lab. Invest.* 33, Suppl. 137: 93–100, 1974.

42. THANNHAUSER, S. J., AND H. MAGENDANTZ. The different clinical groups of xanthomatous disease: a clinical physiological study of 22 cases. *Ann. Internal Med.* 11: 1662–1746, 1938.

43. TÖRSVIK, H. Studies on the protein moiety of serum high density lipoprotein from patients with familial lecithin:cholesterol acyltransferase deficiency. *Clin. Genet.* 3: 188–200, 1972.

44. UTERMANN, G., M. HESS, AND K. H. VOGELBERG. Broad-beta disease (hyperlipoproteinemia type III): genetics, gene frequency and diagnosis without ultracentrifugation). In: *Electrofocusing and Isotachophoresis.* Berlin: Walter de Gruyter, 1976, p. 281–293.

45. UTERMANN, G., M. JAESCHKE, AND J. MENZEL. Familial hyperlipoproteinemia type III: deficiency of a specific apolipoprotein (apoE-III) in very low density lipoproteins. *Fed. European Biochem. Soc. Letters* 56: 352–355, 1975.

13

Hormonal Regulation of Triglyceride Breakdown in Adipocytes

JOHN N. FAIN, RAYMOND E. SHEPHERD,
CRAIG C. MALBON, AND FRANCISCO J. MORENO

*Section of Physiological Chemistry, Division of Biology and Medicine,
Brown University, Providence, Rhode Island*

Coupling of Catecholamine-Receptor Complex to Adenylate Cyclase
Adenosine and Fat Cell Metabolism
Free Fatty Acids as Feedback Regulators of Adenylate Cyclase

LIPID IS MOBILIZED FROM ADIPOSE TISSUE in the form of free fatty acids (FFAs) noncovalently bound to plasma albumin (chapt. 14). The fatty acids are utilized by muscle as a source of energy (chapt. 16). Free fatty acids also are taken up by liver and oxidized, esterified, or converted to ketone bodies (chapt. 15).

The rate of lipolysis is the major factor regulating the release of FFA by adipose tissue since under conditions in which lipolysis is accelerated little α-glycerophosphate is available from glycolysis for fatty acid reesterification. In mammalian fat cells the hydrolysis of the stored triglycerides in adipose tissue is catalyzed by the "hormone-sensitive" lipase that is activated by cyclic AMP (39).

Lipolysis in fat cells is inhibited by insulin, adenosine, and prostaglandins and enhanced by catecholamines, growth hormone, glucocorticoids, and thyroid hormones (9, 11). It is still not clear which hormones are responsible for lipid mobilization during fasting. Lipolysis could be elevated by the drop in plasma insulin that occurs during fasting or by increased release of lipolytic hormones.

There is a lag of 4–6 h before thyroid hormones accelerate lipolysis (9) but only 1–2 h for growth hormone and glucocorticoids (9). In contrast, the lag period for catecholamines is in the order of seconds. Our knowledge of the mechanisms involved in the activation of lipolysis by the various hormones is rather incomplete. Table 1 summarizes the key differences in these mechanisms.

Initially our interest in the hormonal regulation of lipolysis was concerned with the role of cyclic AMP in the action of slow activators of lipolysis such as growth hormone, glucocorticoids, and thyroid hormones. This has turned out to be a difficult problem to address since even for catecholamines cyclic AMP may not be the sole mediator of lipolysis.

TABLE 1. *Agents that increase lipolysis by fat cells*

Agent	Lag Period	Is Protein and RNA Synthesis Involved?	What is Known About Mechanism
Thyroid hormones	4–6 h	Not known	Catecholamine binding is unaffected
Growth hormone	1–2 h	Yes	Increases catecholamine-sensitive adenylate cyclase
Glucocorticoids	1–2 h	Yes	Does not affect cyclic AMP accumulation
Cholera toxin	0.5–1 h	No	Irreversibly activates adenylate cyclase
Catecholamines	s	No	Activate adenylate cyclase
Methylxanthines	s	No	Inhibit cyclic AMP phosphodiesterase and adenosine action
Adenosine deaminase	s	No	Removes adenosine

Incubation of fat cells with growth hormone for 3.5 h prior to the preparation of fat cell ghosts resulted in a 40% increase in the stimulation of adenylate cyclase by norepinephrine (9) while producing no significant effect on basal, ACTH-stimulated, or fluoride-stimulated adenylate cyclase. These results suggest that the lipolytic action of growth hormone involved the synthesis of a protein(s) that increased the sensitivity of fat cell adenylate cyclase to activation by catecholamines.

The lipolytic action of glucocorticoids, like that of growth hormone, appears to be permissive since both hormones increase the sensitivity of fat cells to lipolytic agents such as catecholamines (9, 12). The lipolytic action of glucocorticoids has a lag period and a sensitivity to inhibitors of RNA and protein synthesis similar to those of growth hormone. However, the mode of action of glucocorticoids remains to be elucidated. Even after prolonged incubation either in the absence or presence of growth hormone, glucocorticoids did not alter cyclic AMP (9, 11, 12, 15).

COUPLING OF CATECHOLAMINE-RECEPTOR COMPLEX TO ADENYLATE CYCLASE

Our laboratory has been interested in the mechanisms by which thyroid hormones potentiate catecholamine-stimulated lipolysis in white fat cells (6). Recently Malbon et al. (27) examined the effects of hypothyroidism and thyroid hormone administration on catecholamine binding, cyclic AMP accumulation, and lipolysis. The binding of tritiated dihydroalprenolol was unaffected by thyroid hormone status (Table 2). The total number of binding sites per cell for this beta-adrenergic antagonist was about 100,000 (27). The lipolytic sensitivity of fat cells to catecholamines was decreased in the hypothyroid state but a saturating concentration of epinephrine gave the same maximal activation of lipolysis in fat cells from hypothyrid rats as in cells from hyperthyroid rats (Table 2). However, in fat cells from hypothyroid rats there was no detectable accumulation of cyclic AMP with the high dose of catecholamine. These results suggest that the low level of cyclic AMP accumulation in fat cells from hypothyroid rats is not due to defective catecholamine binding but rather to some further step such as coupling of hormone-receptor complexes to adenylate cyclase. Alternatively, dihydroalprenolol binding may not reflect binding to the receptors involved in catecholamine action (Fig. 1).

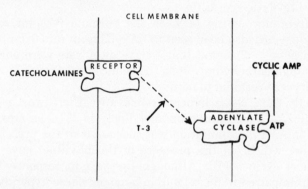

FIG. 1. Regulation of adenylate cyclase by catecholamines and thyroid hormones. Adenylate cyclase in fat cells is activated after binding of catecholamines to a beta-1 receptor in the plasma membrane. There appear to be about 100,000 receptors for catecholamines in rat fat cells and their number is unaffected by thyroid hormone. The hormone-receptor complex is postulated to interact through some sort of coupling mechanism with adenylate cyclase located on the inner surface of the fat cell plasma membrane. The model postulates that 3,5,3'-triiodothyronine (T_3) is involved in coupling of the catecholamine-receptor complex to adenylate cyclase. Amount of fluoride-activatable adenylate cyclase appears to be relatively unaffected by thyroid hormone.

TABLE 2. *Effect of thyroid status on catecholamine binding, cyclic AMP accumulation, and lipolysis in rat fat cells*

	Binding Sites for [³H]Dihydroalprenolol, fmol/mg of Protein			Cyclic AMP Accumulation + Epinephrine, pmol/10⁶ Cells		Glycerol Release + Epinephrine, μmol/10⁶ Cells	
	1 nM	10 nM	100 nM	3.3 μM	100 μM	3 μM	100 μM
Hypothyroid	16	67	236	<5	<5	0.9	9.7
Control	20	71	222	25	100	3.0	8.4
Hypothyroid + T_3				120	275	3.4	9.9
Control + T_3	28	78	261	135	200	3.3	5.6

Wet weight of parametrial adipose tissue from hypothyroid rats was about threefold greater than that of control rats treated with T_3. However, total fat cell count was unaffected by thyroid status as was the yield of membrane protein. Specific binding of (−)-[³H]dihydroalprenolol is in femtomoles per milligram of membrane protein. Cyclic AMP accumulation was measured after 2 min and glycerol release after 15 min in the absence of methylxanthine. Hypothyroidism was produced by feeding rats for 20–24 days a low-iodine diet with 0.006% propylthiouracil added to the drinking water. 3,5,3',-Triiodothyronine (T_3)-treated rats were given 30 μg/100 g body wt of T_3 daily for 5 days prior to the experiments. [Data taken from Malbon et al. (27).]

The adenylate cyclase activity of ghosts prepared from hypothyroid rats demonstrated a marked shift in the sensitivity of these ghosts to catecholamine (27). However, the maximal catalytic activity measured in the presence of sodium fluoride was unaffected by thyroid status. The sensitivity of adenylate cyclase to catecholamine stimulation was increased by guanyl-5′-yl imidodiphosphate [Gpp(NH)p] to a much greater extent in ghosts from normal compared with hypothyroid rats (27). The coupling of the catecholamine-receptor complex to adenylate cyclase, as well as that of other hormones, was altered by thyroid hormones. Hypothyroid animals have a poor response to all lipolytic agents (9).

An apparent uncoupling between the hormone-receptor complex and adenylate cyclase has also been seen in fat cells from rats fed a high-fat diet (22). Gorman et al. (22) found that 3 days after rats were shifted from a high-fat to a high-carbohydrate diet the reduced catecholamine-responsive cyclase activity was restored to normal.

In fat cells from obese hyperglycemic mice there was a dissociation between cyclic AMP accumulation and lipolysis (37), as summarized in Table 3. Cyclic AMP accumulation was measured in the presence of 1 μM norepinephrine, which (in the presence of theophylline) gave a maximal accumulation of cyclic AMP. Although lipolysis in response to catecholamines was unimpaired in fat cells from 5-mo-old obese hyperglycemic mice (*ob/ob* strain), there was no rise in cyclic AMP. The adenylate cyclase activity of fat cell ghosts prepared from 5-mo-old obese hyperglycemic mice was also unresponsive to catecholamines. There was no reduction in Gpp-(NH)p-activated adenylate cyclase. However, there was a small drop in fluoride-stimulated activity (Table 3). These data indicate that the catalytic

TABLE 3. *Uncoupling between adenylate cyclase and cyclic AMP accumulation in fat cells from obese hyperglycemic mice*

	Fat Cells Incubated with 1 μM Norepinephrine + 100 μM Theophylline			Adenylate Cyclase Activity of Fat Cell Ghosts		
					+Gpp(NH)p, 10 μM	
	FFA release	Glycerol release	Cyclic AMP accumulation	Without	+1 μM NE	+Fluoride
	μmol/10^6 Cells		*nmol/10^6 Cells*	*nmol/mg of Protein*		
Lean mice						
5 wk	9.0	3.5	11.5	14	23	14
5 mo	9.3	6.5	0.6	16	19	9
Obese mice						
5 wk	12.5	4.7	2.2	13	14	8
5 mo	8.0	5.7	<0.1	12	12	5

Measurements of lipolysis and cyclic AMP accumulation were based on values obtained after incubation of mouse fat cells for 60 and 5 min, respectively. Values are means of 6 paired experiments done in presence of 100 μM theophylline. Adenylate cyclase activity was measured with the use of fat cell ghosts and results are based on 4 experiments. Adenylate cyclase activity was no greater in the presence of both fluoride and Gpp(NH)p than with fluoride alone. Basal adenylate cyclase activity over the 10-min assay period was 3.2 and 2.5 nmol/mg for ghosts from lean controls at 5 wk and 5 mo, respectively. In ghosts from obese mice basal cyclase was 1.2 at either 5 wk or 5 mo. [Data taken from Shepherd et al. (38)]

activity of adenylate cyclase is relatively unimpaired by obesity. We have not measured catecholamine binding in membranes from mouse fat cells because of the large amount of membranes required for these studies.

It seems unlikely that an increase in cyclic AMP phosphodiesterase activity might account for the impaired cyclic AMP accumulation in fat cells from obese mice or hypothyroid rats. Soluble cyclic AMP phosphodiesterase was higher in fat cells from obese mice, whereas the particulate activity was virtually unchanged (37). In contrast Armstrong et al. (1) reported that soluble cyclic AMP phosphodiesterase was unaltered by thyroid status but the particulate activity was increased.

ADENOSINE AND FAT CELL METABOLISM

Sahyoun et al. (35) recently reported the presence of an inhibitor of adenylate cyclase in tissue extracts that they identified as 2'-deoxy, 3'-AMP. The data in Figure 2 demonstrate that 2'-deoxy, 3'-AMP was ineffective at concentrations up to 100 μM in inhibiting cyclic AMP accumulation or lipolysis by intact fat cells. Thus it is unlikely that this compound is a regulator of lipolysis or cyclic AMP accumulation that is released by fat cells to the medium. In studies with fat cell ghosts we have found that 2'-deoxy,

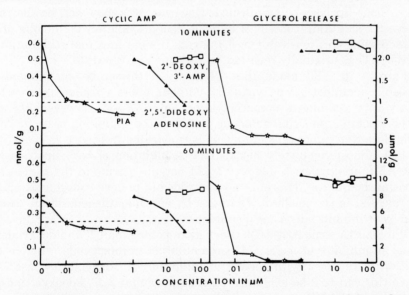

FIG. 2. Comparison of effects of N^6-(phenylisopropyl)adenosine, 2',5'-dideoxyadenosine, and 2'-deoxy, 3'-AMP on cyclic AMP accumulation and lipolysis in the presence of norepinephrine and adenosine deaminase. Fat cells (50 mg/tube) were incubated for 10 or 60 min in the presence of 0.1 μM norepinephrine plus 1 μg/ml of adenosine deaminase. N^6-(phenylisopropyl)adenosine (stars), 2',5'-dideoxyadenosine (triangles), and 2'-deoxy, 3'-AMP (squares) were added with lipolytic agents at indicated concentrations. Dashed line at the bottom of each graph represents the basal value for cyclic AMP accumulation in the absence of added agents. Values are means of 3 paired replications.

3'-AMP was equipotent to 2', 5'-dideoxyadenosine as an inhibitor of hormone-activated adenylate cyclase (Moreno and Fain, unpublished observations).

A concentration of 5 μM 2',5'-dideoxyadenosine produced about 50% inhibition of adenylate cyclase activity in fat cell ghosts (Moreno and Fain, unpublished observations). This concentration produces a similar inhibition of cyclic AMP accumulation in intact rat fat cells (Fig. 2). However, 2',5'-dideoxyadenosine was ineffective as an inhibitor of lipolysis despite the fact than an equivalent inhibition of lipolysis by N^6-(phenylisopropyl)adenosine (PIA) resulted in a complete blockade of catecholamine-induced lipolysis. These results agree with prior studies by Fain et al. (13) where concentrations of 2',5'-dideoxyadenosine as high as 85 μM were completely ineffective in inhibiting lipolysis. The data illustrate another condition besides obesity and hypothyroidism in which measurable cyclic AMP accumulation can be dissociated from lipolysis. Our conclusion from the dideoxyadenosine data is that either there is something else besides adenylate cyclase that is activated by catecholamine binding to membrane receptor or there is compartmentation of adenylate cyclase.

The problem with compartmentation is that it is a refuge to which we retreat when the data do not fit the hypothesis currently in fashion. It is difficult to understand how all the measurable cyclic AMP accumulation occurs in a separate compartment and can be blocked by 2',5'-dideoxyadenosine without lipolysis being affected. However, this may well be the case. The basal cyclic AMP content of fat cells is approximately 0.2 nmol/g of fat and increasing this to a value of 0.3 results in near-maximal stimulation of lipolysis (11) as originally reported by Butcher and Baird (5).

Fain et al. (13) found that PIA, which cannot be deaminated by adenosine deaminase, was virtually without effect on adenylate cyclase activity of fat cell ghosts at concentrations up to 73 μM. However, PIA was the most potent adenosine analogue tested in the inhibition of cyclic AMP accumulation in intact cells (10). This is illustrated in Figure 2, where 0.01 μM PIA almost completely blocked the stimulation of both lipolysis and cyclic AMP accumulation due to 0.1 μM norepinephrine in the presence of adenosine deaminase. This enzyme was added to remove endogenous adenosine released to the medium. Neither PIA nor dideoxyadenosine is deaminated by or inhibits adenosine deaminase.

Why is PIA some 2000–5000 times more potent than 2',5'-dideoxyadenosine as an inhibitor of cyclic AMP accumulation in intact cells, whereas the situation is reversed with regard to inhibition of adenylate cyclase? We believe this can best be explained by assuming that 2',5'-dideoxyadenosine and 2'-deoxy,3'-AMP (in broken-cell preparations only) inhibit adenylate cyclase at a site different from that for adenosine and PIA. This could be either a different site on the same enzyme complex or separate cyclases. Possibly most of the adenylate cyclase molecules within rat fat cells are readily inhibited by 2',5'-dideoxyadenosine and the cyclic AMP produced has little to do with lipolysis. This hypothesis suggests that there is a small pool of adenylate cyclase molecules that generate the cyclic AMP involved in the regulation of lipolysis. This pool of adenylate cyclase is readily inhibited by adenosine in intact cells. In broken-cell preparations this sensitivity to adenosine and PIA may be either lost or masked by the large number of physiologically unimportant adenylate cyclase molecules. This hypothesis may seem rather radical, but the alternative is to assume that the catechol-amine-receptor complex activates some other membrane enzyme, which regulates lipolysis, and that the stimulation of adenylate cyclase is only an amplification signal.

Low levels of hormone may stimulate lipolysis without measurably affecting cyclic AMP accumulation. The converse would explain why $2',5'$-dideoxyadenosine inhibited cyclic AMP accumulation but not lipolysis. However, the problem with this hypothesis is that nearly all inhibitors of lipolysis, except for insulin, also inhibit cyclic AMP accumulation and this is certainly true for PIA. We are left with the possibility of two distinct populations of adenylate cyclase molecules with only those sensitive to adenosine and PIA being involved in regulation of lipolysis.

Fain et al. (13) suggested that adenosine might be a feedback regulator of cyclic AMP accumulation released during incubation of fat cells with stimulators of adenylate cyclase. Schwabe et al. (36) found that an inhibitory substance accumulated in the medium during incubation of rat fat cells, which they identified as adenosine. However, they were unable to find any acceleration of adenosine release by hormones (36). Despite several years of effort we have been unable to find any consistent effect of hormones on adenosine release (17). Fredholm (18) came to a similar conclusion in studies on perfused dog adipose tissue; the only instance in which adenosine release was accelerated was when hypoxia occurred as a result of vasoconstriction. It is well established in other tissues such as heart and skeletal muscle that adenosine release is accelerated by anoxia (2).

We believe that the site of action for adenosine is on the external surface of the fat cell plasma membrane. The best evidence has come from studies with adenosine bound to stachyose. Approximately 3 mol of adenosine can be coupled per mole of stachyose to give a large water-soluble derivative that mimicked the action of adenosine on coronary blood flow after intracoronary infusion into dogs (31). On a molar basis the adenosine bound to stachyose was as potent as adenosine in inhibiting cyclic AMP accumulation by fat cells (17).

Our studies indicated that adenosine is always present and there is little accumulation during incubation of rat fat cells. This suggests that enough adenosine is present in fat cells to partially restrain adenylate cyclase. The large increases in cyclic AMP seen after the addition of methylxanthines to fat cells in the presence of catecholamines might be due to reversal of the inhibitory effect of adenosine on adenylate cyclase. Figure 3 shows that the inhibitory effect of 10 nM PIA on both cyclic AMP accumulation and lipolysis by rat fat cells was reversed by the addition of theophylline. A low concentration of PIA (3.3 nM) inhibited cyclic AMP accumulation but not lipolysis. In contrast the inhibition of cyclic AMP

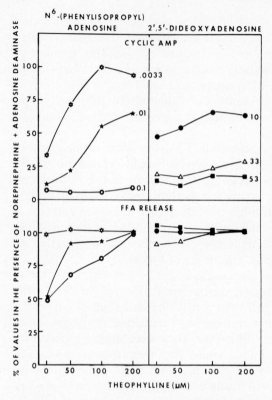

FIG. 3. N^6-(phenylisopropyl)adenosine and 2′,5′-dideoxyadenosine versus methylxanthines. Fat cells (50 mg/tube) were incubated in the presence of 2 μM norepinephrine and 1 μg of adenosine deaminase/ml for 10 min. N^6-(phenylisopropyl)adenosine (left) or 2′,5′-dideoxyadenosine (right) were added with the lipolytic agents at the micromolar concentration listed to right of symbols. Values in the presence of adenosine analogues are shown for 2 paired experiments. Cyclic AMP accumulation due to norepinephrine and adenosine deaminase was 3 nmol/g and FFA release was 0.35 μmol/ml after 10 min in the absence of theophylline.

accumulation caused by 100 nM PIA was not reversed by the addition of theophylline. However, the inhibition of lipolysis by 100 nM PIA was reversed by theophylline. These data illustrate again the lack of correlation between total cyclic AMP accumulation and lipolysis and suggest that either there is dissociation between cyclic AMP and lipolysis or the pool of cyclic AMP involved in lipolysis is rather small.

The addition of 2′,5′-dideoxyadenosine at concentrations between 10 and 53,000 nM gave an inhibition of cyclic AMP accumulation equivalent to 3.3–100 nM PIA. However, the inhibitory effect of 2′,5′-dideoxyadenosine was not reversed by theophylline addition, which supports the hypothesis that dideoxyadenosine does not act at the same site as adenosine. We conclude that dideoxyadenosine inhibits an adenylate cyclase that is not involved in the regulation of lipolysis and is unaffected by methylxanthines.

Inhibition of adenosine action by methylxanthines might result from the interference with adenosine binding to a regulatory site on plasma membrane. The total uptake of tritiated adenosine by isolated fat cells was inhibited markedly by concentrations of theophylline that affect cyclic AMP accumulation (Fig. 4). 1-Methyl, 3-isobutylxanthine was more potent than theophylline in inhibiting the total uptake of adenosine by white fat cells (Fig. 4) and in activating lipolysis by fat cells (9). Uptake was measured by a filtration procedure in which fat cells were incubated with adenosine for only 20 s (the methylxanthines were added 5 s before the adenosine) and then rapidly filtered onto glass fiber disks. Uptake represents label that was not readily removed by washing the cells.

There was a near-maximal uptake or binding of free adenosine at the zero-time value (Fig. 5), which represents the time required to rapidly filter

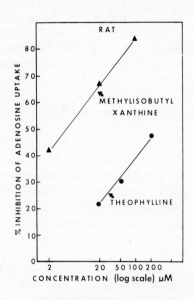

FIG. 4. Inhibition of adenosine uptake by 1-methyl, 3-isobutylxanthine and theophylline. Rat fat cells (37 mg/0.1 ml) were incubated for 20 s in buffer containing 0.1 μM tritiated adenosine. Xanthines were added 5 s before adenosine. Values are shown as percentage inhibition of total adenosine uptake and incorporation into fat cells and are the means of 3 paired experiments. Total uptake of adenosine label by fat cells was 1.8% of the amount present in the medium. Uptake was measured by a rapid filtration procedure in which the cells were diluted with 3 ml of ice-cold buffer at the end of incubation and immediately poured onto the middle of a prewetted 55-mm glass fiber filter disk in a filter holder mounted on a vacuum flask connected to a rotary vacuum pump. Loosely bound label was removed by rapid washing with 6 ml of buffer.

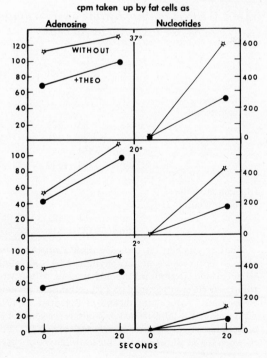

FIG. 5. Effect of temperature on adenosine uptake. Rat fat cells (45 mg/0.1 ml) were incubated for the times indicated at 2, 20, or 37°C. Theophylline (200 μM) was added 5 s prior to 10 μM [2-^{3}H]adenosine. Counts per minute present as adenosine or nucleotides (ATP, ADP, IMP, and AMP) were determined after thin-layer chromatography on PEI cellulose of perchloric acid extracts concentrated on Norit-A columns. Perchloric acid extracts were obtained by extracting cells, filtered onto glass fiber disks as described in Figure 4, with 1 N perchloric acid. Extracts were added to 3 x 75-mm columns containing equal parts of acid-washed charcoal (Norit A) and Celite. Nucleotides and nucleosides were eluted with 50% pyridine after the columns were washed twice with two 3-ml aliquots of water.

the fat cells onto the disks and wash them. If the temperature at which the fat cells were incubated was reduced to 2°C there was only a 30% reduction in free adenosine binding at the zero-time value. Theophylline added 5 s before the labeled adenosine inhibited its binding to cells at the zero-time value. Theophylline was just as effective at 2 or 37°C.

The uptake of adenosine into nucleotides at 20 s was depressed by theophylline at all temperatures and greatly reduced by lowering of the temperature (Fig. 5). No incorporation of adenosine into nucleotides was detectable in the zero-time controls. However, by 20 s at 37°C there was 4–5 times more label present in nucleotides than there was free adenosine (Fig. 5 and Table 4).

The inhibitory effect of theophylline on free adenosine accumulation was transitory and disappeared at 1 min (Table 4). An inhibition of adenosine incorporation into nucleotides, particularly AMP, was seen at all time intervals from 10 s to 5 min. Thus, in intact cells there is a rapid accumulation of adenosine that is transiently inhibited by methylxanthines.

In the experiments shown in Figure 4 the concentration of adenosine was 0.1 μM; in those shown in Figure 5 and Table 4 it was 10 μM. Table 5 indicates that after 5 min of incubation the total uptake of labeled adenosine was linear between adenosine concentrations of 0.1 and 10 μM. The accumulation of free adenosine was a small part of total uptake and was not saturated by raising the adenosine concentration to 1000 μM (Table 5). This indicates that after 5 min of incubation there is apparently equilibration between external and internal adenosine pools. The falloff in uptake at

TABLE 4. *Effect of theophylline on distribution of labeled [2-³H]adenosine taken up by fat cells*

	Time	Without					+ Theophylline, 200 μM				
		ATP, ADP, IMP	AMP	Inosine	HX	Adeno-sine	ATP, ADP, IMP	AMP	Inosine	HX	Adeno-sine
Rat fat cells, counts/min											
	10 s	66	225	16	67	182	23	92	4	10	93
	20 s	120	401	10	28	125	49	155	15	7	78
	1 min	254	657	32	36	153	143	362	32	43	142
	5 min	1206	1540	53	71	152	1037	924	74	79	229
Chicken fat cells, counts/min											
	1 min	84	131	169	137	190	59	101	161	157	183
	5 min	527	612	252	209	201	396	376	193	216	163

Rat or chicken fat cells (50 mg/0.1 ml) were incubated for 10, 20, 60, or 300 s in the absence or presence of theophylline (200 μM) added 5 s prior to addition of 10 μM [2-³H]adenosine. Counts per minute present as the various compounds were determined after thin-layer chromatography on PEI cellulose of perchloric acid extracts concentrated on Norit-A columns. Values are means of 2 paired experiments. Counts per minute present as adenosine in rat fat cells at 1 or 5 min represented 0.3% uptake of medium adenosine. Uptake of 3-O-methylglucose after 30 min was also 0.3%, indicating that adenosine had equilibrated between the medium and the intracellular water space.

TABLE 5. *Effect of varying adenosine concentration in medium on uptake of labeled adenosine by rat fat cells*

Concentration of Added Adenosine, μM	Total Label Taken Up, counts/min	Adenosine Uptake, counts/min
0.1	960	40
1.0	820	36
10.0	840	28
100.0	370	32
1000.0	270	38

Rat fat cells (50 mg/tube) were incubated for 5 min in 0.1 ml of buffer containing 0.10, 1, 10, 100, or 1000 μM adenosine and 10,000 counts/min [2-^{3}H]adenosine. The counts per minute present as adenosine were determined by thin-layer chromatography on PEI cellulose of extracts concentrated on Norit-A columns.

adenosine concentrations of 100 and 1000 μM probably reflects saturation of the enzymatic processes for metabolism of adenosine. Uptake of adenosine after 20 s at adenosine concentrations between 0.1 and 1000 μM displays the same percentage inhibition as that due to theophylline (data not shown).

Recently we have developed a new approach to the study of adenosine action by measuring adenosine binding to rat fat cell membrane fractions. These studies can only be done in the presence of an inhibitor of adenosine deaminase because of appreciable deamination of adenosine by fat cell membrane preparations. There appear to be the same number of binding sites for adenosine as for tritiated dihydroalprenolol (putative β-adrenergic receptors) when either is added at a concentration of 10 or 100 nM. No competition for binding between the two compounds is demonstrable. There was an 18% inhibition of adenosine binding by 1 μM theophylline and a 43% inhibition by 10 μM theophylline (26).

Further support for the hypothesis that methylxanthines might act as adenosine antagonists comes from studies with chicken fat cells. Figure 6 illustrates that neither theophylline nor adenosine deaminase activated chicken fat cell lipolysis under conditions where there was a marked acceleration of rat fat cell lipolysis. Previously it was shown that theophylline at various concentrations had little effect on lipolysis or cyclic AMP accumulation in chicken fat cells (3). Glucagon alone maximally activated cyclic AMP accumulation in chicken fat cells and there was little further acceleration by methylxanthines or adenosine deaminase. Our hypothesis is that in chicken fat cells there is no adenosine for methylxanthines to antagonize or for adenosine deaminase to remove.

We found that chicken fat cells rapidly metabolized added adenosine to inosine and released little adenosine compared with rat fat cells (17). This is also illustrated in Table 4, where adenosine conversion to inosine and hypoxanthine was considerably greater in chicken than in rat fat cells.

Another possibility is that chicken fat cells are insensitive to adenosine, but this is not the case. The addition of PIA or adenosine bound to stachyose, neither of which can be deaminated, reduced cyclic AMP accumulation by chicken fat cells incubated with glucagon (17). Chicken fat cells were just as sensitive to these analogues of adenosine as rat fat cells (17), indicating that

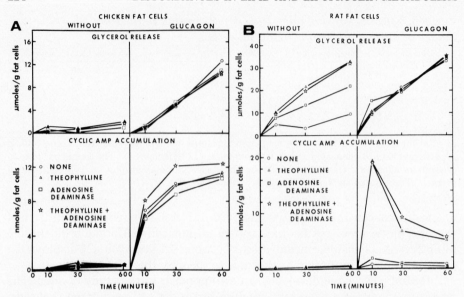

FIG. 6. Time course of effects of glucagon, theophylline, and adenosine deaminase on cyclic AMP accumulation and glycerol release in chicken and rat fat cells. Fat cells from chickens (*A*, 23 mg/tube) or rats (*B*, 16 mg/tube) were incubated for either 10, 30, or 60 min with the addition of 1000 ng/ml glucagon, 100 μM theophylline, or 0.5 μg adenosine deaminase/ml. Values shown are means of 3 experiments done in duplicate.

chicken fat cells respond to adenosine when it is present. Furthermore, there was a reversal by methylxanthines of the decrease in cyclic AMP accumulation due to the adenosine analogues (17).

Our conclusion is that adenosine is always present in rat fat cells and restrains adenylate cyclase, which accounts for the inability of lipolytic agents alone to maximally increase cyclic AMP. The large potentiations of cyclic AMP by methylxanthines may be due to reversal of adenosine restraint of adenylate cyclase by competition with adenosine for binding to a site that regulates adenylate cyclase.

FREE FATTY ACIDS AS FEEDBACK REGULATORS OF ADENYLATE CYCLASE

Adenosine apparently is not the major feedback regulator of cyclic AMP accumulation released during incubation of rat fat cells with lipolytic agents. Fain and Shepherd (16) found that a potent inhibitor of cyclic AMP accumulation was released to the medium in the presence of lipolytic agents that was not inactivated by adenosine deaminase. This inhibitor also differed from adenosine in that it was nondialyzable.

Ho and Sutherland (24) and Manganiello et al. (29) reported that incubation of rat fat cells with lipolytic agents resulted in the formation of antagonists that blocked the ability of cells to elevate cyclic AMP in response to a second addition of hormone. The antagonists that accumulated in the presence of epinephrine were not hormone specific since they blocked the subsequent response to ACTH and glucagon. The response of cells incubated with lipolytic agents was restored by washing the cells and incubating them in fresh buffer (24, 29). The antagonists do not affect cyclic AMP phosphodiesterase activity (32), in agreement with the initial report of Manganiello et al. (30).

Illiano and Cuatrecasas (25) postulated that prostaglandins were physiologically important feedback regulators of lipolysis based on studies with indomethacin. This drug has been shown to effectively block prostaglandin formation in rat fat cells by Dalton and Hope (8). However, Fain et al. (14), Dalton and Hope (7), and Fredholm and Hedquist (19) were unable to find any potentiation of lipolysis or cyclic AMP accumulation by indomethacin in studies with rat fat cells. The available data do not support the hypothesis that prostaglandins are important feedback regulators of lipolysis and cyclic AMP accumulation by rat fat cells.

Gorman (20) suggested that prostaglandin endoperoxide intermediates rather than prostaglandins act as feedback regulators of cyclic AMP accumulation. Gorman et al. (21) reported that prostaglandin H_2 (PGH$_2$: 15-hydroxy-9-peroxidoprosta-5, 13-dienoic acid) at 0.28–28 μM inhibited adenylate cyclase activity of fat cell ghosts. The real question is whether indomethacin also inhibits the formation of prostaglandin endoperoxides. In the tissues tested, indomethacin blocked endoperoxide formation as well as that of prostaglandins (23).

The fatty acids released to the medium during the activation of lipolysis by hormones appear to be the major feedback regulators of adenylate cyclase (16, 28). The important factor is the ratio of FFA to albumin in the medium. Rodbell (33) first demonstrated that lipolysis by isolated fat cells in the presence of hormones virtually ceases when the ratio of FFA to albumin exceeds 3. Only recently have we realized that if the primary binding sites on medium albumin are saturated with FFAs there is an inhibition of both adenylate cyclase and triglyceride lipase.

Burns et al. (4) first reported inhibition of cyclic AMP accumulation by free fatty acids. They incubated human fat cells with medium containing enough added sodium oleate to give an FFA:albumin ratio of 2.3–3 and found marked inhibition of cyclic AMP accumulation. There was little stimulation of cyclic AMP accumulation in human fat cells by lipolytic agents unless albumin was present in the medium.

Medium in which rat fat cells had previously been incubated with lipolytic agents or added free fatty acids markedly inhibited cyclic AMP accumulation by a fresh batch of fat cells (16). Sodium oleate added to the medium in amounts sufficient to raise the FFA:albumin ratio above 2 also inhibited cyclic AMP accumulation, with the maximal inhibition occurring at a ratio of 6 (16).

The inhibition of cyclic AMP accumulation by FFA:albumin ratios above 2 was rapid in onset, with near-maximal effects after only 30 s (16). This suggested that fatty acids directly inhibit adenylate cyclase. Fain and Shepherd (16) reported a direct inhibition of hormone-sensitive adenylate cyclase activity of rat fat cell ghosts by dialyzed medium previously incubated with fat cells in the presence of lipolytic agents. The effects of the medium could be mimicked by addition of oleate to fat cell ghosts in amounts sufficient to raise the fatty acid:albumin ratio above 2 and maximal inhibition was seen at a ratio of 6 (Fig. 7).

Rodbell (34) demonstrated that Gpp(NH)p is a potent activator of adenylate cyclase in fat cells. The increase in cyclase due to Gpp(NH)p is slow in onset and irreversible after prolonged incubation. Interestingly, we found that oleate enhanced the activation of adenylate cyclase by Gpp(NH)p under conditions in which it inhibited activation due to norepinephrine and had little effect on that due to fluoride (Fig. 8). The most striking differences were seen during the first 5 min of incubation. Oleate reduced the lag period required before cyclase was activated by the guanine nucleotide. Possibly oleate interferes with the binding of catecholamines to their receptor or interferes with the activation of adenylate cyclase by the catecholamine-receptor complex.

Further support for the hypothesis that FFAs can be important feedback regulators of adenylate cyclase comes from studies with chicken fat cells (28). In chicken fat cells glucagon alone produced a large rise in cyclic AMP that was maintained over incubation periods of up to 1 h (Fig. 6). This suggested that chicken fat cells might not show the feedback regulation of cyclic AMP accumulation by lipolytic agents that is observed readily in rat fat cells.

The addition of enough sodium oleate to raise the FFA:albumin ratio to 7 did not affect the level of cyclic AMP in chicken fat cells under conditions in which cyclic AMP accumulation by rat fat cells was markedly reduced (28). Furthermore, FFA:albumin ratios as high as 12 did not inhibit adenylate cyclase activity of chicken fat cell ghosts (Fig. 7).

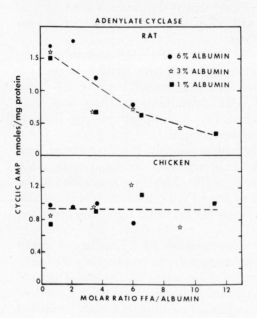

FIG. 7. Failure of oleate to inhibit adenylate cyclase activity of chicken fat cell ghosts. Rat fat cell ghosts (76 μg of protein/tube) and chicken fat cell ghosts (24 μg of protein/tube) were isolated on the same day. Ghosts were incubated for 10 min in the presence of 5 μg of glucagon/ml. Cyclic AMP accumulation in the absence of glucagon was less than 0.1 nmol/mg of protein. Medium contained 15 μl of 6% albumin (filled circles), 3% albumin (stars), or 1% albumin (filled squares) without or with added oleate plus 85 μl of other additions in albumin-free buffer. Values are means of 3 experiments with rat ghosts and 2 with chicken fat cell ghosts. [From Malgieri et al. (28).]

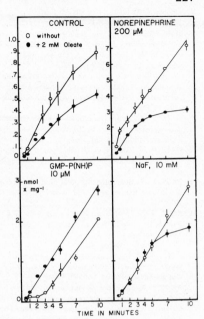

FIG. 8. Effect of oleate on activation of adenylate cyclase. Fat cell ghosts (46 μg of protein/tube) were incubated at 37°C without or with 200 μM norepinephrine, 10 μM Gpp(NH)p, or 10 mM NaF in the absence (open squares) or presence (filled squares) of 2 mM oleate for designated times. Values are expressed as nanomoles of cyclic AMP formed per milligram of protein and represent means of 3 experiments. [Data from Shepherd and Fain, unpublished observations.]

This chapter has reviewed the hormonal activation of lipolysis in fat cells with particular emphasis on the role of cyclic AMP. There is adequate evidence that cyclic AMP can activate lipolysis (38), but there is no proof that it is the sole regulator of lipolysis. Three aspects of the regulation of cyclic AMP accumulation and lipolysis have been emphasized: *1*) the lack of correlation between maximal cyclic AMP accumulation and lipolysis; *2*) the possibility that adenylate cyclase is ordinarily restrained by adenosine in rat fat cells and that some of the methylxanthine effects are due to antagonism of adenosine; *3*) the evidence that FFAs released during lipolysis act as product inhibitors of triglyceride lipase and feedback regulators of adenylate cyclase when the primary FA-binding sites on albumin are saturated.

The authors' work is supported by Research Grant AM 10149 from the National Institute of Arthritis, Metabolism, and Digestive Diseases. C. C. Malbon is the recipient of a postdoctoral fellowship (AM05425) from the National Institute of Arthritis, Metabolism, and Digestive Diseases. F. J. Moreno is the recipient of a Fulbright Fellowship from the Spanish government; his permanent address is: Departamento de Bioquimica y Biologia Molecular, Univ. Autonoma, Madrid, Spain.

REFERENCES

1. ARMSTRONG, K. J., J. E. STOUFFER, R. G. VAN INWEGEN, W. J. THOMPSON, AND G. A. ROBISON. Effect of thyroid hormone deficiency on cyclic adenosine 3'5'-monophosphate and control of lipolysis in fat cells. *J. Biol. Chem.* 249: 4226–4231, 1974.

2. BERNE, R. M., R. RUBIO, AND R. C. DULING. Vasoactive substances affecting the coronary circulation. In:

Myocardial Ischemia. Amsterdam: Excerpta Med. Found., 1971, p. 28–43.

3. BOYD, T. A., P. B. WEISER, AND J. N. FAIN. Lipolysis and cyclic AMP accumulation in isolated fat cells from chicks. *Gen. Comp. Endocrinol.* 26: 243–247, 1975.

4. BURNS, T. W., P. E. LANGLEY, AND G. A. ROBISON. Site of free-fatty-acid inhibition of lipolysis by human

adipocytes. *Metabolism* 24: 265–276, 1975.

5. BUTCHER, R. W., AND C. E. BAIRD. The regulation of cyclic AMP and lipolysis in adipose tissue by hormones and other agents. In: *Drugs Affecting Lipid Metabolism*, edited by W. L. Holmes, L. A. Carlson, and R. Paoletti. New York: Plenum, 1969, p. 5–23..

6. CALDWELL, A., AND J. N. FAIN. Triiodothyronine stimulation of cyclic adenosine 3′5′-monophosphate accumulation in white fat cells. *Endocrinology* 89: 1195–1204, 1971.

7. DALTON, C. AND H. R. HOPE. Inability of prostaglandin synthesis inhibitors to affect adipose tissue lipolysis. *Prostaglandins* 4: 641–651, 1973.

8. DALTON, C., AND W. C. HOPE. Cyclic AMP regulation of prostaglandin biosynthesis in fat cells. *Prostaglandins* 6: 227–242, 1974.

9. FAIN, J. N. Biochemical aspects of drug and hormone action on adipose tissue. *Pharmacol. Rev.* 25: 67–118, 1973.

10. FAIN, J. N. Inhibition of adenosine cyclic 3′,5′-monophosphate accumulation in fat cells by adenosine, N^6 (phenylisopropyl) adenosine, and related compounds. *Mol. Pharmacol.* 9: 595–604, 1973.

11. FAIN, J. N. Cyclic nucleotides in adipose tissue. In: *Cyclic Nucleotides: Mechanisms of Action*, edited by H. Cramer and J. Schultz. London: Wiley, 1977, p. 207–228.

12. FAIN, J. N. Inhibition of glucose transport in fat cells and activation of lipolysis by glucocorticoids. In: *Mechanisms of Glucocorticoid Hormone Action*, edited by J. D. Baxter and G. G. Rousseau. Berlin: Springer-Verlag, in press.

13. FAIN, J. N., R. H. POINTER, AND W. F. WARD. Effects of adenosine nucleotides on adenylate cyclase, phosphodiesterase, cyclic adenosine monophosphate accumulation, and lipolysis in fat cells. *J. Biol. Chem.* 247: 6866–6872, 1972.

14. FAIN, J. N., S. PSYCHOYOS, A. J. CZERNIK, S. FROST, AND W. D. CASH. Indomethacin, lipolysis and cyclic AMP accumulation in white fat cells. *Endocrinology* 93: 632–639, 1973.

15. FAIN, J. N., AND R. SAPERSTEIN. The involvement of RNA synthesis and cyclic AMP in the activation of fat cell lipolysis by growth hormone and glucocorticoids. In: *Adipose Tissue: Regulation and Metabolic Functions*, edited by B. Jeanrenaud and D. Hepp. New York: Academic, 1970, p. 20–27.

16. FAIN, J. N., AND R. E. SHEPHERD. Free fatty acids as feedback regulators of adenylate cyclase and cyclic 3′:5′-AMP accumulation in rat fat cells. *J. Biol. Chem.* 250: 6586–6592, 1975.

17. FAIN, J. N., AND R. E. SHEPHERD. Hormonal regulation of lipolysis: role of cyclic nucleotide, adenosine and free fatty acids. In: *Proceedings of the Midwest Regional Conference on Endocrinology and Metabolism*. New York: Plenum, in press.

18. FREDHOLM, B. B. Release of adenosine-like material from isolated perfused dog adipose tissue following sympathetic nerve stimulation and its inhibition by adrenergic α-receptor blockade. *Acta Physiol. Scand.* 96: 422–430, 1976.

19. FREHDOLM, B. B., AND P. HEDQVIST. Indomethacin and the role of prostaglandins in adipose tissue. *Biochem. Pharmacol.* 24: 61–66, 1975.

20. GORMAN, R. R. Prostaglandin endoperoxides: possible new regulators of cyclic nucleotide metabolism. *J. Cyclic Nucleotide Res.* 1: 1–9, 1975.

21. GORMAN, R. R., M. HAMBERG, AND B. SAMUELSSON. Inhibition of basal and hormone-stimulated aden-

ylate cyclase in adipocyte ghosts by the prostaglandin endoperoxide prostaglandin H_2. *J. Biol. Chem.* 250: 6460–6463, 1975.

22. GORMAN, R. R., H. M. TEPPERMAN, AND J. TEPPERMAN. Epinephrine binding and the selective restoration of adenylate cyclase activity in fat-fed rats. *J. Lipid Res.* 14: 279–285, 1973.

23. HAMBERG, M., AND B. SAMUELSSON. Prostaglandin endoperoxides. Novel transformations of arachidonic acid in human platelets. *Proc. Natl. Acad. Sci. U.S.* 71: 3400–3404, 1974.

24. HO, R. J., AND E. W. SUTHERLAND. Formation and release of a hormone antagonist by rat adipocytes. *J. Biol. Chem.* 246: 6822–6827, 1971.

25. ILLIANO, G., AND P. CUATRECASAS. Endogenous prostaglandins modulate lipolytic processes in adipose tissue. *Nature New Biol.* 234: 72–74, 1971.

26. MALBON, C. C., AND J. N. FAIN. Binding of [³H]adenosine to crude rat adipocyte membranes: inhibition by theophylline. *Federation Proc.* 36: 710, 1977.

27. MALBON, C. C., F. J. MORENO, R. J. CABELLI, AND J. N. FAIN. Fat cell beta-adrenergic receptors and adenylate cyclase in altered thyroid states. *J. Biol. Chem.* In press.

28. MALGIERI, J. A., R. E. SHEPHERD, AND J. N. FAIN. Lack of feedback regulation of cyclic 3′:5′-AMP accumulation by free fatty acids in chicken fat cells. *J. Biol. Chem.* 250: 6593–6598, 1975.

29. MANGANIELLO, V., F. MURAD, AND M. VAUGHAN. Effects of lipolytic and antilipolytic agents on 3′:5′-adenosine monophosphate in fat cells. *J. Biol. Chem.* 246: 2195–2202, 1971.

30. MANGANIELLO, V., AND M. VAUGHAN. An effect of insulin on cyclic adenosine 3′:5′-monophosphate phosphodiesterase activity in fat cells. *J. Biol. Chem.* 248: 7164–7170, 1973.

31. OLSSON, R. A., C. J. DAVIS, E. M. KHOURI, AND R. E. PATTERSON. Evidence for an adenosine receptor on the surface of dog coronary myocytes. *Circulation Res.* 39: 93–98, 1976.

32. PAWLSON, L. G., C. J. LOVELL-SMITH, V. C. MANGANIELLO, AND M. VAUGHAN. Effects of epinephrine, adrenocorticotrophic hormone, and theophylline on adenosine 3′:5′-monophosphate phosphodiesterase activity in fat cells. *Proc. Natl. Acad. Sci. US* 71: 1639–1642, 1974.

33. RODBELL, M. Modulation of lipolysis in adipose tissue by fatty acid concentration in fat cell. *Ann. N.Y. Acad. Sci.* 131: 302–333, 1965.

34. RODBELL, M. On the mechanism of activation of fat cell adenylate cyclase by guanine nucleotides. *J. Biol. Chem.* 250: 5826–5834, 1975.

35. SAHYOUN, H., C. J. SCHMITGES, M. I. SIEGEL, AND P. CUATRECASAS. Inhibition of fat cell membrane adenylate cyclase by 2′-deoxyadenosine-3′-monophosphate. *Life Sci.* 19: 1971–1980, 1976.

36. SCHWABE, U., R. EBERT, AND H. C. ERBLER. Adenosine release from isolated fat cells and its significance for the effects of hormones on cyclic 3′:5′-AMP levels and lipolysis. *Arch. Pharmacol.* 276: 133–148, 1973.

37. SHEPHERD, R. E., C. C. MALBON, C. J. SMITH, AND J. N. FAIN. Lipolysis and adenosine 3′5′-cyclic AMP metabolism in isolated fat cells from obese hyperglycemic mice (*ob/ob*). *J. Biol. Chem.* In press.

38. STEINBERG, D. L. Interconvertible enzymes in adipose tissue regulated by cyclic AMP-dependent protein kinase. *Advan. Cyclic Nucleotide Res.* 7: 157–198, 1976.

14

Transport of Fatty Acid in the Circulation

ARTHUR A. SPECTOR AND JOHN E. FLETCHER

Department of Biochemistry and Arteriosclerosis Specialized Center of Research, University of Iowa, Iowa City, Iowa; and Laboratory of Applied Studies, Division of Computer Research and Technology, National Institutes of Health, Bethesda, Maryland

TWO CLASSES OF FATTY ACIDS are present in the circulation. One is the covalently bonded form, in which the carboxyl group is chemically linked with another molecule. Examples of this class are the esterified fatty acids present in triacylglycerols, phosphoglycerides, and cholesteryl esters and the amide-linked fatty acids present in sphingolipids. Essentially all the covalently bonded fatty acids are contained in the plasma lipoproteins. The second class of circulatory fatty acid is the unesterified form, in which the carboxyl group is not covalently combined and exists almost entirely in anionic form. This class is known commonly as free fatty acid (FFA). The terminology implies that the carboxyl group is free and not that the fatty acid exists freely dissolved in the aqueous solution. In fact, more than 99% of the FFA present in the circulation exists as a complex physically bound to components of the circulation. For the most part, the FFAs are bound to plasma albumin (47). Free fatty acid is the form in which fat is released from adipocytes for utilization elsewhere in the body. Some FFA also is released into the circulation during the hydrolysis of lipoprotein triglycerides. Although present in the plasma in relatively low concentrations, it is a major source of fat for many tissues. This is due to the fact that the half-life of the plasma FFA is only about 1–2 min. In addition to its role in energy metabolism and in supplying fatty acids for membrane production and replacement, the plasma FFA may produce pathological effects when present in abnormally high concentrations. It also appears to be an important source of fat for many tumors (48). Because of these important physiological and pathological considerations, FFA transport in the circulation is a topic of continuing interest and active investigation.

Fatty acids bind to many components of the blood. For example, they bind to plasma lipoproteins of $d < 1.019$ and 1.019–1.063 (17). They also bind to erythrocytes, platelets, and leukocytes (5, 16, 49, 51). Under the usual circumstances, however, all these components make only a very minor contribution to FFA transport, and plasma albumin carries essentially all the FFA present in the circulation (47).

ALBUMIN STRUCTURE

Plasma albumin is composed of a single polypeptide chain and has a molecular weight of about 66,200. The primary amino acid sequence is known for both human and bovine albumin (4). A schematic representation of the structure of human albumin, adapted from the work of Brown (4) and Peters (33), is shown in Figure 1. Except for a few minor differences, the overall structures of human and bovine albumin are nearly identical, and much of the data obtained with one of these proteins should be applicable to the other. An important exception is spectroscopic data based on tryptophan emissions or absorbance. As seen in Figure 1, human albumin contains only one tryptophan residue, this being at position 213. Bovine albumin has two tryptophan residues, at positions 134 and 212. Therefore, fluorescence results with bovine and human albumins often are different (38, 39, 52). The advantage of the use of human albumins for these types of studies is that any event that causes a change in tryptophan fluorescence must be associated with a structural change in the region of the protein containing the tryptophan residue.

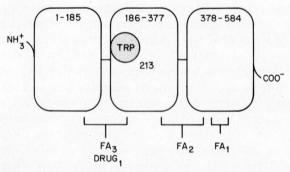

FIG. 1. Schematic representation of tertiary structure of human plasma albumin. This model is an adaptation of the work of Brown (4). The suggested localization of the major fatty acid- and drug-binding sites is based on the fragment studies with bovine albumin by Peters (33).

An important insight gained from the structural studies was the recognition that albumin contains many repeating sequences. From the standpoint of tertiary structure, the protein behaves as if it were composed of three cylindrical subunits. These are not true subunits, for they are joined together by the continuous polypeptide chain. In order to make this distinction, they have been called domains (4). Domain 1 comprises the amino-terminal region of the protein, domain 2 the central region, and domain 3 the carboxyl-terminal region. According to the tertiary structure postulated by Brown (4), the single tryptophan residue of human albumin is in domain 2, located in such a way that it forms part of the interfacial region between domains 1 and 2.

Based on this tertiary structure, several conjectures might be made about the binding properties of plasma albumin. First, the subunit-type structure suggests that the protein may have more than one binding site for a given compound. Second, because of the repeating structure, two or more of the sites may have similar properties, enabling them to be separated into a functionally similar group or class. Finally, because more than one site is present, it may be possible for the protein to bind small amounts of two different substances in a fairly independent manner so that the presence of one would have little effect on the binding of the other. As described, later all these properties actually can be demonstrated for plasma albumin.

FATTY ACID BINDING

Figure 2 illustrates the binding of a long-chain fatty acid (oleic) to human plasma albumin defatted by charcoal treatment (6). These data are displayed in the form of a Scatchard plot. Several important conclusions can be drawn from these results. One is that an albumin molecule has many sites that can bind fatty acid, for more than 10 mol of oleate were bound per mole of albumin in this experiment. This agrees with the observations concerning the protein tertiary structure and the expectation that the molecule would contain multiple binding sites. Another concerns the negative curvature of the Scatchard plot. Electrostatic interactions are too small to account for the nonlinearity (46). Therefore, the nonlinearity indicates

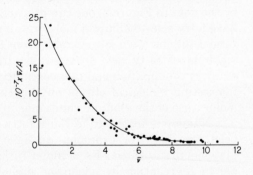

FIG. 2. Scatchard plot of oleate binding to defatted human serum albumin. These measurements were made at 37°C in a buffer solution containing 122 mM NaCl, 4.9 mM KCl, 1.2 mM MgSO$_4$, and 16 mM Na$_2$HPO$_4$ adjusted to pH 7.4 with 0.1 N HCl. Abbreviations are $\bar{\nu}$, molar ratio of oleate to albumin, and A, unbound oleate concentration in molarity. A represents total unbound oleate concentration, and no corrections have been made for the presence of either the undissociated acid form or aggregated forms such as dimers.

that the binding sites must be heterogeneous. On the other hand, these data can be represented by a sum of terms, each of which represents a class or group of similar sites. Each term in this representation would itself produce a straight line in Figure 2, but no single term would necessarily fit a given segment of the binding data (11, 53). This led to the concept that albumin contains groups of similar binding sites. With this type of analysis, there is general agreement that at least three classes of sites are required to fit the binding data obtained with long-chain fatty acids (15, 53). There is some uncertainty, however, as to the number of sites within each of the three classes. The earlier data were interpreted to indicate the presence of two primary and four or five secondary sites (15). Our data indicated that a slightly better fit was obtained with a model having three primary and three secondary sites (53). Based on our subsequent studies with a series of fatty acids, we believe that any grouping of the binding sites in this manner is somewhat arbitrary and, from a mechanistic standpoint, that it makes little difference which of the models is accepted. The final general conclusion from these data concerns the fact that the Scatchard plot of the binding curve is decreasing everywhere. This establishes that strong positive cooperative binding effects, such as occur when oxygen binds to hemoglobin, do not occur when long-chain fatty acids bind to albumin. It is entirely possible, however, that small positive cooperative effects or negative cooperative effects may be associated with the molecular mechanism of binding. We have demonstrated mathematically that these various possibilities cannot be identified unequivocally from equilibrium binding data like those presented in Figure 2 (11, 13).

BIOLOGICAL EFFECTS OF FREE FATTY ACIDS

Most of the fatty acids in animals contain 16 or more carbon atoms. Therefore, most biological studies with fatty acids require the use of these long-chain compounds. These fatty acids, however, are extremely insoluble in the aqueous media employed for biological work. In order to overcome this difficulty, the fatty acids usually are bound to albumin. This enables the investigator to dissolve large quantities of long-chain fatty acids such as palmitate or oleate into all types of aqueous buffer solutions. As suggested by the data in Figure 2, one can prepare stable, optically clear solutions that have fatty acid-to-albumin molar ratios of 5 or more. The use of high-molar-ratio solutions often is preferable from the experimental standpoint, for the amounts of fatty acid incorporated by the tissues are greater and the analysis is simplified and more accurate (46). On the other hand, some very interesting biological effects have been produced by fatty acids when the molar ratio of the albumin solution is in the range of 3–6 or higher.

Numerous instances of these fatty acid-induced biological effects have been reported. For example, we have observed that exposure of human platelets to saturated FFA of molar ratios above 2 made them more susceptible to aggregation by adenosine diphosphate (21). When the molar ratio exceeded 3, FFA were found to be feedback regulators of adenylate cyclase in rat adipocytes (10). Free fatty acids also are reported to act as modulators of adenylate cyclase in turkey erythrocytes (32) and to stimulate guanylate cyclase (60). Palmitate at molar ratios between 4 and 8 inhibits chemotaxis and depresses phagocytosis and bactericidal ability of human neutrophils (19). Chemotaxis was 50% inhibited even at a molar ratio of 2. Oleate at molar ratios of 4 and above has been shown to alter the electrophoretic mobility of β-lipoproteins (18). Palmitate at a molar ratio of 5 enhances lactate dehydrogenase release from the perfused working rat heart (9), and linoleate at a molar ratio of about 3 depresses the contractility of rat papillary muscle preparations during hypoxia (20). Moreover, total plasma FFA concentrations of 4–5 meq/liter cause ventricular extrasystoles after myocardial infarction (22). Finally, FFAs added in an ethanol solution inhibit the Na^+-K^+-ATPase of rat brain (1). All these effects occurred in perfused organs, intact cells, or membrane preparations – that is, in systems ordinarily exposed to circulating FFA.

Membrane-Bound Free Fatty Acids

Our studies with ascites tumor cells and platelets suggest a mechanism for these effects. Fatty acids are transferred rapidly to cells when they are exposed to solutions containing FFA and albumin (46). A schematic representation of this process is shown in Figure 3. Most of the newly taken up fatty acid is either incorporated into cell lipid esters or oxidized as a source of energy. A small amount, however, remains associated with the cell in unesterified form. This cell FFA fraction undergoes continuous turnover and is constantly replaced by new FFA taken up from the extracellular fluid, provided that sufficient amounts of FFA are available to the cell (56). In this way, the amount present in the form of FFA remains in a relatively steady state. About 70% of the cell FFA content can be released rapidly if the cells are exposed to an albumin solution, suggesting that the bulk of this material is present in a location readily available to the extracellular fluid (46). Based on these considerations, we have postulated that this releasable fraction of the cell FFA is associated with the plasma membrane (57). Much of this material probably is embedded in the lipid bilayer of the membrane, although some may be associated with membrane proteins that contain

FIG. 3. Schematic representation of mechanism by which cells take up FFA from a solution containing plasma albumin. Abbreviations are: FA, free fatty acid; PL, phospholipids; CE, cholesteryl esters; GSL, glycosphingolipids; TG, triglycerides.

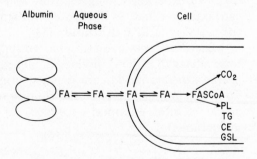

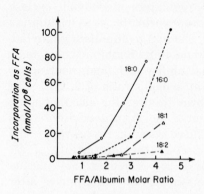

FIG. 4. Incorporation of fatty acids into the cell FFA pool. Ehrlich ascites cells were incubated in a solution containing 113 mM NaCl, 4 mM KCl, 1 mM $MgSO_4$, and 28 mM Na_2HPO_4 adjusted to pH 7.4 with 1 N HCl. The medium also contained 125 μM defatted bovine plasma albumin, 10 mM glucose, and various amounts of a radioactive fatty acid. Incubations were carried out at 37°C with air as the gas phase. Each flask contained 8×10^7 cells. After 60 min of incubation, cells were isolated from the medium by centrifugation and washed 3 times by dispersal in 40 ml of phosphate-buffered saline followed by centrifugation. Lipids were extracted with a chloroform-methanol solution and then separated by thin-layer chromatography. Radioactivity contained in the FFA band of the chromatogram was measured. Graph shows amount of radioactive FFA associated with the cells as a function of the FFA-to-albumin molar ratio in the incubation medium. This is a steady-state amount of cell radioactive FFA that remains relatively constant as incubation progresses, as long as the fatty acid content of the medium is not depleted excessively (19, 31). Specific radioactivity of the fatty acid added to the incubation medium was utilized to convert the isotope data into nanomoles of fatty acid. Each fatty acid tested is abbreviated as chain length:number of double bonds—i.e., 16:0, palmitate; 18:0, stearate; 18:1, oleate, 18:2 linoleate.

nonpolar binding sites. The demonstration of two classes of binding sites in human erythrocytes supports an interpretation involving a small number of strong protein sites and a very large number of weaker lipid sites (49).

Several factors regulate the amount of FFA that associates with the cell in unesterified form. As shown in Figure 4, one factor is the structure of the fatty acid. In general, the amount increases as the fatty acid chain length increases, and it decreases as the number of double bonds increases. Another factor is the molar ratio of FFA to albumin. In most cases, the accumulation is not appreciable until the molar ratio exceeds 3. Even with stearate, the cell FFA content is fairly low until the molar ratio exceeds 2. A third factor is the pH of the extracellular fluid. As the pH decreases below 7.4, the uptake as FFA at a given molar ratio increases (45). Other factors such as metabolic inhibitors or various energy substrates appear to have little influence on the uptake (57). The values in Figure 4 are steady-state quantities and should not be taken as rates of uptake for the various FFAs. In this system, the rates of uptake are too rapid to be measured accurately (57). Our experiments suggest that very rapid turnover of the cell FFA pool can occur and that, as illustrated in Figure 3, this pool is an intermediate in the pathway of FFA utilization (56).

Based on these observations, we suggest that many of the regulatory or toxic effects that FFAs produce in biological systems are due to the presence of excessive fatty acid in unesterified form associated with the cell membrane. The FFA may either alter the fluidity of the lipid bilayer or influence the action of vital enzymes, receptors, or transport systems located in the membrane.

Cytoplasmic Free Fatty Acids

As noted above, only about 70% of the newly incorporated FFA that remains in unesterified form can be removed rapidly when a cell is exposed to an albumin solution (46, 57). The remainder either is present at very strong binding sites within the membrane (49) or is actually inside the cell. Cytoplasmic proteins that are able to bind FFA exist in many cells. These have been given various names, including fatty acid-binding protein (30, 64) or Z protein (26). Their role in cellular metabolism is not completely understood. One idea is that they may be involved in FFA transport in the cell cytoplasm, much like albumin functions in the circulation (31). Another is that they actually may be binding proteins for intracellular nonpolar metabolites and coincidentally bind FFA because of structural similarities. In this context, the Z protein may be a regulator of long-chain acyl coenzyme A availability inside the cell (27). Likewise, at least one form of the sterol carrier protein is able to bind FFA (35). It is possible that the function of these or other intracellular proteins is compromised if they are overloaded with fatty acid, such as might occur when a cell is exposed to fatty acid bound to albumin at high molar ratios. Therefore, these cytoplasmic proteins also may be involved in certain of the toxic effects produced by high concentrations of FFA.

Physiological Range of Free Fatty Acid Concentrations

As shown in Figure 4, appreciable amounts of FFA do not accumulate in most cases unless the molar ratio of FFA to albumin is above 3. Furthermore, 65% of the plasma FFA usually is composed of unsaturated fatty acids (37), making it most unlikely that the pronounced effect of stearate is manifest under physiological conditions. Therefore, the crucial question in terms of physiological relevance of these effects is whether the molar ratio ever reaches high levels in the body. The available evidence indicates that this rarely occurs. Assuming that the plasma albumin concentration is 4 g/dl, the FFA concentration would have to be higher than 1.8 μeq/ml in order to exceed a molar ratio of 3. Most investigators report plasma FFA concentrations of about 0.5 μeq/ml in the basal state. After a carbohydrate load, the concentration decreases to 0.09–0.17 μeq/ml (41). The opposite extreme occurs after prolonged fasting, when values of about 1.2 μeq/ml have been measured (40). We have observed values as high as 2.4 μeq/ml between 5 and 15 min after the intravenous injection of heparin into patients with hypertriglyceridemia, but this is quite abnormal.

In summary, it is our interpretation that FFA concentrations in man hardly ever reach the levels at which injurious biological effects have been observed. Therefore, we think it unlikely that FFA exerts these kinds of regulatory actions under ordinary physiological conditions. Even in pathological situations, it is rare to have FFA concentrations rise to a level where they might be harmful. For these reasons, we feel that experimentally observed regulatory actions of FFA should be interpreted with extreme caution, at least in terms of physiological significance. Alternatively, as suggested by Orly and Schramm (32), it is perfectly reasonable to use the membrane-binding property of FFA as a probe to investigate various aspects of membrane function.

CALCULATION OF BINDING CONSTANTS

We have analyzed fatty acid binding to bovine and human albumin in terms of a model that describes the process by a series of multiple equilibrium reactions. This has been termed the stepwise equilibrium model (12) and is described by *equation 1*:

$$\nu = \frac{K_1[A] + 2K_1K_2[A]^2 + \cdots + NK_1K_2 \cdots K_n[A]^n}{1 + K_1[A] + K_1K_2[A]^2 + \cdots + K_1K_2 \cdots K_n[A]^n} \qquad (1)$$

In this formulation, ν is the molar ratio of fatty acid to albumin, K_i's are the individual binding constants, and A is the unbound fatty acid concentration in molarity at any given value of ν. The results of this type of analysis for the binding of several fatty acids to defatted human plasma albumin are listed in Table 1. More extensive data for both human and bovine albumins have been reported (2, 3, 50).

Several conclusions can be drawn from these data. First, the stoichiometric binding constants (K_i) for a given fatty acid generally occur in decreasing order of magnitude. This indicates that strong positive cooperative binding effects do not occur. However, the presence of some positive cooperativity or more likely some strong negative cooperative effects cannot be excluded. A similar conclusion is drawn from the Scatchard plot shown in Figure 2. Second, there are no large changes in magnitude in the adjacent constants K_{i-1}, K_i, and K_{i+1} among the derived values. This suggests that cooperative effects or dissimilar classes of sites do not produce abrupt

TABLE 1. *Stepwise association constants for fatty acid binding to defatted human plasma albumin*

Bound Fatty Acid	K_i, M^{-1}				
	Laurate	Palmitate	Stearate	Oleate	Linoleate
1	2.4×10^6	6.2×10^7	1.5×10^8	2.6×10^8	7.9×10^7
2	1.1×10^6	2.3×10^7	5.3×10^7	9.4×10^7	8.7×10^6
3	4.9×10^5	1.2×10^7	1.9×10^7	2.9×10^7	5.1×10^6
4	2.5×10^5	3.1×10^6	5.6×10^6	2.1×10^7	3.1×10^6
5	1.9×10^5	1.5×10^6	4.5×10^6	1.1×10^7	6.8×10^5
6	6.2×10^4	9.6×10^5	3.7×10^6	2.4×10^6	3.4×10^5

Values were obtained at 37°C in a solution containing 122 mM NaCl, 4.9 mM KCl, 1.2 mM MgSO$_4$, and 16 mM Na$_2$HPO$_4$ adjusted to pH 7.4 with 0.1 N HCl. Values are calculated assuming that no fatty acid association occurs in the aqueous solution and that the pK_a of the fatty acids is 4.8.

changes in the molecular mechanism of binding. Based on structural considerations (Fig. 1), however, there is reason to suspect that groups of similar binding sites may indeed exist. Finally, binding is dependent on the structure of the fatty acid hydrocarbon chain. The strength of binding increases as the chain length increases (lauric < palmitic < stearic). At a given chain length, the insertion of a single *cis* double bond increases the strength of binding (oleate > stearate). Insertion of a second double bond, however, reduces the strength of binding below that of the corresponding saturated fatty acid (linoleate < stearate).

These binding constants were obtained with a heptane-aqueous buffer partition system (53). Because of the possibility that hydrocarbon binding to albumin might interfere in some way with fatty acid binding, we compared the binding of decanoate using this method and the more widely used equilibrium-dialysis technique. Decanoate is the longest fatty acid for which we are able to obtain accurate results by equilibrium dialysis. Within the range of experimental error, we could not detect any difference in the decanoate binding results by the two methods (3). Any effect of the hydrocarbon should be more apparent with decanoate than with the longer chain fatty acids because the K_i values for decanoate are smaller (2). Based on this observation, it appears that the two-phase partition method does not introduce any serious error into the binding measurements.

All the values in Table 1 were calculated on the assumption that self-association of unbound fatty acid in the aqueous phase does not occur. As described below, this assumption may not be correct. If so, the magnitude of the individual K_i will change, but the qualitative relationships that have been presented probably will still be valid.

Fatty Acid Association in Aqueous Solutions

In order to present binding data in the form of the graph shown in Figure 2 or derive the constants listed in Table 1, two values are required, ν and A. These values can be derived from experimental binding measurements. The value of A that should be used is the unbound activity of the species that actually binds to the protein. What actually is measured is the total concentration of unbound material. In the case of fatty acids, it is the fatty acid anion that binds to albumin as shown in Figure 5. Therefore, the value needed for A in *equation 1* is the unbound fatty acid anion activity. It was thought previously that substitution of the total unbound fatty acid concentration for the unbound anion activity would not introduce serious errors for two reasons. First, the concentration value is not much different from the activity, which is much more difficult to measure. Second, it was assumed that the only other unbound species is the undissociated acid, abbreviated as *HA* in Figure 5. This assumption was based on the fact that the unbound fatty acid concentrations that were in equilibrium with the albumin complex were below the critical micellar concentration. Furthermore, the *HA* concentration should be negligibly small relative to the A^- concentration at the pH of the circulatory fluids, for the pK_a for this dissociation is about 4.8. Therefore, the assumption that the total unbound fatty acid concentration is an accurate approximation of the unbound A^- activity appeared to be acceptable in theory.

Actual distribution measurement, however, deviated systematically from the accepted partition theory (14). One possible explanation for this is the formation of anionic dimers (28), depicted as $A_2^=$ in Figure 5. Subsequently, other investigators have confirmed systematic deviations from the partition theory (42, 43), but their explanations have differed. Smith and Tanford (43) believe that the explanation involves the presence of aggregated species in the aqueous solution, but they were not able to identify the exact nature of these aggregated forms. Our data also could not be fitted to any precise combination of aggregated forms. Furthermore, we could not justify on theoretical grounds the formation of the postulated aggregates at these premicellar concentrations. Although we could not exclude the possibility that aggregation occurs, we suggested that the deviation from partition theory may be an artifact of the two-phase system in which the measurements were made (42). Therefore, the question of whether or not premicellar association actually occurs probably cannot be answered definitively at present.

This question needs to be resolved, for it has important consequences. For example, Table 2 lists the constants for the binding of palmitate and stearate to human albumin, assuming that fatty acid self-association in the aqueous phase occurs. The dimerization constants used in making these calculations for palmitate and stearate are 3.09×10^3 and 2.47×10^3, respectively (42). The albumin binding constants are about 4 times larger for palmitate and 8 times larger for stearate than the corresponding constants calculated without accounting for dimerization (Table 1). These large corrections would have a profound quantitative effect on comparisons of FFA binding constants with those of other ligands and on the calculation of membrane binding constants for long-chain FFA. They also would have qualitative importance, for tissues would be exposed to species such as $A_2^=$ and A^-HA if strong premicellar self-association actually occurs. In fact, possibly the very high uptake of fatty acid in the form of FFA that occurs when cells are exposed to palmitate or stearate at molar ratios above 3 (Fig. 4) may be due to the presence of large amounts of $A_2^=$ or A^-HA. Likewise, many of the injurious actions of FFA, which we suggest are due in part to FFA binding to the cell membrane, may result from the presence of associated forms in the aqueous solution. In terms of albumin binding, however, the qualitative patterns are not affected appreciably whether or

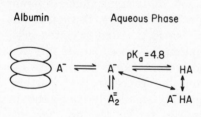

FIG. 5. Schematic representation of fatty acid binding to plasma albumin showing forms of unbound fatty acid postulated to exist in aqueous solution. Abbreviations are A^-, fatty acid anions; HA, undissociated fatty acid; A_2^-, fatty acid anionic dimer; A^-HA, mixed dimer of fatty acid anion and undissociated acid.

TABLE 2. *Stepwise association constants for fatty acid binding to defatted human plasma albumin in the presence of aqueous phase association*

Bound Fatty Acid	K_i, M^{-1}	
	Palmitate	Stearate
1	2.55×10^8	9.14×10^8
2	9.77×10^7	3.58×10^8
3	5.39×10^7	1.34×10^8
4	1.36×10^7	4.31×10^7
5	7.36×10^6	3.45×10^7
6	4.43×10^6	2.87×10^7

Conditions are the same as those described in Table 1.

not premicellar association occurs (3). Only the magnitude of the binding constants is affected. Therefore, the binding models described below are valid whether or not fatty acid self-association occurs.

FLUORESCENCE STUDIES

Human plasma albumin contains only one tryptophan residue located at position 213. Figure 1, based on the structural hypothesis suggested by Brown (4), illustrates that the tryptophan residue is thought to lie in the cleft between the first and second structural domains. Previous work indicates that this tryptophan residue forms a part of one of the strong anion binding sites of the protein (58). Studies with bovine serum albumin fragments also indicate that one of the strong fatty acid-binding sites is located in this region (33). Therefore, it should be possible to monitor certain aspects of the fatty acid-binding process by following the tryptophan fluorescence of the protein. The advantage of using human albumin is that, because it has only one tryptophan, any changes can be localized to a single region of the polypeptide chain.

When fatty acids are added to human albumin, there is a small blue shift in the wavelength of maximum fluorescence. No change in fluorescence intensity occurs, however, until the molar ratio exceeds 3. Thereafter, a small increase in fluorescence intensity is observed (52). Even though fatty acids themselves do not have much effect on the tryptophan fluorescence, they do influence the region of the protein containing the tryptophan residue. This is illustrated in Figure 6, which shows a portion of the tryptophan emission spectrum of defatted human plasma albumin. The emission is quenched considerably when KI is added to the solution. When palmitate also is added, the quenching produced by KI is reduced considerably. In the experiment shown in Figure 6, the molar ratio of palmitate to albumin was 5 and the KI was 100 mM.

Figure 7 shows the effects of KI concentration on this process. As the KI concentration is increased from 10 to 200 mM, quenching increases from 14 to 53% of the tryptophan fluorescence. Palmitate is effective in reducing

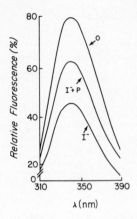

FIG. 6. Tryptophan fluorescence spectrum of human plasma albumin. Wavelength of excitation was 295 nm, and temperature of the cuvette was maintained at 25°C with a circulating water bath. All solutions contained 50 mM Na_2HPO_4 and 10 μM fatty acid-extracted albumin adjusted to pH 7.4. In addition, the media contained: O, 200 mM NaCl; I⁻, 100 mM NaCl, 100 mM KI; I⁻ + P, 100 mM NaCl, 100 mM KI, and 50 μM palmitate.

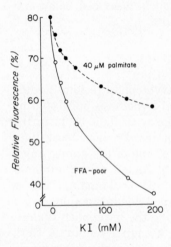

FIG. 7. Protective effect of fatty acid against quenching of tryptophan fluorescence of human albumin relative to iodide ion concentration. Conditions were the same as those described in Figure 6. In those media containing palmitate (filled circles), the molar ratio of FFA to albumin was 4. Each medium contained sufficient KI and NaCl to total 200 mM, NaCl being decreased as KI concentration was raised. Excitation wavelength was 295 nm, and fluorescent emission was recorded at 342 nm.

quenching by about 50% at each of the KI concentrations tested. The molar ratio of palmitate to albumin was 4 in this experiment.

Figure 8 contains additional information about the effects of fatty acids on this process. First, other long-chain saturated and unsaturated fatty acids are about as effective as palmitate in protecting against the quenching produced by KI. By contrast, the 8- and 10-carbon atom acids have essentially no protective effect. Protection is described in terms of the percentage of the tryptophan fluorescence available for quenching, a value obtained from modified Stern-Volmer plots (23). Second, protection increases in an almost linear fashion as the molar ratio of FFA to albumin is raised from 0 to 5. Since there is only one tryptophan residue in the molecule, it is somewhat surprising that protection is progressive as more fatty acid is added.

One possibility is that the nonpolar cleft in which the tryptophan residue is buried serves as a binding site for several moles of fatty acid and that the site gradually fills up as more fatty acid is added to the protein. Fluorine magnetic resonance studies, however, tend to exclude this possibil-

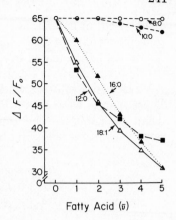

FIG. 8. Effect of molar ratio of FFA to albumin on quenching of fluorescence produced by iodide ions. Conditions were the same as those described in Figures 6 and 7 except that the KI concentration in each medium was 100 mM. Value plotted on the ordinate, $\Delta F/F°$, is a measure of the quenching of tryptophan fluorescence. Quenching decreases as the numerical value becomes smaller, illustrating the progressively greater protective effect with certain fatty acids as the molar ratio of FFA to albumin ($\bar{\nu}$) is raised. Fatty acid abbreviations used are: 8:0, octanoate; 10:0, decanoate; 12:0, laurate; 16:0, palmitate; 18:1, oleate.

ity (29). These experiments indicate that within the physiological concentration range 2 mol of a long-chain hydrocarbon ligand are not present at the same location on the albumin molecule. A second possibility is that the binding of fatty acids at other locations on the albumin molecule causes conformational changes in the region of the tryptophan residue, progressively decreasing its accessibility to iodide ions. For example, suppose that fatty acid-binding sites were located within the structural domains. The filling up of these sites with fatty acid might compress the clefts between the domains, making it more difficult for iodide to penetrate into the cleft containing the tryptophan residue. Such a conformational mechanism has been evoked to explain certain effects of fatty acids on drug binding to albumin (54). This mechanism remains a viable alternative, but presents several problems. First, even though some conformational changes have been shown to accompany fatty acid binding, these are minimal until the molar ratio exceeds 3 (44). Second, one of the strong binding sites appears to be located in the region of the tryptophan residue (33, 58), and yet there is no abrupt change in the protective effect against iodide quenching when up to 5 mol of laurate, palmitate, or oleate are added (Fig. 8). A final possibility, which we believe plays at least some role in the process, involves fatty acid distribution over a number of different binding sites in a population of albumin molecules.

DISTRIBUTION ANALYSIS

A priori, one might expect that essentially all the fatty acid would be located at the strongest binding site when an albumin solution contains only 1 mol of fatty acid. Information concerning this point can be obtained from the stepwise equilibrium binding constants (Tables 1 and 2). The constants indicate that fatty acid probably is not confined to the specific number of sites that correspond to the total number of moles of fatty acid in the solution. In other words, not all the fatty acid is likely to be present at the strongest albumin-binding site when only 1 mol of fatty acid is contained in the solution. The stoichiometric constants suggest that the fatty acid is distributed, or spread, over several sites. A schematic representation of this concept, which is a direct mathematical consequence of the observed binding constants, is illustrated in Figure 9.

Figure 9 shows the distribution of the various human albumin complexes contained in a solution when the molar ratio of total oleate to albumin is 2. These results were calculated with the stepwise binding constants for oleate listed in Table 1. The concentrations of the various fatty acid-albumin complexes in the solution are derived by means of the following equations:

$$[PA_1] = K_1[P][A],$$
$$[PA_2] = K_2[PA_1][A] = K_1K_2[A]^2[P],$$
$$[PA_n] = K_n[PA_{n-1}][A] = K_1K_2\cdots K_n[A]^n[P] \tag{2}$$

The total concentration af albumin $[P_T]$ is related to the albumin-bound species $[PA_i]$ by equation 3.

$$[P_T] = [P] + [PA_1] + \cdots + [PA_n] \tag{3}$$

Then, by substituting from equation 2, one obtains equation 4, which relates the binding parameters $[P]$ and $[P_T]$.

$$[P] = \frac{[P_T]}{1 + K_1[A] + K_1K_2[A]^2 + \cdots + K_1 \cdots K_n[A]^n} \tag{4}$$

By the use of equations 2 and 3, equation 5 is derived, which gives the fraction of the total albumin (FP_i) present in each form of the fatty acid-albumin complex.

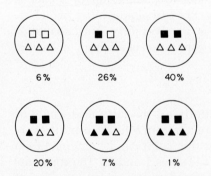

6%   26%   40%

20%   7%   1%

FIG. 9. Schematic representation of distribution of oleate-albumin complexes in a human plasma albumin solution. For this calculation, the albumin concentration was assumed to be 0.58 mM and the oleate concentration 1.16 mM, the molar ratio $(\bar{v})$ of total oleate to albumin being 2. Each of the 6 circular structures represents a species of albumin in the solution. Squares and triangles represent fatty acid-binding sites. Each square is a binding site that is specific for fatty acids, whereas triangles are sites that can bind either fatty acids or other organic compounds. Unfilled squares and triangles do not contain any fatty acid; those that are filled contain bound fatty acid. Under each albumin species is listed the percentage of total albumin in the solution that is present in that particular form. For example, 6% of the albumin molecules contain no fatty acids under these conditions and 1% contain 5 mol of fatty acid. Sites in each complex need not be occupied in the order illustrated, but space and clarity considerations preclude listing all such possibilities.

$$FP_i = \frac{[PA_i]}{[P_T]} = \frac{K_1 K_2 \cdots K_i [A]^i}{1 + K_1[A] + K_1 K_2 [A]^2 + \cdots + K_1 \cdots K_n[A]^n} \tag{5}$$

In this equation, FP_i is the fraction the total albumin that has i molecules of fatty acid attached.

As shown in Figure 9, six different complexes of albumin are predicted by these equations when the albumin concentration is 0.58 mM and the oleate concentration is 1.16 mM. Actually, this diagram is an oversimplification in terms of specific sites that are occupied. The stepwise binding constants are not site specific (13). Therefore, the albumin molecules containing 1 mol of bound oleate possibly may have that 1 mol present at different binding sites. For example, some of these albumin molecules may have the fatty acid at the FA_1 site in Figure 1, others at the FA_2 site, and still others at the FA_3 site. The 26% value in Figure 9 only indicates the fraction of the total albumin complexes that contain one bound fatty acid molecule. These formulas do not indicate whether the fatty acid is bound to a strong or a weak site. The same is true for each of the other albumin species. This greatly increases the complexity in terms of occupancy of individual binding sites. Even if this further complexity is disregarded, the distribution of the various species is somewhat surprising and may have important implications for certain biological interpretations. Note that only 40% of the albumin molecules contain two oleate molecules even though the molar ratio of total oleate to albumin is 2. Moreover, 28% of the albumin molecules contain more than two oleate molecules, and 32% contain less than two.

Similar distributions have been calculated for various concentrations of oleate (Table 3). The data when the molar ratio of total oleate to albumin is 2, presented in Figure 9, are included in Table 3 for completeness. At each oleate concentration, the same type of result as that noted in Figure 9 occurs. There are a large number of albumin species present in the solution so that a distribution of oleate-containing complexes is present. Even when the molar ratio of total oleate to albumin is only 1, about 4% of the albumin in the solution will contain three or more oleate molecules. Likewise, when

TABLE 3. *Percentage of total albumin in solution containing various amounts of oleate*

Total Oleate Concentration, mM	Oleate-Albumin Molar Ratios	Percentage of Albumin,*%							
		0†	1	2	3	4	5	6	7
0.29	0.5	58.3	34.0	7.2	0.5	0	0	0	0
0.58	1.0	30.8	43.1	22.1	3.6	0.4	0	0	0
1.16	2.0	6.2	25.8	40.0	19.5	7.1	1.3	0.1	0
1.74	3.0	1.0	8.0	27.4	29.4	23.7	9.7	0.8	0.1
2.32	4.0	0	1.3	9.1	20.3	34.1	29.2	5.2	0.8

* Total albumin concentration is 0.58 mM in each case.   † Number of fatty acids per albumin molecule.

the molar ratio of total oleate to albumin is 3, 9% of the albumin will contain less than two oleate molecules.

A similar analysis, using the stepwise binding constants that we have reported (3), has been carried out by Wosilait and Soler-Argilaga (61–63). These investigators have computed the palmitate distributions for bovine as well as human albumin (61, 63). In addition, they have worked out the distributions for five other long-chain fatty acids in human albumin solutions (62). Their general conclusions concerning the distribution of fatty acid-albumin complex are in complete agreement with our results.

Biological Implications

Wosilait and Soler-Argilaga (61–63) have employed the distribution analysis to describe the role of albumin in delivering FFA to the tissues. Cunningham et al. (8) also have utilized this concept to explain the effect of FFA on the binding of tryptophan to serum albumin. This analysis also helps to explain several other observations about the interaction between FFA and plasma albumin. For example, the progressive protective effect against iodide quenching of fluorescence (Fig. 8) can be explained by the distribution analysis. Quenching results from iodide binding to the region of the tryptophan residue. As shown in Figure 1, this region is believed to contain one of the strong fatty acid-binding sites (58). According to the work of Peters and his colleagues (33) with bovine albumin, this site ranks third with respect to affinity for palmitate. Therefore, one would expect fatty acids to have a greater tendency to interact with the sites abbreviated as FA_1 and FA_2 in Figure 1. Yet, although this site ranks third in terms of strength, the distribution analysis predicts that it could contain fatty acid even when the molar ratio of total fatty acid to albumin is in the range of 1–2. This would provide some fatty acid to shield the tryptophan residue from iodide even at relatively low molar ratios. Moreover, the distribution analysis predicts that, as the molar ratio is increased, progressively more of the albumin molecules in the solution would contain three or more bound fatty acids. This would lead to a progressively greater probability of having fatty acid present at the FA_3 site in Figure 1 and hence progressively greater shielding and protection of the tryptophan. In this way, it is possible to account for the progressive protection of FFA against iodide quenching as the molar ratio of FFA to albumin is raised (Fig. 8).

Role in Competitive Binding

The distribution analysis also helps to explain several puzzling aspects about the interaction between organic compounds and fatty acids when both are bound to albumin. The constants for long-chain FFA binding to albumin are 100–10,000 times larger than those for the binding of other organic compounds (47, 54). Yet, according to equilibrium-dialysis measurements,

FFAs do not displace appreciable amounts of other organic compounds until the molar ratio of FFA to albumin exceeds 2 (7, 15, 36). The currently held view, illustrated in Figure 1, is that albumin contains two very strong binding sites that are specific for FFA. Extrapolating from the localization studies with bovine serum albumin (32, 34), we have conceptually localized these sites as FA_1 and FA_2 in Figure 1. Other organic compounds, presumably because of structural differences, are thought not to be able to penetrate into these two sites (15). By contrast, the site labeled FA_3 is thought to be available to all organic anions, including FFA. This site is located in the region of the tryptophan residue of human albumin. The FFA will begin to displace a second organic ligand only when enough fatty acid is available to effectively compete for the weaker FA_3 site. Our binding studies using equilibrium dialysis are consistent with this model involving separate types of binding sites (38, 39, 54). Yet, using more sensitive fluorescent compounds, we find that some binding interactions occur between FFA and a second ligand even when the molar ratio of total FFA to albumin is in the range of 1–2 (38, 39). This has been explained on the basis of a fatty acid-induced conformational change in the FA_3 binding site (54).

Although this remains a possibility, a second explanation based on fatty acid distribution over several binding sites within the population of albumin molecules is equally plausible. The distributional analysis predicts, as indicated in Table 3 and Figure 9, that some albumin molecules contain 3 mol of FFA or more even when the molar ratio of total FFA to albumin is only 1 or 2. Since the FA_3 site has a strong affinity for FFA (33), one would expect that fatty acid would be present at this site in a high percentage of the albumin complexes that contain 3 mol of FFA or more. The presence of some fatty acid at the FA_3 site could account for the effects on 1-anilino-8-naphthalenesulfonate (ANS) fluorescence that we have observed when the molar ratio of total FFA to albumin is low (38, 39). Even if a conformational mechanism is involved, the distributional effect is still a factor in the binding process. Conversely, the entire process can be explained satisfactorily by the distributional effect alone without having to invoke any conformational mechanism.

Finally, several unexplained effects of the drug chlorophenoxyisobutyrate (CPIB) on FFA binding to albumin might be explained by the distribution analysis. Albumin binds the first 2 mol of FFA about 1000 times more tightly than it binds CPIB (54). This, together with the separation of the first two strong FFA-binding sites from the drug-binding sites (Fig. 1), makes it seem very unlikely that CPIB could displace FFA from albumin when the concentrations of both are low. Yet, this explanation of the hypolipidemic effects of the drug was advanced by Thorp (59). Surprisingly, recent experiments show that CPIB can indeed displace a small amount of palmitate from albumin. In the presence of the drug, palmitate uptake by ascites cell suspensions is enhanced (55). Likewise, the release of palmitate into heptane is enhanced when the drug is added (25). These effects occur even when the molar ratio of palmitate to albumin is less than 2. They are difficult to explain if the first 2 mol of palmitate are completely isolated at separate sites that do not interact with the drug-binding sites. The distribution analysis predicts, however, that albumin complexes containing 3 mol of palmitate or more would be present in the solution even when the molar ratio of total FFA to albumin is between 1 and 2. If so, interactions between CPIB and FFA could take place in these higher complexes. Such interactions might facilitate the release of a small quantity of palmitate located at lower affinity sites.

In summary, we believe that the distributional analysis can provide a great deal of new insight into the regulation of FFA transport in the circulation. However, the distributional predictions are based on a theoretical analysis (curve fitting) of the fatty acid-binding data. Actual complexes containing the predicted quantities of bound FFA have not yet been isolated from albumin solutions. Until such chemical verification is obtained, the concept must be treated as a hypothesis.

SUMMARY AND CONCLUSIONS

Free fatty acid is transported in the circulation primarily as a physical complex with plasma albumin. This protein has a molecular weight of about 67,000 and is composed of a single polypeptide chain. The chain contains many repeating sequences and folds up into three very similar cylindrical regions or domains. This repeating, subunitlike structure provides multiple binding sites for FFA. Because of this, albumin solution can be prepared to contain 5 mol of fatty acid or more. When the molar ratio of FFA to albumin is high, a number of potentially important biological effects are produced. These include effects on platelet aggregation, granulocyte function, and enzymatic activities. A common mechanism for these effects is suggested by studies with ascites tumor cells. This involves the binding of FFA in unesterified form on or within the cell. Accumulation of fatty acid in the form of FFA produces abnormal effects by altering either the lipid bilayer of the cell membranes, protein components associated with the membranes, or cytoplasmic binding proteins. With all the fatty acids tested except stearate, accumulation of appreciable quantities of FFA in the cell occurs only when the molar ratio of FFA to albumin exceeds 3. Under the usual physiological conditions, the molar ratio of FFA to albumin is between 0.5 and 2, and stearate comprises less than 20% of the circulating FFA. Therefore, it is likely that many of the injurious actions of FFA take place at molar ratios that hardly ever occur in vivo. Although these effects may be important in certain pathological states, it is difficult to see how they could play a major role as physiological regulatory mechanisms.

The binding of FFA to albumin has been described in terms of a series of multiple equilibrium reactions. Stoichiometric constants are available for the binding of all the physiologically important fatty acids to both human and bovine albumin. The results are generally similar with both proteins, in agreement with the similarities of the two proteins in terms of amino acid sequence and tertiary structure. The binding constants occur in a monotone descending order, suggesting that strong positive cooperative effects do not accompany the binding process. There also is no evidence for the existence of distinct groups of equivalent binding sites, but this could be due in part to negative cooperativity associated with binding. The values of the stoichiometric constants remain in doubt because of the uncertainties in the available binding models (11, 12), and the question of fatty acid self-association in aqueous solution is unresolved. If association occurs, the numerical value of each constant would be increased, but the qualitative relationship between the various constants for a given fatty acid should not change appreciably. Therefore, qualitative conclusions about the binding process probably are not affected appreciably by this uncertainty.

With the use of the stoichiometric binding constants, the distribution of fatty acids among the various albumin-binding sites has been calculated at different FFA concentrations. These calculations suggest that, even when the molar ratio is low, some of the albumin molecules in a solution will bind three or more molecules of fatty acid. Such a distribution can explain how FFA in low concentrations progressively protects the single tryptophan residue of human albumin from quenching by iodide ions. It also provides an explanation for certain binding interactions observed between FFA and other organic compounds. Previously, these observations could be explained only on the basis of conformational changes even though such changes have not been demonstrated conclusively by physical measurement. Although a conformational mechanism remains a possibility, the distributional analysis offers a potential alternative. The latter explanation must be considered as a hypothesis, for the presence of albumin complexes containing varying amounts of FFA in a solution remains to be demonstrated by a chemical assay.

Future Directions

As indicated in this brief overview, although a great deal already is known at the molecular level about fatty acid transport in the circulation, additional studies would seem to be profitable in several areas. First, the question of fatty acid association in aqueous solutions needs to be settled definitively. Second, the FFA-binding sites should be localized in the intact albumin molecule. Elucidation of the complete amino acid sequence (4), together with recent advances in X-ray crystallography (24), offers exciting possibilities in this area. Attempts also should be made to verify the distributional analysis, by use of a chemical method to demonstrate the existence of multiple albumin complexes in a solution containing FFA. Finally, the physiological significance of many of the regulatory and toxic effects produced by FFA should be assessed carefully. Sensitive assay systems will be needed to test for subtle effects at FFA-to-albumin molar ratios between 0.5 and 2. In this regard, we believe that careful study of the interaction of FFA with biological and artificial membrane preparations might be a useful area for further exploration. Finally, the role of FFA in influencing the action of certain cytoplasmic proteins that bind nonpolar compounds is another area where additional investigation might be profitable.

These studies were supported in part by research grants from the National Institutes of Health (HL 14,230 and HL 14,781) and the American Heart Association (74-689).

REFERENCES

1. AHMED, K., AND B. S. THOMAS. The effects of long-chain fatty acids on sodium plus potassium ion-stimulated adenosine triphosphatase of rat brain. *J. Biol. Chem.* 246: 103–109, 1971.
2. ASHBROOK, J. D., A. A. SPECTOR, AND J. E. FLETCHER. Medium-chain fatty acid binding to human plasma albumin. *J. Biol. Chem.* 247: 7038–7042, 1972.
3. ASHBROOK, J. D., A. A. SPECTOR, E. C. SANTOS, AND J. E. FLETCHER. Long-chain fatty acid binding to human plasma albumin. *J. Biol. Chem.* 250: 2333–2338, 1975.
4. BROWN, J. R. Structural origins of mammalian albumin. *Federation Proc.* 35: 2141–2144, 1976.
5. BURNS, C. P., I. R. WELSHMAN, AND A. A. SPECTOR. Differences in free fatty acid and glucose metabolism of human blood neutrophils and lymphocytes. *Blood* 47: 431–437, 1976.
6. CHEN, R. F. Removal of fatty acids from serum albumin by charcoal treatment. *J. Biol. Chem.* 242: 173–181, 1967.
7. COGIN, G. E., AND B. D. DAVIS. Competition in the binding of long-chain fatty acids and methyl orange to bovine serum albumin. *J. Am. Chem. Soc.* 73: 3135–3138, 1951.
8. CUNNINGHAM, V. J., L. HAY, AND H. B. STONER. The binding of L-tryptophan to serum albumins in the presence of non-esterified fatty acids. *Biochem. J.* 146: 636–658, 1975.
9. DELEIRIS, J., L. H. OPIE, AND W. F. LUBBE. Effects of free fatty acid and glucose on enzyme release in experimental myocardial infarction. *Nature* 253: 746–747, 1975.
10. FAIN, J. N., AND R. E. SHEPHERD. Free fatty acids as feedback regulators of adenylate cyclase and cyclic 3':5'-AMP accumulation in rat fat cells. *J. Biol. Chem.* 250: 6586–6592, 1975.
11. FLETCHER, J. E. A generalized approach to equilibrium models. *J. Phys. Chem.* In press.
12. FLETCHER, J. E., J. D. ASHBROOK, AND A. A. SPECTOR. Computer analysis of drug-protein binding data. *Ann. N.Y. Acad. Sci.* 226: 69–81, 1973.
13. FLETCHER, J. E. AND A. A. SPECTOR. Alternative models for the analysis of drug-protein binding. *Mol. Pharmacol.* 13: 387–399, 1977.
14. GOODMAN, D. S. The distribution of fatty acids between n-heptane and aqueous phosphate buffer. *J. Am. Chem. Soc.* 80: 3887–3892, 1958.
15. GOODMAN, D. S. The interaction of human serum albumin with long-chain fatty acid anions. *J. Am. Chem. Soc.* 80: 3892–3898, 1958.
16. GOODMAN, D. S. The interaction of human erythrocytes with sodium palmitate. *J. Clin. Invest.* 37: 1729–1735, 1958.
17. GOODMAN, D. S. AND E. SHAFRIR. The interaction of human low-density lipoproteins with long-chain fatty acid anions. *J. Am. Chem. Soc.* 81: 364–370, 1959.
18. GORDON, R. S., JR. Interaction between oleate and the lipoproteins of human serum. *J. Clin. Invest.* 34: 477–484, 1955.
19. HAWLEY, H. P., AND G. B. GORDON. The effects of long-chain free fatty acids on human neutrophil function and structure. *Lab. Invest.* 34: 216–222, 1976.
20. HENDERSON, A. H., A. S. MOST, AND E. H. SONNENBLICK. Depression of contractility in rat heart muscle by free fatty acids during hypoxia. *Lancet* 2: 825–826, 1969.
21. HOAK, J. C., A. A. SPECTOR, G. L. FRY, AND E. D. WARNER. Effect of free fatty acids on ADP-induced platelet aggregation. *Nature* 228: 1330–1332, 1970.
22. KURIEN, V. A., P. A. YATES, AND M. F. OLIVER. Free fatty acids, heparin, and arrhythmias during experimental myocardial infarction. *Lancet* 2: 185–187, 1969.
23. LEHRER, S. S. Solute perturbation of protein fluorescence. The quenching of the tryptophyl fluorescence of model compounds and of lysozyme by iodide ions. *Biochemistry* 10: 3254–3263, 1971.
24. McCLURE, R. J., AND B. M. CRAVEN. X-ray data for four crystalline forms of serum albumin. *J. Mol. Biol.* 83: 551–555, 1974.
25. MEISNER, H. Displacement of palmitate from albumin by chlorophenoxyisobutyrate. *Biochem. Biophys. Res. Commun.* 66: 1134–1140, 1975.
26. MISHKIN, S., L. STEIN, Z. GATMAITAN, AND I. M. ARIAS. The binding of fatty acids to cytoplasmic proteins: binding to Z protein in liver and other tissues of the rat. *Biochem. Biophys. Res. Commun.* 47: 997–1003, 1972.
27. MISHKIN, S., AND R. TURCOTTE. The binding of long-chain fatty acid CoA to Z, cytoplasmic protein present in liver and other tissues of the rat. *Biochem. Biophys. Res. Commun.* 57: 917–926, 1974.
28. MUKERJEE, P. Dimerization of anions of long-chain fatty acids in aqueous solutions and the hydrophobic properties of the acids. *J. Phys. Chem.* 69: 2821–2827, 1965.
29. MULLER, N., AND R. J. MEAD, JR. Fluorine magnetic resonance study of the binding of long-chain trifluoroalkyl sulfate ions by bovine serum albumin. *Biochemistry* 12: 3831–3835, 1973.
30. OCKNER, R. K. AND J. A. MANNING. Fatty acid binding protein. Role in esterification of absorbed long-chain fatty acid in rat intestine. *J. Clin. Invest.* 58: 632–641, 1976.
31. OCKNER, R. K., J. A. MANNING, R. B. POPPENHAUSEN, AND W. K. L. HO. A binding protein for fatty acids in cytosol of intestinal mucosa, liver, myocardium and other tissues. *Science* 177: 56–58, 1972.
32. ORLY, J., AND M. SCHRAMM. Fatty acids as modulators of membrane functions: catecholamine-activated adenylate cyclase of the turkey erythrocyte. *Proc. Natl. Acad. Sci. US* 72: 3433–3437, 1975.
33. PETERS, T., JR. The plasma proteins. In: *Structure,*

Function, and Genetic Control (2nd ed.), edited by F. W. Putnam. New York: Academic, 1975, vol. 1, p. 133–181.

34. REED, R. G., R. C. FELDHOFF, O. L. CLUTE, AND T. PETERS, JR. Fragments of bovine serum albumin produced by limited proteolysis. Conformation and ligand binding. *Biochemistry* 14: 4578–4583, 1975.

35. RITTER, M. C., AND M. E. DEMPSEY. Squalene and sterol carrier protein: structural properties, lipid-binding, and function in cholesterol biosynthesis. *Proc. Natl. Acad. Sci. US* 70: 265–269, 1973.

36. RUDMAN, D., T. J. BIXLER II, AND A. E. DEL RIO. Effect of free fatty acids on binding of drugs by bovine serum albumin, by human serum albumin, and by rabbit serum. *J. Pharmacol Exptl. Therap.* 176: 261–272, 1971.

37. SAIFER, A., AND L. GOLDMAN. The free fatty acid bound to human serum albumin. *J. Lipid Res.* 2: 268–270, 1961.

38. SANTOS, E. C., AND A. A. SPECTOR. Effect of fatty acids on the binding of 1-anilino-8-naphthalenesulfonate to bovine serum albumin. *Biochemistry* 11: 2299–2302, 1972.

39. SANTOS, E. C., AND A. A. SPECTOR. Effects of fatty acids on the interaction of 1-anilino-8-naphthalenesulfonate with human plasma albumin. *Mol. Pharmacol.* 10: 519–528, 1974.

40. SAWIN, C. T., AND D. A. WILLARD. Normal rise in plasma free fatty acids during fasting in patients with hypopituitarism. *J. Clin. Endocrinol.* 31: 233–234, 1970.

41. SHAFRIR, E., AND A. GUTMAN. Patterns of decrease of free fatty acids during glucose tolerance tests. *Diabetes* 14: 77–83, 1965.

42. SIMPSON, R. B., J. D. ASHBROOK, E. C. SANTOS, AND A. A. SPECTOR. Partition of fatty acids. *J. Lipid Res.* 15: 415–422, 1974.

43. SMITH, R., AND C. TANFORD. Hydrophobicity of long-chain n-alkyl carboxylic acids, as measured by their distribution between heptane and aqueous solutions. *Proc. Natl. Acad. Sci. US* 70: 289–293, 1973.

44. SOETEWEY, F., M. ROSSENEU-MOTREFF, R. LA-MOTE, AND H. PEETERS. Size and shape determination of native and defatted bovine serum albumin monomers. II. Influence of the fatty acid content on the conformation of bovine serum albumin monomers. *J. Biochem., Tokyo* 71: 705–710, 1972.

45. SPECTOR, A. A. Influence of pH of the medium on free fatty acid utilization by isolated mammalian cells. *J. Lipid Res.* 10: 207–215, 1969.

46. SPECTOR, A. A. Metabolism of free fatty acids. *Progr. Biochem. Pharmacol.* 6: 130–176, 1971.

47. SPECTOR, A. A. Fatty acid binding to plasma albumin. *J. Lipid Res.* 16: 165–179, 1975.

48. SPECTOR, A. A. Fatty acid metabolism in tumors. *Progr. Biochem. Pharmacol.* 10: 42–75, 1975.

49. SPECTOR, A. A., J. D. ASHBROOK, E. C. SANTOS, AND J. E. FLETCHER. Quantitative analysis of uptake of free fatty acid by mammalian cells: lauric acid and human erythrocytes. *J. Lipid Res.* 13: 445–451, 1972.

50. SPECTOR, A. A., J. E. FLETCHER, AND J. D. ASHBROOK. Analysis of long-chain free fatty acid binding to bovine serum albumin by determination of stepwise equilibrium constants. *Biochemistry* 10: 3229–3232, 1971.

51. SPECTOR, A. A., J. C. HOAK, E. D. WARNER, AND G. L. FRY. Utilization of long-chain free fatty acids by human platelets *J. Clin. Invest.* 49: 1489–1496, 1970.

52. SPECTOR, A. A., AND K. M. JOHN. Effects of free fatty acid on the fluorescence of bovine serum albumin. *Arch. Biochem. Biophys.* 127: 65–71, 1968.

53. SPECTOR, A. A., K. JOHN, AND J. E. FLETCHER. Binding of long-chain fatty acids to bovine serum albumin. *J. Lipid Res.* 10: 56–67, 1969.

54. SPECTOR, A. A., E. C. SANTOS, J. D. ASHBROOK, AND J. E. FLETCHER. Influence of free fatty acid concentration on drug binding to plasma albumin. *Ann. N.Y Acad. Sci.* 226: 247–258, 1973.

55. SPECTOR, A. A., AND J. M. SOBOROFF. Effect of chlorophenoxyisobutyrate on free fatty acid utilization by mammalian cells. *Proc. Soc. Exptl. Biol. Med.* 137: 945–947, 1971.

56. SPECTOR, A. A., AND D. STEINBERG. The utilization of unesterified palmitate by Ehrlich ascites tumor cells. *J. Biol. Chem.* 240: 3747–3753, 1965.

57. SPECTOR, A. A., D. STEINBERG, AND A. TANAKA. Uptake of free fatty acids by Ehrlich ascites tumor cells. *J. Biol. Chem.* 240: 1032–1041, 1965.

58. SWANEY, J. B., AND I. M. KLOTZ. Amino acid sequence adjoining the lone tryptophan of human serum albumin. A binding site of the protein. *Biochemistry* 9: 2570–2574, 1970.

59. THORP, J. M. An experimental approach to the problem of disordered lipid metabolism. *J. Atherosclerosis Res.* 3: 351–360, 1963.

60. WALLACH, D., AND I. PASTAN. Stimulation of guanylate cyclase of fibroblasts by free fatty acids. *J. Biol. Chem.* 251: 5802–5809, 1976.

61. WOSILAIT, W. D., AND C. SOLER-ARGILAGA. A theoretical analysis of the multiple binding of palmitate by bovine serum albumin: the relationship to uptake of free fatty acid by tissues. *Life Sci.* 17: 159–166, 1975.

62. WOSILAIT, W. D., AND C. SOLER-ARGILAGA. A comparative analysis of the binding of different long-chain free fatty acids by human serum albumin. *Fed. European Biochem. Soc. Letters* 73: 72–76, 1977.

63. WOSILAIT, W. D., C. SOLER-ARGILAGA, AND P. NAGY. A theoretical analysis of the binding of palmitate by human serum albumin. *Biochem. Biophys. Res. Commun.* 71: 419–426.

64. WU-RIDEOUT, M. Y. C., C. ELSON, AND E. SHRAGO. The role of fatty acid binding protein on the metabolism of fatty acids in isolated rat hepatocytes. *Biochem. Biophys. Res. Commun.* 71: 809–816, 1976.

15

Regulation of Hepatic Metabolism of Free Fatty Acids: Interrelationships Among Secretion of Very-Low-Density Lipoproteins, Ketogenesis, and Cholesterogenesis

MURRAY HEIMBERG, EDWARD H. GOH, HOWARD A. KLAUSNER,[†]
CARLOS SOLER-ARGILAGA, IRA WEINSTEIN, AND HENRY G. WILCOX

Department of Pharmacology, University of Missouri
School of Medicine, Columbia, Missouri

THE ALTERNATE PATHWAYS FOR METABOLISM of free fatty acid (FFA) by the liver are determined in part by the quantity and structure of the substrate FFA available to the liver. Equally important, however, are the underlying hormonal and nutritional conditions in the animal that affect the subsequent metabolism of the FFA by the liver. It has been shown repeatedly that uptake of FFA by the liver is proportional to the concentration of FFA in the plasma in vivo or in the medium perfusing the isolated liver in vitro (29). The influence of concentration on FFA uptake by the liver in vitro, moreover, can be modulated by the rate of flow of the perfusate and by the ratio of FFA to albumin in the medium (48). Furthermore, uptake of FFA is probably not altered substantially by many hormonal actions that drastically affect the subsequent utilization of the fatty acid. Clearly, uptake of FFA by the liver in vitro does not appear to be an important rate-limiting factor in the subsequent metabolism of the fatty acid. For example, FFA uptake is not altered by glucagon (28), insulin (62), diabetes (61, 62), estrogens (56), and cyclic AMP (34), all of which affect the subsequent metabolism of FFA by the liver. The FFA available to the liver in the intact animal can be derived from exogenous or endogenous sources. In the animal in the fasting state, or on a fat-free diet, or stimulated under certain endocrinopathies, the major source of plasma FFA is probably adipose tissue triglycerides; however, in

---

† Deceased September 17, 1974.

the fed state, when neutral fats are provided in the diet in man and animals, the primary source of plasma FFA probably is dietary triglycerides (25). When man or animals are fed neutral fats of a particular fatty acid composition, the plasma FFA and plasma and hepatic triglycerides within a short time become enriched with the fed fatty acid. The triglyceride fatty acids of adipose tissue appear to turn over at a much slower rate than do those of liver or plasma (8, 12, 20, 31). The composition of the plasma FFA, which may affect subsequent hepatic metabolism of the FFA, is therefore a reflection of the composition of the ingested triglyceride.

The metabolism of the fatty acid taken up by the liver varies with the hormonal and nutritional state of the animal. The FFA taken up by the liver will be esterified primarily to triglyceride and to a lesser extent to phospholipid, diglyceride, and cholesteryl esters or will be oxidized to CO_2 and ketone bodies. The triglyceride is stored in the liver or is secreted into the plasma (or perfusate) as the major component of the very-low-density lipoproteins (VLDL), in conjunction with other lipid moieties of the VLDL (phospholipid, cholesterol, and cholesteryl esters) and the apoprotein components. When triglyceride is not secreted—for example, when blocked by various hepatotoxins or in several pathogenic states—or when the maximal rate of triglyceride output has been exceeded because of a large available pool of FFA, triglyceride accumulates in the liver, producing hepatic steatosis. When equivalent quantities of FFA are available to the liver, hepatic output of triglyceride, and therefore of the VLDL, is reduced and ketogenesis is accelerated by fasting (27, 37, 41), experimental diabetes (24, 41, 42, 62), glucagon (28, 42), dibutyryl cyclic AMP [DBcAMP (28, 34)], monobutyryl cyclic GMP [MBcGMP (49)], and also to some extent by epinephrine (26). Conversely, hepatic output of triglyceride and the VLDL is increased and ketogenesis is reduced by feeding (27, 37, 41), by treatment of the diabetic animal with insulin (24, 61, 62), and by estrogens (56). The hepatic output of triglyceride can also be reduced by a number of hepatotoxins, resulting in a fatty liver. These hepatotoxins, which are not discussed further here, include $CHCl_3$, CCl_4, tetracyclines, inhibitors of protein synthesis (e.g., puromycin, ethionine, cycloheximide), microtubule inhibitors (e.g., colchicine), and many others. Generally, formation and secretion of triglyceride and ketogenesis are regulated in a reciprocal manner by various hormonal and nutritional conditions. This brief presentation does not pretend to be an exhaustive review of the literature, but rather is primarily a discussion of some recent work from our laboratory. We therefore limit the discussion to catabolic effects of cyclic nucleotides, anabolic effects of estrogens, and regulation of hepatic cholesterogenesis by fatty acids. Most of this work was done with the isolated perfused rat liver in vitro.

EFFECTS OF CYCLIC NUCLEOTIDES

N^6-2'-O-Dibutyryl Adenosine-3',5'-Monophosphate

The observation that fasting stimulated ketogenesis and reduced the output of triglyceride by the isolated perfused rat liver was reported from our laboratory a number of years ago (27). Since that time, it was observed that experimental diabetes, produced with alloxan or with anti-insulin serum, and glucagon also stimulated ketogenesis and diminished secretion of triglyceride. Dibutyryl cyclic AMP, added directly to the medium perfusing livers from normal fed rats, had similar effects. These latter experiments are summarized in Table 1. The uptake of FFA and the concentration of FFA in the perfusate were unaffected by addition of DBcAMP to the medium. The subsequent metabolism of the FFA, however, was altered radically by the nucleotide. The net output of triglyceride by the liver was reduced by DBcAMP, but there was a time lag before the effects of the nucleotide became pronounced (34). The effects on output of triglyceride after 1 h of perfusion were relatively small, but had become extensive by the 2nd h. Not only were formation and output of triglyceride reduced by DBcAMP, but net uptake from the perfusate (negative values) of triglyceride that had been present in the plasma of the initial medium, or had been added to the perfusate by hepatic secretion, was also observed. This lag phase, observed even at a concentration of 1×10^{-5} M DBcAMP suggests that a finite period of time is required either to increase intracellular concentrations of cAMP, or for cAMP to exert its action on output of triglyceride, or both. This delay contrasts with the more rapid effects exerted on ketogenesis and glycogenolysis (34).

The effects of varying concentrations of DBcAMP on output of ketone bodies by the liver are also shown in Table 1. Clearly, rates of ketogenesis were stimulated by DBcAMP. The simultaneous effect of DBcAMP on output of glucose by the liver was also measured and, as reported by numerous laboratories (9, 10, 15, 28), the stimulatory effect of the nucleotide was evident. The reciprocal relationship between inhibition of triglyceride output and stimulation of ketogenesis by DBcAMP is striking, reminiscent of the effects of treatment of the animal with anti-insulin serum or alloxan, effects of fasting, or action of glucagon. The effects of the nucleotide appear to be quite sensitive to concentration, were detectable at 0.4×10^{-5} M nucleotide, were prominent at 1×10^{-5} M, and were maximal at 3×10^{-5} M. The effects of DBcAMP on the disposition of infused [1-^{14}C]oleate by the isolated perfused

TABLE 1. *Effects of dibutyryl adenosine-3',5'-monophosphate on hepatic metabolism of free fatty acids*

Treatment Group	FFA Uptake, µmol/g liver	Output, µmol/g liver		
		Triglyceride	Ketone bodies	Glucose
Control	49.9 ± 4.5	2.90 ± 0.31	36.4 ± 10.8	104.2 ± 9.0
DBcAMP				
0.4 × 10⁻⁵ M	60.9 (2)	2.69 (2)	92.4 (2)	140.7 (2)
1.0 × 10⁻⁵ M	60.7 ± 2.8	0.88 ± 0.09	110.0 ± 2.9	224.0 ± 17.3
4.0 × 10⁻⁵ M	52.9 ± 2.6	−0.17 ± 0.06	126.0 ± 33.3	410.8 ± 57.8
10.0 × 10⁻⁵ M	53.5 ± 4.0	−0.04 ± 0.21	122.7 ± 2.5	372.5 ± 46.2

Data are cumulative means ± SE for a 4-h perfusion period. Experimental conditions have been described (34). Percentage uptake of infused FFA by the liver was 87.9–91.8% for all groups. Three perfusions were carried out in each group unless indicated otherwise in parentheses.

liver were also investigated. Dibutyryl cAMP stimulated oxidation of oleate, increasing incorporation of ^{14}C into both CO_2 and ketone bodies (Table 2). The increase in oxidation was primarily at the expense of reduction in the quantity of [^{14}C]oleate esterified to triglyceride, in both the liver and the perfusate. Again, in these experiments, uptake of oleate from the medium was unaltered by the nucleotide (9.3 ± 0.1 vs. 10.6 ± 0.5 μmol/g liver per h for control and experimental, respectively).

In related experiments, perfusate was centrifuged by flotation in a zonal ultracentrifuge. As can be seen in Figure 1, the output of VLDL, the transport form for the triglyceride secreted by the liver, was reduced by the nucleotide. Therefore, secretion of the other components of VLDL (cholesterol and cholesteryl esters, phospholipid, and apoprotein) were also reduced by the action of DBcAMP, in addition to triglyceride.

Possible Mechanisms of Action of Dibutyryl cAMP

The metabolism of FFA can be altered dramatically by DBcAMP and the metabolism of FFA by the liver does not merely passively reflect the flow of fatty acid from dietary sources or adipose tissue to the liver. The actions of the cyclic nucleotides on hepatic synthesis of triglyceride and ketone bodies probably are indicative of a physiologic regulatory role for cAMP in hepatic metabolism of FFA, since these effects were observed at reltively low perfusate concentrations of DBcAMP and were dose dependent. The effects of DBcAMP, moreover, were similar to those of glucagon, which can increase hepatic concentration of cAMP by activation of adenylate cyclase (10).

TABLE 2. *Effects of dibutyryl adenosine-3′,5′-monophosphate on infused [1-^{14}C]oleate by perfused liver*

Analysis	FFA Uptake, %	
	Control (4)	DBcAMP (3)
Incorporation into esterified lipids:		
In liver		
TG	36.3 ± 5.7	11.1 ± 2.0
DG, PL, CE	13.8	11.1
In perfusate		
TG	25.8 ± 2.1	8.0 ± 1.3
DG, PL, CE	1.6	1.6
Incorporation into oxidation products:		
CO_2	15.7 ± 2.6	26.9 ± 0.9
Ketone bodies	3.1 ± 0.8	40.3 ± 2.6
Recovery	96.4 ± 5.5	99.1 ± 5.9

Data are mean percent of FFA taken up by the liver found in each fraction; numbers of experiments are indicated in parentheses. Concentration of DBcAMP was 2×10^{-5} M. TG, triglyceride; DG, diglyceride; PL, phospholipid; CE, cholesteryl ester. Experimental conditions have been described (34).

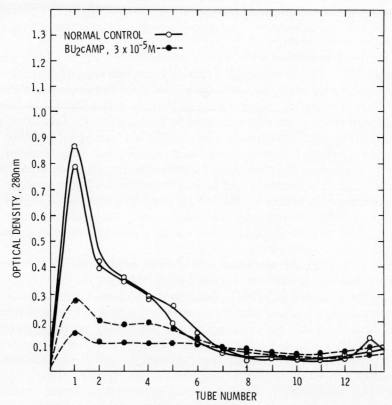

FIG. 1. Isolation of perfusate VLDL by ultracentrifugation in zonal rotors. Data are from 4 individual control and experimental perfusions. Perfusate plasma was centrifuged in a Spinco Ti-14 zonal rotor for 1 h at 37,000 rpm. Gradient volume was 480 ml ($d = 1.0$–1.4) and water-overlay volume was 100 ml. Density of sample was adjusted to 1.4 with NaBr, and EDTA was added to all solutions to make a final concentration of 1 mM. [From Klausner, Soler-Argilaga, and Heimberg (34).]

The mechanism(s) of action by which DBcAMP (and presumably cAMP) diminishes hepatic output of triglyceride and increases rates of ketogenesis may include inhibition of esterification of long-chain fatty acid acyl-CoA to triglyceride; depression of formation and release of the VLDL associated with transport of triglyceride; increase in the rate of transport of fatty acids from the cytoplasm into the mitochondria by altering the activity of acylcarnitine-CoA transferase, or by increasing the availability of free carnitine, or both; direct stimulation of the mitochondrial pathways for oxidation of fatty acids and for formation of ketone bodies; and any combination of these factors (28).

It is evident that FFA taken up by the liver is channeled preferentially into oxidative pathways by the cyclic nucleotides while the quantity of oleate esterified to triglyceride is reduced. We do not know, however, whether changes in the partition of fatty acids result from dual reciprocal control over synthesis of triglyceride and oxidation of fatty acids. To evaluate synthesis, we measured rates of incorporation of sn-[^{14}C]glycerol-3-phosphate into triglyceride, diglyceride, and phosphatidic acid and the activities of phosphatidate phosphohydrolase and diglyceride acyltransferase in microsomes obtained from livers perfused in a nonrecycling system in the presence or absence of 2×10^{-5} M DBcAMP. Under these conditions, FFA uptake was unchanged, triglyceride output was diminished, and ketogenesis and glucose output were stimulated; incorporation of [^{14}C]glycerol-3-phosphate into diglyceride and triglyceride was decreased by prior perfusion of the liver with DBcAMP (Table 3). Activities of phosphatidic acid phosphohydrolase and diglyceride acyltransferase actually were accelerated after exposure to DBcAMP, suggesting that the block in synthesis of triglyceride occurs prior to formation of phosphatidate and perhaps may be at the glycerophosphate acyltransferase step (Table 4). Clearly, a block in synthesis of triglyceride can, in part, reduce secretion of the VLDL, divert fatty acid into oxidative pathways, and be synergistic with any effect of the nucleotide to stimulate mitochondrial fatty acid oxidation.

Since DBcAMP did not affect synthesis of triglyceride in the hepatic microsome directly, it was necessary to consider at least one other additional signal in the sequence of events. Because it had been suggested that the metabolic response to cAMP might be associated with movements of calcium ion within the cell (45), we investigated the role of Ca^{2+} on the microsomal synthesis of glycerolipids from α-glycerophosphate. In several very preliminary experiments, we observed that calcium inhibited the microsomal synthesis of various glycerolipids (triglyceride, diglyceride, phosphatidate), measured by incorporation of radioactive sn-glycerol-3-phosphate. A similar effect was observed with the 400-g supernatant prior to isolation of microsomes. In these experiments, the calcium that accumulated in the microsomes was the result of passive transport, and relatively high concentrations (millimolar range) were required. The physiological role of these data therefore is highly questionable. Recently, a MgATP-dependent calcium-sequestering activity of rat liver microsomes was characterized by Moore et al. (43). In preliminary experiments, we observed that the active accumula-

TABLE 3. *Incorporation of sn-[^{14}C]glycerol-3-phosphate into glycerolipids by microsomes from livers perfused with or without exogenous DBcAMP*

Metabolite	G3P Incorporation, nmol/mg protein	
	Control	DBcAMP
Phosphatidate	39.4 ± 9.6	35.9 ± 8.2
Diglyceride	10.2 ± 1.6	8.3 ± 1.4*
Triglyceride	6.9 ± 1.3	4.9 ± 1.1*

Assay system consisted of 15 mM Tris-HCl (pH 7.5), 35 mM ATP, 50 mM CoA, 0.75 mM dithiothreitol, 35 mM MgCl$_2$, 0.5 mM sn-[^{14}C]glycerol-3-phosphate (0.1 μCi), 25 mM sucrose, 1.5 mM palmitic acid, 4.5 mg bovine serum albumin, and ~0.5 mg of the microsomal preparation. Incubations were carried out at 37°C in a volume of 0.45 ml for 30 min essentially as described by Fallon et al. (11). * Significantly different from controls, $P < 0.05$ for paired data.

tion of calcium mediated by the ATP-dependent system was reciprocally related to the rate of incorporation of radioactive sn-glycerol-3-phosphate into phosphatidate (Table 5). Whether and how the effects of Ca^{2+} on biosynthesis of triglycerides are related causally to the actions of the cyclic nucleotides remains to be determined. The inhibitory effect of DBcAMP on hepatic triglyceride synthesis and output also may conceivably result from a limitation of substrate for synthesis of triglyceride by suppression of lipogenesis. Under our experimental conditions, however, and perhaps in some

TABLE 4. *Effects of DBcAMP on microsomal phosphatidate phosphohydrolase and diglyceride acyltransferase*

Treatment	Phosphatidate Phosphohydrolase, nmol DG formed/mg protein per min	Diglyceride Acyltransferase, nmol TG formed/mg protein per min
Control	0.73 ± 0.19	0.49 ± 0.10
DBcAMP	1.19 ± 0.23*	0.81 ± 0.16*

Assay system for phosphatidate phosphohydrolase contained 15 mM Tris-HCl (pH 7.5), 50 mM sucrose, 0.1 mM dithiothreitol, and microsomal-bound [^{14}C]phosphatidate (~0.5 mg protein); incubations were carried out in 1.0 ml at 37°C for 10 min. Assay system for diglyceride acyltransferase contained 50 mM KPO$_4$ buffer (pH 6.5), 2 mM dithiothreitol, 2.5 mg bovine albumin, 0.1 mM MgCl$_2$, 50 mM NaF, 35 nmol palmitoyl-CoA, 35 nmol oleoyl-CoA, and microsomal-bound [^{14}C]diglyceride (0.1–0.3 mg protein); incubations were carried out in 0.45 ml at 37°C for 4 min. Assays of activity of phosphatidate phosphohydrolase and diglyceride acyltransferase with microsomal-bound substrate were carried out as described by Lamb and Fallon (35) and by Fallon and co-workers (11), respectively.   * Significantly different from controls, $P < 0.05$ for paired data.

TABLE 5. *Reciprocal relationship between ATP-dependent active uptake of Ca^{2+} and biosynthesis of phosphatidate from glycerol-3-phosphate by rat liver microsomes*

Incubation for Active Uptake of Ca²⁺ by Microsomes, min	Ca²⁺ Uptake, nmol/mg protein	G3P Incorporation into Phosphatidate, nmol/mg protein per 30 min
ATP omitted		
0	1.2	27.0 (100)
10	2.2	26.8 (99.2)
20	2.3	25.0 (92.6)
ATP added		
0	1.6	26.6 (100)
10	35.5	21.4 (80.5)
20	68.4	18.3 (68.8)

Microsomes (1.3 mg protein/ml) were incubated with or without 5 mM ATP in a medium containing 30 mM imidazole histidine buffer (pH 6.8), 100 mM KCl, 5 mM NH$_4$ oxalate, 5 mM NaN$_3$, 5 mM MgCl$_2$, and 0.1 mM ^{45}CaCl$_2$ (0.1 μCi/ml). Incubations were performed in a total volume of 3.0 ml at 37°C. Samples were removed at 0, 10, and 20 min. At each time period, aliquots were taken (in duplicate) for measurement of Ca^{2+} uptake by Millipore filtration technique (43). Simultaneously, other aliquots were removed (in triplicate) and used as the source of enzyme for measurement of incorporation of sn-[^{14}C]glycerol-3-phosphate into phosphatidate, which was measured as described in Table 3. Incubations were carried out with 0.26 mg microsomal protein in a final volume of 1.0 ml at 37°C for 30 min.

physiological conditions in vivo, reduced lipogenesis may be of minor importance because most of the fatty acid released as triglyceride was derived
from exogenous sources.

The stimulation of ketogenesis by DBcAMP reported here and elsewhere
(34, 61) agrees with observations of other investigators using isolated rat
hepatocytes (6, 32) or perfused livers (38). Raskin et al. (44), however, did
not observe any significant effect of DBcAMP and glucagon on hepatic
ketogenesis. The reason for this discrepancy is unknown. In the studies of
Raskin et al. incubations or perfusions were done with [1-^{14}C]acetate or [1-
^{14}C]octanoate rather than with long-chain fatty acids. If the carnitine
acyltransferase reaction is the rate-limiting step in long-chain fatty acid
oxidation, and is activated in the livers from fasting or ketotic animals (34),
it is conceivable that stimulation by DBcAMP may not be observed in the
absence of long-chain fatty acids. Octanoic acid can cross the mitochondrial
membrane without the necessity of the carnitine transport mechanism;
octanoate, furthermore, is oxidized to acetyl-CoA at the same rate in livers
from fed, fasted, and diabetic animals (39, 40). In contrast to long-chain
fatty acids, octanoate is not utilized for synthesis of triglyceride, so that
differences in the synthesis of triglyceride cannot be responsible for a
preferential oxidation of fatty acids. Most probably, increased transport of
fatty acids from cytoplasm into mitochondria is important in the stimulation
of ketogenesis by DBcAMP. The cyclic nucleotides, however, do not appear
to have a direct effect on ketone body production by isolated rat liver
mitochondria (2). The data of Amatruda et al. (2) in fact suggest that the
stimulation of ketogenesis by cyclic nucleotides results from nonmitochon-
drial events leading to altered disposition of hepatic fatty acids. The increased
entry of fatty acid into the mitochondria, however, may alter the distribution
of fatty acid between oxidation to carbon dioxide and ketogenesis. The
stimulation of ketogenesis by DBcAMP in livers from normal fed rats
perfused in the absence of added FFA may result primarily from increases
in intrahepatic lipolysis (4, 21). When sufficient exogenous FFA is provided
the liver, as in the experiments reported here, such effects may be obscured.
Regardless of the molecular mechanism, however, DBcAMP reciprocally
inhibits hepatic secretion of triglyceride and VLDL and stimulates ketogenesis by shunting fatty acids into catabolic pathways.

O^2-Monobutyryl Guanosine-3',5'-Monophosphate

We also investigated the effects of MBcGMP on the liver, with the
nucleotide infused directly into the medium perfusing livers from normal fed
rats (49). Hepatic output of triglyceride was depressed by 10^{-4} M nucleotide
but was unaffected at 10^{-5} M, with [1-^{14}C]oleate used as the substrate.
Under these conditions, uptake of oleic acid was not affected by the MBcGMP
and the specific radioactivity of the FFA taken up by the liver was constant
throughout the experiment. Conversely, the output of ketone bodies by the
liver was stimulated by 10^{-4} M MBcGMP but not by a concentration of 10^{-5}

M. Output of glucose by the liver was stimulated by 10^{-4} M MBcGMP, but not by 10^{-5} M. Clearly, although effects of MBcGMP on hepatic metabolism of FFA are qualitatively similar to those of DBcAMP, cGMP is much less potent than the cAMP derivative and may be operative through different mechanisms, if at all, physiologically.

EFFECTS OF ESTROGENS

Estrogens have an anabolic effect on metabolism of FFA, in contrast to the catabolic effects of the cyclic nucleotides. An increased interest in the metabolic actions of estrogens may be the result of the awareness of elevated concentrations of serum triglyceride observed in humans (3, 14, 23, 63) and rats (54) and decreased concentrations of serum cholesterol (1, 13, 54) after treatment with estrogenic drugs. Perhaps more fundamental are the observations suggesting major differences in hepatic metabolism of FFA in male and female animals. Our laboratory reported previously that the output of triglyceride and the VLDL by livers from female animals exceeded that of livers from male animals in vitro (29, 47, 50, 53) and in vivo (46). Furthermore, triglyceride output by perfused livers from ovariectomized female rats was reduced, but was restored to control levels by treatment of the ovariectomized rats with estrogens (53 , 55). Livers from female animals esterified a larger proportion of [1-^{14}C]oleate, primarily to the triglyceride, and oxidized less to CO_2 and ketone bodies than did livers from male animals (47). Of particular interest also was the observation that the VLDL secreted by the female in vitro (50, 59) or in vivo (46) were larger particles, had a faster rate-zonal mobility in the ultracentrifuge, and contained less cholesterol and phospholipid per mole of triglyceride than did livers from male animals. This difference became less in experiments in vitro as the quantity of FFA (oleate) provided the liver increased and the rate of output of triglyceride increased (50). It appears from these and other experiments that the particle size of the VLDL increased (rate-zonal mobility increased) as the amount of oleate or palmitoleate provided the liver increased (50, 58). It soon became apparent from the experimental work of our laboratory and others that the concentration (30) and output of triglyceride and VLDL by the liver increased in vivo (33, 51, 52) and in vitro (53, 54, 56) when the animal was treated with estrogens. To obtain more definitive information about the actions of estrogens on hepatic metabolism of FFA, rats were treated with ethynylestradiol, and the disposition of [1-^{14}C]oleate by the perfused rat liver isolated from these animals was studied. We also evaluated effects of the drugs on serum lipoproteins in vivo. Some of the results from the in vivo experiments are presented in Table 6. Ethynylestradiol depressed the concentration of total cholesterol and increased that of triglyceride in the serum of female rats. In agreement with data reported previously (54), similar observations were made in male animals. In the present studies, no differences were observed in the concentration of total serum cholesterol of control rats; ethynylestradiol, however, reduced total serum cholesterol in both sexes. The rate of hepatic secretion of triglyceride in vivo was greater in the female than the male animal (Table 6), as reported previously from this laboratory. Despite these important differences in secretion rate, the serum concentrations of triglyceride in untreated male and female animals were generally similar. Ethynylestradiol clearly stimulated the secretion of VLDL triglyceride and the basal and stimulated rates of triglyceride secretion in the female exceeded those in the male rat. Although the concentration of total cholesterol in the serum decreased on treatment with ethynylestradiol, the concentration (51, 52) and the rate of secretion of VLDL cholesterol actually were increased by the estrogen. The decrease in serum cholesterol with estrogen treatment resulted primarily from a decrease in the concentration of high-density lipoprotein (HDL) sterol. These data indeed suggest that estrogens not only increased hepatic production of VLDL but also stimulated utilization of the various classes of lipoprotein lipids.

The effect of pretreatment of the female rat with estrogens in the subsequent disposition of [1-^{14}C]oleate by the isolated liver is presented in Table 7. Ethynylestradiol did not affect the rate of uptake of oleate, but stimulated the output of triglyceride and VLDL and reduced the rates of ketogenesis. The proportion of [1-^{14}C]oleate esterified to triglyceride in liver and perfusate was stimulated. The proportion oxidized to ketone bodies was reduced severely, while CO_2 production from oleate was essentially unchanged. It was of particular interest that output of glucose by livers from female rats treated with ethynylestradiol was impaired (25.0 ± 4.0 µmol/g per h for the control vs. 3.5 ± 3.5 for the treated animals) even though hepatic glycogen stores were increased. The biochemical mechanisms by which these changes in hepatic metabolism of FFA are brought about by estrogen remain to be determined. It has been reported that synthesis of VLDL apoprotein is increased by treatment with estrogens (5, 36). It may be also that the enzymes of triglyceride biosynthesis are induced or activated

TABLE 6. *Effects of ethynylestradiol on concentration of serum lipids and secretion of serum VLDL lipids in male and female rats*

Treatment	Concentration of Lipids, µmol/ml serum		Secretion of VLDL lipids, µmol/h per 100 g body wt	
	Triglyceride	Total cholesterol	Triglyceride	Free cholesterol
Female				
Control	0.26 ± 0.02	1.87 ± 0.12	4.70	1.28
Ethynylestradiol	0.57 ± 0.04	1.31 ± 0.03	9.01	2.10
Male				
Control	0.19 ± 0.04	1.66 ± 0.04	1.94	1.00
Ethynylestradiol	0.29 ± 0.04	1.28 ± 0.06	4.02	1.82

Data are means ± SE (n = 8) for concentration of serum lipids. Experimental data are all significantly different from controls, with $P < 0.05$ or better. Animals received 15 µg ethynylestradiol/kg body wt, in sesame oil, daily for 14 days by subcutaneous injection. Food was removed 12–14 h before sacrifice on the 15th day. Secretory rates for VLDL were calculated as described previously (46), after treatment with Triton WR-1339 on *day 15,* on VLDL isolated from pooled samples of sera in 2 separate experiments.

TABLE 7. *Effects of ethynylestradiol on disposition of infused [1-^{14}C]oleate by perfused liver*

Analysis	FFA Uptake, %	
	Control (4)	Ethynylestradiol (5)
Incorporation into esterified lipids:		
In liver		
TG	14.9 ± 0.4	32.9 ± 6.0*
DG, PL, CE	9.7	11.1
In perfusate		
TG	13.8 ± 1.8	36.1 ± 1.4*
DG, PL, CE	1.1	1.5
Incorporation into oxidation products:		
CO_2	28.9 ± 2.7	25.4 ± 3.8
Ketone bodies	25.7 ± 2.6	4.0 ± 1.0*
Recovery	93.8 ± 2.0	111.0 ± 3.3

Data are expressed as mean percent of FFA taken up by the liver found in each fraction. Animals were treated with ethynylestradiol as indicated in Table 6.   * Significantly different from controls, $P < 0.05$.

by estrogen and that rates of microsomal synthesis of triglyceride and other VLDL lipids are increased by estrogens, while pathways of mitochondrial oxidation of fatty acids are inhibited. These data, however, are not yet available.

Recently, in collaboration with Dr. H. Werner, we examined the utilization of [1-^{14}C]oleate by hepatocytes isolated from livers of normal female rats and from animals treated with ethynylestradiol (as described in Table 5). Cells were incubated with 0.3, 0.6, or 1.2 μmol oleate/ml containing 0.25, 0.5, or 1.0 μCi, respectively, for 1 h at 37°C. Cells from animals treated with ethynylestradiol secreted significant amounts of triglyceride into the medium, measured colorimetrically or by determination of radioactivity in triglyceride; cells from control rats secreted quantites of triglyceride that were not detectable by our methods of chemical analysis, while radioactivity in triglyceride was about 10% of that secreted by cells from estrogen-treated female rats. In confirmation of the perfusion studies, ethynylestradiol directed oleate into anabolic pathways of synthesis of triglyceride and reduced the fraction oxidized to ketone bodies. These data suggested to us a possible interrelationship between estrogens and cyclic nucleotides. In one preliminary experiment, hepatocytes from female rats were incubated with glucagon (4.2 nmol/flask) and oleic acid (4.8 μmol/flask) for 0, 2, 5, and 10 min. The reaction was stopped by the addition of perchloric acid and cyclic AMP was determined (by Dr. L. R. Forte) by the method of Harper and Brooker (22). Cells from estrogen-treated rats contained 208, 1262, 1061, and 988 pmol cAMP/mg DNA at the end of 0, 2, 5, and 10 min of incubation; cells from control rats contained 473, 1384, 2016, and 1880 pmol/mg DNA, respectively. These data are most exciting and suggest that estrogens, directly or by some indirect mechanism, reduce the response of the liver to stimuli that ordinarily increase the concentration of cAMP in the hepatocyte.

REGULATION OF HEPATIC CHOLESTEROGENESIS BY FREE FATTY ACIDS

Triglyceride is secreted by the liver as a moiety of the VLDL, and phospholipid and cholesterol quite clearly are secreted in certain specific proportions to the quantity of triglyceride secreted. The phospholipid and cholesterol are necessary presumably, along with the VLDL apoprotein, to help stabilize the nonpolar triglyceride in the aqueous environment of the serum (29). The specific molar ratios of phospholipid and cholesterol relative to triglyceride in the VLDL were reported from our laboratory to be altered by structure and quantity of the FFA substrate (57, 58), by rate of output of triglyceride (50, 58), by sex of the animal (46, 50, 59), by fat feeding (7), and presumably by other influences. Clearly, however, triglyceride is not secreted without concomitant output of cholesterol as a component of the VLDL. These observations prompted us to suggest that factors that stimulate output of triglyceride and the VLDL by the liver would, since cholesterol is an obligate requirement for secretion of triglyceride, stimulate biosynthesis of cholesterol. Since exogenous FFAs are prime stimulants of VLDL output we studied initially the effects of oleate on cholesterol synthesis by isolated perfused livers from normal rats. Synthesis of cholesterol was estimated in those initial experiments by incorporation of tritium from ^3H_2O into the cholesterol of perfusate and liver (Table 8). Addition of oleate to the perfusate stimulated output of triglyceride and cholesterol, as expected, and also stimulated incorporation of ^3H into cholesterol (17). Simultaneously, biosynthesis of fatty acid, measured by incorporation of ^3H into fatty acids, was diminished by the exogenous oleate. Oleic acid not only stimulated incorporation of ^3H_2O into cholesterol, but also stimulated activity of hepatic 3-hydroxy-3-methylglutarate (HMG)-CoA reductase (EC 1.1.1.34), the rate-limiting enzyme in cholesterol biosynthesis (18, 19). Furthermore, when exogenous cholesterol was added to the medium along with oleate, HMG-CoA reductase activity was depressed while output of triglyceride continued with little change (18; Table 9). Within limits, stimulation of hepatic HMG-CoA reductase activity was also proportional to the quantity of oleate added. When equimolar concentrations of palmitate (16:0), oleate (18:1), or linoleate

TABLE 8. *Rate of synthesis of hepatic lipids*

Lipid Components	Rate of Synthesis, μmol/g liver per h	
	Oleic acid omitted	Oleic acid added
Total fatty acid	1.53 ± 0.27 (3)	0.37 ± 0.05 (3)
Free cholesterol	0.12 ± 0.02 (7)	0.26 ± 0.03 (5)
Esterified cholesterol	0.01 ± 0.001 (7)	0.07 ± 0.001 (5)

Data calculated as described by Windmueller and Spaeth (60); for additional details, see Goh (16). Livers from normal fed male rats were perfused as previously reported (17–19). Oleic acid (166 μmol/h) or the albumin alone was infused for 4 h at a constant rate. Biosynthesis was estimated by incorporation of radioactivity from ^3H_2O into lipids of liver plus perfusate. Data with oleic acid are significantly different from controls in all cases ($P < 0.02$ or better).

TABLE 9. *Effects of free fatty acids on activity of*
hepatic microsomal HMG-CoA reductase

Fatty Acid Infused, μmol/h	Enzyme Activity, nmol mevalonate/min per mg protein
None (nonperfused)	0.49 ± 0.12 (6)
None (after perfusion)	1.08 ± 0.11 (5)
Oleate, 83	1.61 ± 0.13 (6)
Oleate, 166	2.29 ± 0.11 (8)
Oleate, 166, + cholesterol, 55	0.63 ± 0.03 (4)
Oleate, 332	4.28 ± 0.32 (4)
Palmitate, 166	0.96 ± 0.12 (7)
Linoleate, 166	1.28 ± 0.27 (6)

Conditions of perfusion have been described previously (17–19). Fatty acid or albumin alone was added as a pulse dose and then infused at a constant rate for 4 h. Complex with cholesterol was prepared as indicated previously (18).

(18:2) were infused into the medium perfusing livers from normal fed animals, activity of HMG-CoA reductase was generally proportional to the output of triglyceride and total cholesterol by the liver (19). More specifically, however, output of cholesterol was in the order 18:1 > 18:2 > 16:0, enzyme activity was in the order 18:1 > 18:2 = 16:0, and output of triglyceride was in the order 18:1 = 18:2 > 16:0, such that the molar ratio of cholesterol to triglyceride in the secreted particle was greater when 16:0 was the substrate than when either 18:1 or 18:2 was infused. These observations are in substantial agreement with the properties (lipid class composition, rate-zonal mobility) reported previously for the VLDL in response to different FFA substrates (57). In later experiments, the VLDL were isolated from the medium after perfusion in the presence or absence of oleic acid. Output of the VLDL lipids and activity of microsomal HMG-CoA reductase were stimulated by addition of oleate to the medium (Table 9). Clearly, the increase in output of VLDL triglyceride and cholesterol is associated with increased rates of cholesterogenesis. Finally, to determine whether HMG-CoA reductase activity varied with output of the VLDL lipids in vivo as well as in vitro, we compared the activity of the enzyme with the output of the VLDL during the diurnal cycle in the rat (Table 10). The increased activity of HMG-CoA reductase under these conditions coincided with increased output of VLDL triglyceride and cholesterol in vivo as it did with the isolated perfused liver in vitro.

These data and others suggest that hepatic cholesterogenesis can be stimulated by plasma FFA and inhibited by cholesterol [perhaps in VLDL and chylomicron remnants, low-density lipoproteins (LDL), and HDL] and that the net rate of cholesterogenesis may be determined by the relative strengths of these negative-feedback and positive-feedback signals. How the free fatty acids stimulate cholesterogenesis is not clear at this time. If we may be permitted to speculate on the biochemical mechanisms involved, the following hypothesis may be proposed. If the activity of HMG-CoA reductase is regulated by end-product inhibition by free cholesterol, FFA may remove free cholesterol from an inhibitory site on the enzyme either by stimulation of conversion of cholesterol to cholesteryl esters, by utilization of the cholesterol for synthesis and secretion of the VLDL or for conversion to biliary cholesterol and bile acids, or by a combination of these processes. Cholesteryl esters are not likely to inhibit cholesterogenesis since they can accumulate in the liver when large quantities of FFA are available to the liver, under conditions that secretion of VLDL can be stimulated and cholesterogenesis increased. Whether oleate or other fatty acids (or derivatives) may act directly on HMG-CoA reductase to alter its activity is not known currently. Clearly, this area needs much further study.

Whether the effects of FFA on the activity of HMG-CoA reductase and cholesterogenesis and on the secretion of the VLDL observed with the isolated perfused liver are indeed important physiological mechanisms in vivo must be established. The simultaneous increase in activity of HMG-CoA reductase and hepatic secretion of VLDL during the diurnal cycle suggests an important physiological mechanism for cholesterogenesis related to the quantity and composition of the diet consumed by the animal. One may hypothesize that various nutrients that directly or indirectly stimulate the formation and secretion of the VLDL by the liver also stimulate hepatic cholesterogenesis, although dietary cholesterol as well as endogenous lipoprotein cholesterol would be expected to reduce de novo synthesis and supply some of the sterol required for the formation and secretion of the VLDL. Since the composition of dietary fats affects the composition of the plasma

TABLE 10. *Relationship between output of VLDL lipids and activity of HMG-CoA reductase in vitro and in vivo*

Analysis	In Vitro		In Vivo	
	− Oleate (4)	+ Oleate (6)	Noon (4)	Midnight (4)
VLDL, μmol/g liver per h				
TG	0.52 ± 0.04	1.37 ± 0.09	0.98 ± 0.06	1.20 ± 0.09
Cholesterol	0.16 ± 0.01	0.22 ± 0.01	0.07 ± 0.01	0.11 ± 0.01
HMG-CoA reductase, nmol mevalonate formed/min per mg microsomal protein	0.93 ± 0.12	2.24 ± 0.22	0.14 ± 0.01	0.79 ± 0.07

Data are means ± SE; numbers in parentheses indicate number of experiments. Differences between + oleate (166 μmol/h) and − oleate and between midnight and noon are statistically significant for all parameters ($P < 0.02$ or better). Conditions for perfusion have been reported previously (17–19). Output of VLDL in vivo was estimated with Triton WR-1339 (46). Male rats were maintained on a light (0500–1700 h)-dark cycle for 10–21 days prior to sacrifice. Purina rat chow and water were fed ad libitum. For in vitro experiments, animals were killed between 0800 and 1000 h. For in vivo experiments, animals killed at 1200 or 2400 h received Triton WR-1339 or 0.9% NaCl 2 h prior.

FAA and subsequently the properties and composition of the VLDL secreted by the liver, the mechanisms by which the amount and kind of fat in the diet may affect rates of hepatic cholesterogenesis may be regulated partly through some of the processes discussed here. It is also conceivable that the kind and quantity of carbohydrate in the diet, by being substrates for lipogenesis, can give rise to plasma or hepatic fatty acids and stimulate secretion of the VLDL and cholesterogenesis by some of the proposed mechanisms.

CONCLUSION

Hepatic metabolism of FFA can be altered dramatically by hormones and certainly is modulated by the quantity and structure of the plasma FFA available to the liver. Clearly, the composition and quantity of the plasma VLDL, and ketogenesis and ketonemia, are under hormonal and substrate regulation. It may also be postulated that hormonal factors that stimulate formation and secretion of the VLDL are conducive to hepatic cholesterogenesis, whereas factors that reduce output of the VLDL should reduce cholesterogenesis, providing other factors, such as the supply of FFA and cholesterol available to the liver, are equal. It also is evident that our current knowledge of the regulation of various aspects of hepatic lipid metabolism and ketogenesis is most incomplete, is quite complex, and at times is most confusing.

This work was supported in part by grants from the National Institutes of Health (AM-18125 and GRS RR05387-14) and from the Missouri Heart Association.

REFERENCES

1. AFTERGOOD, L., AND R. B. ALFIN-SLATER. Effect of an oral contraceptive steroid mixture on some aspects of lipid metabolism in the rat. In: *Metabolic Effects of Gonadal Hormones and Contraceptive Steroids*, edited by H. A. Salhanick, D. M. Kipnis, and R. L. Vande Wiele. New York: Plenum, 1969, p. 265–274.

2. AMATRUDA, J. M., S. MARGOLIS, AND D. H. LOCKWOOD. Regulation of ketone body production from [^{14}C]palmitate in rat liver mitochondria: effects of cyclic nucleotides and unlabeled fatty acids. *Biochem. Biophys. Res. Commun.* 67: 1337–1345, 1975.

3. AURELL, M., K. CRAMER, AND G. RYBO. Serum lipids and lipoproteins during long-term administration of an oral contraceptive. *Lancet* 1: 291–293, 1966.

4. BEWSHER, P. D., AND J. ASHMORE. Ketogenic and lipolytic effects of glucagon on liver. *Biochem. Biophys. Res. Commun.* 24: 431–436, 1966.

5. CHAN, L., R. J. JACKSON, B. W. O'MALLEY, AND A. R. MEANS. Synthesis of the very low density lipoproteins in the cockerel. *J. Clin. Invest.* 58: 368–379, 1976.

6. COLE, R. A., AND S. MARGOLIS. Stimulation of ketogenesis by dibutyryl cyclic AMP in isolated rat hepatocytes. *Endocrinology* 94: 1391–1396, 1974.

7. DUNN, G. D., H. G. WILCOX, AND M. HEIMBERG. Effects of dietary triglyceride on the properties and composition of plasma lipoproteins: acute experiments in rats fed safflower oil. *Lipids* 10: 773–782, 1975.

8. DUNN, G. D., H. G. WILCOX, AND M. HEIMBERG. Temporal relationship between dietary, plasma, hepatic, and adipose tissue lipids after short-term feeding of safflower oil to rats. *J. Lab. Clin. Med.* 86: 369–377, 1975.

9. EXTON, J. H., J. G. HARDMAN, T. F. WILLIAMS, E. W. SUTHERLAND, AND C. R. PARK. Effects of guanosine 3′,5′-monophosphate on the perfused rat liver. *J. Biol. Chem.* 246: 2658–2664, 1971.

10. EXTON, J. H., G. A. ROBISON, E. W. SUTHERLAND, AND C. R. PARK. Studies on the role of adenosine-3′,5′-monophosphate in the hepatic actions of glucagon and catecholamines. *J. Biol. Chem.* 246: 6166–6177, 1971.

11. FALLON, H. J., J. BARWICK, R. G. LAMB, AND H. VAN DEN BOSCH. Studies of rat liver microsomal diglyceride acyltransferase and cholinephosphotransferase using microsomal-bound substrate: effects of high fructose intake. *J. Lipid Res* 16: 107–115, 1975.

12. FLEISCHMAN, A. I., T. HAYTON, AND M. L. BIERENBAUM. Variation in composition of serum free fatty acid with dietary change under isocaloric conditions. *Am. J. Clin. Nutr.* 15: 299–302, 1964.

13. FURMAN, R. H. Gonadal steroid effects on serum lipids. In: *Metabolic Effects of Gonadal Hormones and Contraceptive Steroids*, edited by H. A. Salhanick, D. M. Kipnis, and R. L. Vande Wiele. New York: Plenum, 1969, p. 247–264.

14. GERSHBERG, H., M. HULSE, AND A. JAVIER. Hypertriglyceridemia during treatment with estrogen and oral contraceptives. *Obstet. Gynecol.* 31: 186–189, 1968.

15. GLINSMANN, W. H., E. P. HERN, L. G. LINARELLI, AND R. V. FARESE. Similarities between effects of adenosine 3′,5′-monophosphate and guanosine 3′,5′-monophosphate on liver and adrenal metabolism. *Endocrinology* 85: 711–719, 1969.

16. GOH, E. H. *Stimulation of Hepatic Cholesterol Biosynthesis by Oleic Acid in the Perfused Liver* (PhD Thesis). Nashville, Tenn.: Vanderbilt Univ., 1974.

17. GOH, E. H., AND M. HEIMBERG. Stimulation of hepatic cholesterol biosynthesis by oleic acid. *Biochem. Biophys. Res. Commun.* 55: 382–388, 1973.

18. GOH, E. H., AND M. HEIMBERG. Effect of oleic acid and cholesterol on the activity of hepatic hydroxymethylglutaryl coenzyme A reductase. *Fed. European Biochem. Soc. Letters* 63: 209–210, 1976.

19. GOH, E. H., AND M. HEIMBERG. Effect of free fatty acids on activity of hepatic microsomal 3-hydroxy-3-methylglutaryl coenzyme A reductase and on secretion of triglyceride and cholesterol by liver. *J. Biol. Chem.* 252: 2822–2826, 1977.

20. GORDIS, E. The long-term stability of triglyceride molecules in adipose tissue. *J. Clin. Invest.* 44: 1978–1985, 1965.

21. GUDER, W., J. FROHLICH, C. PATZELT, AND O. WIELAND. The effect of glucagon on the state of lysosomal enzymes in isolated perfused rat liver. *Fed. European Biochem. Soc. Letters* 10: 215–218, 1970.

22. HARPER, J. F., AND G. BROOKER. Femtomole sensitive radioimmunoassay for cyclic AMP and cyclic GMP after 2′-O acetylation by acetic anhydride in aqueous solution. *J. Cyclic Nucleotide Res.* 1: 207–218, 1975.

23. HAZZARD, W. R., M. J. SPIGER, J. D. BAGDADE, AND E. L. BIERMAN. Studies on the mechanism of increased plasma triglyceride levels induced by oral contraceptives. *New Engl. J. Med.* 280: 471–474, 1969.

24. HEIMBERG, M., A. DUNKERLEY, AND T. O. BROWN. Hepatic lipid metabolism in experimental diabetes. I. Release and uptake of triglycerides by perfused livers from normal and alloxan-diabetic rats. *Biochim. Biophys. Acta* 125: 252–264, 1966.

25. HEIMBERG, M., G. D. DUNN, AND H. G. WILCOX. The derivation of plasma free fatty acids from dietary neutral fat in man. *J. Lab. Clin. Med.* 83: 393–402, 1974.

26. HEIMBERG, M., N. B. FIZETTE, AND H. KLAUSNER. The action of adrenal hormones on hepatic transport of triglycerides and fatty acids. *J. Am. Oil Chem. Soc.* 41: 774–779, 1964.

27. HEIMBERG, M., I. WEINSTEIN, H. KLAUSNER, AND M. L. WATKINS. Release and uptake of triglycerides by isolated perfused rat liver. *Am. J. Physiol.* 202: 353–358, 1962.

28. HEIMBERG, M., I. WEINSTEIN, AND M. KOHOUT. The effect of glucagon, dibutyryl cyclic adenosine-3′,5′-monophosphate and concentration of free fatty acid on hepatic lipid metabolism. *J. Biol. Chem.* 244: 5131–5139, 1969.

29. HEIMBERG, M., H. G. WILCOX, G. D. DUNN, W. F. WOODSIDE, K. J. BREEN, AND C. SOLER-ARGILAGA. Studies on the regulation of secretion of the very low density lipoprotein and on ketogenesis by the liver. In: *Regulation of Hepatic Metabolism*, edited by F. Lundquist and N. Tygstrup. Copenhagen: Munksgaard, 1974, p. 119–143.

30. HILL, P., AND W. G. MARTIN. Effect of estrogens on rat serum lipoproteins. *Can. J. Biochem.* 50: 474–483, 1972.

31. HIRSCH, J., J. W. FARQUHAR, E. H. AHRENS, M. L. PETERSON, AND W. STOFFEL. Studies of adipose tissue in man. *Am. J. Clin. Nutr.* 8: 499–511, 1960.

32. HOMCY, C. J., AND S. MARGOLIS. Fatty acid oxidation and esterification in isolated rat hepatocytes: regulation by dibutyryl adenosine-3′,5′-cyclic monophosphate. *J. Lipid Res.* 14: 678–687, 1973.

33. KIM, H. K., AND R. K. KALKHOFF. Sex steroid influences on triglyceride metabolism. *J. Clin. Invest.* 56: 888–896, 1975.

34. KLAUSNER, H. J., C. SOLER-ARGILAGA, AND M. HEIMBERG. The effects of dibutyryl adenosine-3′,5′-monophosphate on hepatic metabolism of free fatty acids. *Metabolism* In press.

35. LAMB, R. G., AND H. J. FALLON. Glycerolipid formation from sn-glycerol-3-phosphate by rat liver cell fractions. The role of phosphatidate phosphohydrolase. *Biochim. Biophys. Acta* 348: 166–178, 1974.

36. LUSKEY, K. L., M. S. BROWN, AND J. L. GOLDSTEIN. Stimulation of the synthesis of very low density lipoproteins in rooster liver by estradiol. *J. Biol. Chem.* 249: 5939–5947, 1974.

37. MAYES, P. A., AND J. M. FELTS. Regulation of fat metabolism in the liver. *Nature* 215: 716–718, 1967.

38. MENAHAN, L. A., AND O. WIELAND. Glucagon-like action of N^6-2′-O-dibutyryl cyclic AMP on perfused rat liver. *Biochem. Biophys. Res. Commun.* 29: 880–885, 1967.

39. McGARRY, J. D., AND D. W. FOSTER. The regulation of ketogenesis from octanoic acid. The role of the tricarboxylic acid cycle and fatty acid synthesis. *J. Biol. Chem.* 246: 1149–1159, 1971.

40. McGARRY, J. D., AND D. W. FOSTER. The metabolism of (−)-octanoylcarnitine in perfused livers from fed and fasted rats. Evidence for a possible regulatory role of carnitine acyltransferase. *J. Biol. Chem.* 249: 7984–7990, 1974.

41. McGARRY, J. D., J. M. MEIER, AND D. W. FOSTER. Effects of starvation and refeeding on carbohydrate and lipid metabolism *in vivo* and in the perfused rat liver. *J. Biol. Chem.* 248: 270–278, 1973.

42. McGARRY, J. D., P. H. WRIGHT, AND D. W. FOSTER. Hormonal control of ketogenesis. Rapid activation of hepatic ketogenic capacity in fed rats by anti-insulin serum and glucagon. *J. Clin. Invest.* 55: 1202–1209, 1975.

43. MOORE, L., T. CHEN, H. R. KNAPP, JR., AND E. L. LANDON. Energy-dependent calcium sequestration activity in rat liver microsomes. *J. Biol. Chem.* 250: 4562–4568, 1975.

44. RASKIN, P., J. D. McGARRY, AND D. W. FOSTER. Independence of cholesterol and fatty acid biosynthesis from cyclic adenosine monophosphate concentration in the perfused rat liver. *J. Biol. Chem.* 249: 6029–6032, 1974.

45. RASMUSSEN, H. Cell communication, calcium ion, and cyclic adenosine monophosphate. *Science* 170: 404–412, 1970.

46. SOLER-ARGILAGA, C., A. DANON, H. G. WILCOX, AND M. HEIMBERG. Effects of sex on formation and properties of plasma very low density lipoprotein *in vivo. Lipids* 11: 517–525, 1976.

47. SOLER-ARGILAGA, C., AND M. HEIMBERG. Comparison of metabolism of free fatty acid by isolated perfused livers from male and female rats. *J. Lipid Res.* 17: 605–615, 1976.

48. SOLER-ARGILAGA, C., R. INFANTE, G. RENAUD, AND J. POLONOVSKI. Factors influencing free fatty acid uptake by the isolated perfused rat liver. *Biochimie* 56: 757–761, 1974.

49. SOLER-ARGILAGA, C., R. L. RUSSELL, AND M. HEIMBERG. Effect of O^2-monobutyrylguanosine-3',5'-monophosphate on hepatic metabolism of free fatty acids. *Biochem. Biophys. Res. Commun.* 74: 1340–1347, 1977.

50. SOLER-ARGILAGA, C., H. G. WILCOX, AND M. HEIMBERG. The effect of sex on the quantity and properties of the very low density lipoproteins secreted by the liver *in vitro. J. Lipid Res.* 17: 139–145, 1976.

51. TURNER, F., I. WEINSTEIN, E. GOH, C. SOLER-ARGILAGA, AND M. HEIMBERG. Estrogen effects on hepatic secretion and tissue utilization of serum cholesterol. *Gastroenterology* 70: A137, 1976.

52. TURNER, F., I. WEINSTEIN, AND M. HEIMBERG. Mechanisms for estrogen induced hypertriglyceridemia. *Clin. Res.* 24: 292A, 1976.

53. WATKINS, M. L., N. FIZETTE, AND M. HEIMBERG. Sexual influences on hepatic secretion of triglyceride. *Biochim. Biophys. Acta* 280: 82–85, 1972.

54. WEINSTEIN, I., S. SEEDMAN, AND M. VELDHUIS. Effect of ethynyl estradiol on the secretion of hepatic triglyceride. *Proc. Soc. Exptl. Biol. Med.* 149: 181–184, 1975.

55. WEINSTEIN, I., M. SELTZER, AND R. BELITSKY. The interrelation of glucagon and gonadectomy upon hepatic triglyceride metabolism in rats. *Biochim. Biophys. Acta* 348: 14–22, 1974.

56. WEINSTEIN, I., C. SOLER-ARGILAGA, AND M. HEIMBERG. Effects of ethynyl estradiol on incorporation of [1-^{14}C]-oleate into triglyceride and ketone bodies by the liver. *Biochem. Pharmacol.* 26: 77–80, 1977.

57. WILCOX, H. G., G. D. DUNN, AND M. HEIMBERG. Effects of several common long chain fatty acids on the properties and lipid composition of the very low density lipoprotein secreted by the perfused rat liver. *Biochim. Biophys. Acta* 398: 39–54, 1975.

58. WILCOX, H. G., G. D. DUNN, AND M. HEIMBERG. Effects of a mixture of a saturated with an unsaturated fatty acid on secretion of the very low density lipoprotein by the liver. *Biochem. Biophys. Res. Commun.* 73: 733–740, 1976.

59. WILCOX, H. G., W. F. WOODSIDE, K. J. BREEN, H. R. KNAPP, JR., AND M. HEIMBERG. The effect of sex on certain properties of the very low density lipoprotein secreted by the liver. *Biochem. Biophys. Res. Commun.* 58: 919–926, 1974.

60. WINDMUELLER, H. G., AND A. E. SPAETH. Perfusion in situ with tritium oxide to measure hepatic lipogenesis and lipid secretion. *J. Biol. Chem.* 241: 2891–2899, 1966.

61. WOODSIDE, W. F., AND M. HEIMBERG. Hepatic metabolism of free fatty acid in experimental diabetes. *Israel J. Med. Sci.* 8: 309–316, 1972.

62. WOODSIDE, W. F., AND M. HEIMBERG. Effects of anti-insulin serum, insulin, and glucose on output of triglyceride and on ketogenesis by the perfused rat liver. *J. Biol. Chem.* 251: 13–23, 1976.

63. WYNN, V., J. W. H. DOAR, AND G. L. MILLS. Some effects of oral contraceptives on serum lipid and lipoproteins. *Lancet* 2: 720–723, 1966.

16

Regulation of Uptake and Metabolism of Fatty Acids by Muscle

JANE A. IDELL-WENGER AND JAMES R. NEELY

*Department of Physiology, Milton S. Hershey Medical Center,
Pennsylvania State University, Hershey, Pennsylvania*

Fatty Acid Uptake
Fatty Acid Activation
Acyl Transfer and Transport into Mitochondria
β-Oxidation
Acetyl Transfer and Transport

THE RATE OF FATTY ACID UPTAKE and utilization by peripheral tissues depends to a large extent on the concentration of fatty acids in the blood, but mostly on the metabolic activity of the tissue in question. The fate of the fatty acid taken up depends on the type of tissue. It may be used for synthetic purposes, as in liver and adipose tissue, or for oxidation to produce energy, as in muscle. Cardiac muscle and red skeletal muscle oxidize fatty acids as the principal fuel for ATP production. Synthetic processes account for the metabolism of only a small percent of the total fatty acid taken up by these tissues. Therefore, our discussion of the control of fatty acid utilization by muscle concentrates primarily on the regulation of oxidative processes. Most of the work in this area has been done on heart muscle and therefore we are concerned with this tissue for the most part, although metabolic control in red skeletal muscle apparently is very similar.

Since the overall rate of fatty acid utilization by muscle should be determined primarily by the exogenous supply and by the energy demands of the tissue (25, 28), at a constant rate of energy utilization an increased supply would be expected to have a limited ability to accelerate fatty acid uptake. The upper limit would be reached when the supply exceeds the capacity of the cells to bind the fatty acids and to convert them to CO_2, to complex lipids, or to metabolic intermediates. Binding and conversion to metabolic intermediates can have only a small transient effect on uptake rate and the major determinant of uptake should be oxidation to CO_2. The control of uptake by heart muscle is examined here for three conditions: *1*) increased availability of extracellular fatty acids at both a low and high level of cardiac work to determine the effects of serum fatty acid:albumin ratio; *2*) increased oxidative metabolism by increase in cardiac work; and *3*) decreased oxidative metabolism by restriction of oxygen availability in ischemic muscle. Control of the pathway of fatty acid oxidation is discussed first in major segments that include membrane transport, activation, acyl transfer to carnitine and transport into mitochondria, β-oxidation, and the oxidation of acetyl-CoA by the citric acid cycle. Second, the integrated control of the entire pathway is discussed for the three conditions listed above.

FATTY ACID UPTAKE

Fatty acids are supplied to muscle tissue from the blood, where they are carried either as the free acid bound to albumin or as triglycerides in chylomicrons and lipoproteins (Fig. 1). The free fatty acid (FFA) is the principal form utilized by muscle tissue. The triglycerides are hydrolyzed to FFA by lipoprotein lipases prior to their utilization by muscle tissue (2, 18, 35). The majority of serum FFA is bound to albumin (36). The amount of acid that is free in solution is small and is determined by the FFA:albumin molar ratio. Physiologically, this is probably less than 1% of the total present. The unbound pool of FFA is in equilibrium with albumin-bound serum FFA and a tissue pool of FFA (Fig. 1). The exact nature of the tissue

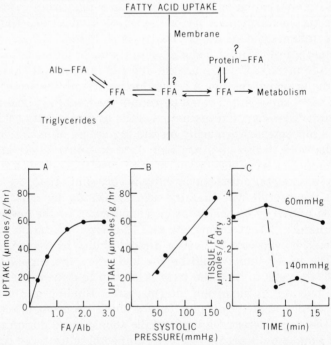

FIG. 1. Fatty acid uptake by heart muscle. Effects of fatty acid:albumin ratio (A) and ventricular pressure development (B) on rates of fatty acid uptake. Effect of increased pressure development on tissue content of fatty acids is shown in C. Rat hearts were perfused with Krebs-Henseleit buffer (27, 28) containing 11 mM glucose and palmitate bound to 3% bovine serum albumin at a ratio as indicated in A or at a concentration of 1.0 mM (B and C).

pool is not known, but it may be composed of FFAs in the cytoplasm as well as those bound to intracellular membranes and soluble proteins. A cytosolic protein has been described (12) that binds fatty acids and may function intracellularly as albumin does extracellularly. The uptake of FFA by cells appears to be an energy-independent process (37) that functions only to maintain an equilibrium between the plasma and cellular pools of FFA. Thus, an increase in the FFA:albumin molar ratio in plasma would elevate the level of FFA outside the cell and increase the concentration gradient for inward diffusion. Studies on FFA uptake have indicated a linear relationship between extracellular levels and initial rates of uptake (38). The effect of altering the FFA:albumin ratio on the rate of uptake in heart muscle (28) is shown in Figure 1A. These measurements were made during steady-state conditions where the rate of oxygen consumption by the tissue was constant. At low FFA:albumin ratios, the supply of fatty acids to the intracellular space was less than the rate of their removal by oxidative metabolism, a concentration gradient for the inward diffusion of FFA was maintained, and the rate of efflux from the cells must have been low. Thus an increase in extracellular levels caused an increase in the rate of uptake. The apparent saturation of uptake at higher FFA:albumin ratios probably occurred when the rate of inward diffusion of FFA exceeded the rate of intracellular utilization by oxidative metabolism. Since these studies were performed in a steady state, the leveling off in uptake rate implies saturation of intracellular metabolism rather than saturation of the transport process.

If the net rate of FFA uptake depends only on the concentration gradient across the cell membrane, then the rate of uptake should be increased when the rate of removal of intracellular FFA is increased by increasing the rate of oxidative metabolism. As shown in Figure 1B, the rate of FFA uptake by isolated rat hearts was linearly related to increased ventricular pressure development, which resulted in increased rates of fatty acid oxidation and oxygen consumption (27). Figure 1C shows that this acceleration in uptake resulted from an increased concentration gradient for inward diffusion (28). Increasing ventricular pressure development from 60 to 140 mmHg resulted in a rapid decrease in the tissue content of fatty acids. Thus, the predominant control of fatty acid uptake in heart muscle appears to be related to the plasma content of unbound fatty acid, which is determined by diet and hormonal control of fatty acid mobilization from liver and adipose tissue, and the level of intracellular fatty acid, which is determined by the rate of FFA removal by cellular metabolism.

FATTY ACID ACTIVATION

The first step in the cellular metabolism of fatty acids is their conversion to long-chain fatty acyl-CoA (FACoA) esters. This process, referred to as activation, is catalyzed by long-chain acyl-CoA synthetases as illustrated by the reaction in Figure 2. In heart muscle these enzymes are located on the outer mitochondrial membrane (7). The K_m of the synthetases for CoA

FATTY ACID ACTIVATION

$$FFA + MgATP + CoASH \longrightarrow FACoA + PPi + AMP$$

mM [0.5]   [11]   [<.02]   [<.02]   [.25]

FIG. 2. Long-chain fatty acid activation in heart muscle. Numbers in parentheses are cytosolic concentrations of substrates and products of the synthetase reaction. K_m values of the synthetase reactions for CoA, ATP, and FFA and K_i for FACoA were determined on whole-tissue homogenates of heart (29).

Acyl—CoA SYNTHETASES

K_m: CoASH = .007 mM —— .024mM
ATP = 4.6 mM
FFA = .04 mM

ACTIVITY INHIBITED BY:

1. FACoA: K_i= .005 mM
2. AMP
3. PPi

REGULATED BY:

$$\frac{FACoA}{CoASH} \quad ; \quad \frac{ATP}{AMP} \quad RATIOS$$

determined on whole-heart homogenate is about 0.007 mM (29). Fatty acyl-CoA, one of the reaction products, is relatively insoluble in water and like fatty acids is probably bound to cellular proteins and lipid membranes (24). The activity of the synthetases is inhibited competitively by FACoA with respect to CoA (K_i = 0.005 mM). The K_m for CoA was increased to 0.024 mM in the presence of FACoA. Other products of the reaction, AMP and PP$_i$, also inhibit synthetase activity (29, 32). The tissue levels of fatty acid and ATP are normally well above the K_m of the synthetases for these substrates (Fig. 2). The concentration of free CoA in the cytosol is unknown. However, the cytosolic content of total CoA represents approximately 5–10% (15, 29) of the whole-tissue level in heart and about 30% of the whole-tissue level in liver. The concentration of total CoA in the cytosol of heart is about 0.025 mM. Since this CoA is distributed among FACoA, acetyl-CoA, and free CoA, the cytosolic concentration of CoA would be less than 0.025 mM and may be either near or below the K_m for acyl-CoA synthetase. The cytosolic concentration of FACoA may also be near the K_i value for inhibition. This creates a favorable situation for control of fatty acid activation by the FACoA:CoA ratio and, as discussed later, much of the feedback control of fatty acid activation may be mediated by changes in this ratio. In addition, the ATP:AMP ratio may be important in some pathological states, i.e., myocardial ischemia.

ACYL TRANSFER AND TRANSPORT INTO MITOCHONDRIA

After FACoA is formed, it can be used either for the synthesis of complex lipids in the cytosolic compartment of the cell or for the production of ATP by oxidation in the mitochondrial compartment. Prior to mitochondrial oxidation, the fatty acyl moiety undergoes reactions that function to move the acyl group from the site of its activation on the outer mitochondrial membrane to the mitochondrial matrix, where it is oxidized (Fig. 3). The first reaction is the transfer of the acyl group from CoA to carnitine (10). The second reaction(s) is transport of the acyl moiety across the inner mitochondrial membrane. Recent studies with heart mitochondria (30, 33, 34) indicate that the transport of acylcarnitine involves an exchange reaction in which acylcarnitine moves across the mitochondrial membrane in exchange for carnitine. This appears to be a 1:1 exchange, which means that the content of carnitine on both sides of the membrane would remain constant under physiological conditions. Exchange transport appears to be driven by concentration gradients and is independent of metabolic energy. The third reaction in this segment is the transfer of the acyl group from carnitine to matrix CoA (10), forming FACoA in the matrix that can be used for β-oxidation. Thus, of the two pathways for metabolizing cytosolic FACoA—complex lipid synthesis and oxidation—oxidation is separated from

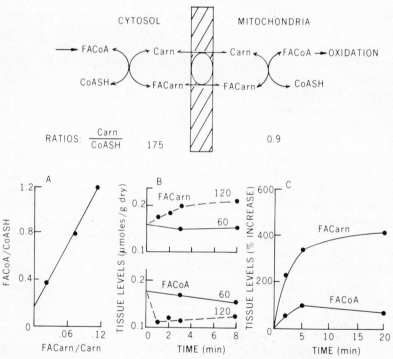

FIG. 3. Acyl transfer and transport. Effect of fatty acid concentration (0–1.2 mM bound to 3% albumin) on mass-action ratio of carnitine palmityltransferase in hearts developing 60 mmHg ventricular pressure is shown in A. Effect of increasing ventricular pressure development from 60 to 120 mmHg on tissue levels of long-chain derivatives of CoA and carnitine in hearts perfused with 1.2 mM fatty acid is shown in B. C illustrates the increase in tissue levels of FACarn and FACoA after induction of ischemia in hearts perfused with 1.2 mM fatty acid.

its source of substrate by an impermeable barrier that must be traversed by a series of reactions involving carnitine.

It seems reasonable to suppose that the insertion of this barrier between the formation and oxidation of FACoA has some physiological function and evidence is accumulating that indicates that the function may be to direct fatty acids toward either lipid synthesis or oxidation. The predominant pathway may vary among different tissues and perhaps within a single tissue, depending on either the ratio of carnitine:CoA in the cytosol or the activity of the carnitine acyltransferase(s). Heart muscle, for example, synthesizes low amounts of complex lipids, but has a high oxidative rate, and this tissue appears to have a high carnitine:CoA ratio in the cytosol (29). At present, an exact value for this ratio is difficult to obtain because the fraction of CoA and carnitine present in their free and esterified forms in the cytosolic and mitochondrial compartments is unknown. However, if one assumes that the transferase reactions are at equilibrium in the cell, this fraction in each cellular compartment should approximate that measured for the whole tissue. A second problem is the lack of knowledge on cellular distribution of total CoA and carnitine in the cytosolic and mitochondrial compartments. Coenzyme A does not penetrate the inner mitochondrial membrane and its cellular distribution can be estimated by cell fractionation and measurements of total CoA in the mitochondrial and supernatant fractions. This approach indicates that CoA is distributed about 95% in the mitochondria and 5% in the cytosol (29). Carnitine, on the other hand, does move across the mitochondrial membranes and one cannot be sure that redistribution does not occur during cellular fractionation. Mitochondria isolated from the tissue contain only small amounts of carnitine, about 5% of the whole-tissue level (15, 33). If the 1:1 exchange transport system for carnitine works in the cell and during cellular fractionation as it does on the isolated mitochondria, this 5% value should represent the amount of carnitine present in mitochondria of intact tissue. Therefore, if one assumes that the fraction of CoA and carnitine in the free form is the same in the cytosol as that measured on whole tissue and that 5% of the whole-tissue CoA and 95% of the whole-tissue carnitine are cytosolic, the carnitine:CoA ratios would be 175 in the cytosol and 0.9 in the mitochondria (Fig. 3). This would establish a condition in which fatty acids activated in the outer mitochondrial spaces of heart muscle would be diverted toward oxidation by the mitochondria rather than to lipid synthesis in the cytosol. For comparison, the liver normally has a much lower carnitine:CoA ratio in the cytosol, about 35 (29), and this tissue synthesizes large amounts of complex lipids (14). Under some pathological conditions, such as diabetes and starvation, levels of carnitine in liver and/or the activity of the transferases increase and fatty acids are directed away from lipid synthesis toward oxidation and ketone body formation (19–21).

There is little evidence for in vivo control of the carnitine acyltransferases or for the acylcarnitine transport system. As shown in Figure 3A, the transferases appear to maintain a constant ratio between the CoA and carnitine derivatives. In hearts perfused with several concentrations of palmitate in the buffer, the ratios of FACoA:CoA and fatty acylcarnitine (FACarn):Carn varied over a wide range, but a linear relationship existed between the fraction of CoA and carnitine in the fatty acyl forms (25). These data were obtained at a low rate of oxidative metabolism (hearts were developing 60 mmHg peak pressure) and may suggest that the transferase and transport systems are in equilibrium in the intact cell. With more rapid rates of oxidative metabolism, however, the tissue level of FACarn increased while that of FACoA decreased, as shown in Figure 3B. For these studies oxidative metabolism was increased by increasing ventricular pressure development at 0 time. The changes in tissue levels of long-chain acylcarnitine and CoA derivatives resulted in an increased FACarn:Carn ratio and a decreased FACoA:CoA ratio. This observation suggests that, with rapid rates of oxidation, β-oxidation removes mitochondrial FACoA faster than either acylcarnitine transport or the inner mitochondrial transferase can replenish the supply and that one of these two reactions becomes the slowest step in fatty acid oxidation. As discussed later, the higher levels of FACarn probably resulted from increased concentrations of free carnitine in the cytosol as acetylcarnitine was used at a faster rate and the higher levels of FACarn may function to accelerate transport into the matrix space.

If β-oxidation is inhibited, as occurs in ischemic hearts, most of the total CoA and carnitine are converted to their long-chain acyl derivatives. The percent increase in the tissue levels of FACoA and FACarn in isolated hearts as a function of perfusion time when the whole heart is made ischemic is shown in Figure 3C. The percent and absolute increase in FACarn was much greater than the increase in FACoA. Normally, tissue levels of both FACoA and FACarn are low while levels of acetyl-CoA and acetylcarnitine are high. However, there is about 10 times as much carnitine as CoA present in the tissue, which probably accounts for the greater increase in acylcarnitine. Under ischemic conditions, the increase in FACoA:CoA was linearly related to the rise in FACarn:Carn, again indicating that the system of transferases, as a whole, remained in equilibrium. Therefore, changes in the rates of these reactions on a short-term basis are most likely brought about by increased levels of substrates and/or faster rates of removal of products. On a longer time scale, the activities of the enzymes involved in these reactions may be increased by synthesis of more enzyme as has been demonstrated in exercising muscle (23).

β-OXIDATION

After production of FACoA in the matrix, the next major sequence of reactions involved in the oxidation of fatty acids is the β-oxidation system (Fig. 4). This sequence of reactions is catalyzed by four separate enzymes, which have been isolated but none show usual control characteristics. The reactions are illustrated on p. 276.

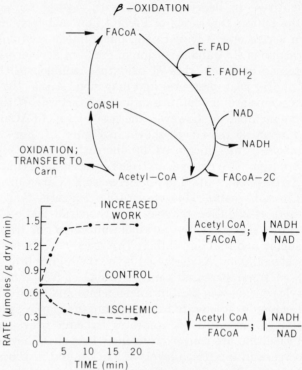

FIG. 4. Effects of increased work and ischemia on rate of β-oxidation and acetyl-CoA:FACoA and NADH:NAD ratios. Rates of β-oxidation were calculated from measurements of $^{14}CO_2$ production from [U-^{14}C]palmitate by correcting for conversion of label to products of palmitate oxidation other than CO_2 (24). With increased cardiac work, both acetyl-CoA and FACoA levels decreased in the tissue, but the change in acetyl-CoA was much larger. In ischemic hearts, levels of acetyl-CoA decreased while FACoA increased.

1) $RCH_2CH_2CO \cdot SCoA + E \cdot FAD \rightarrow RCH{=}CHCO \cdot SCoA + E \cdot FADH_2$
                                                        acyl-CoA dehydrogenase (1, 13)

2) $RCH{=}CHCO \cdot SCoA + H_2O \leftrightharpoons RCHOHCH_2CO \cdot SCoA$
                                                        enoyl-CoA hydratase (40)

3) $RCHOHCH_2CO \cdot SCoA + NAD \leftrightharpoons RCOCH_2CO \cdot SCoA + NADH + H^+$

                                                        3-hydroxyacyl-CoA dehydrogenase (3, 40)

4) $RCOCH_2CO \cdot SCoA + CoA \rightarrow RCO \cdot SCoA + CH_3CO \cdot SCoA$
                                                        3-oxoacyl-CoA thiolase (11, 22)

All the enzymes shown above have been demonstrated in heart extracts. The system is linked very tightly and the intermediates appear to be channeled from one reaction to the next in the sequence (39). No obviously rate-limiting step has been demonstrated under normal conditions. One possible means of controlling these reactions is through the availability of one or more of the substrates: FACoA, CoA, NAD^+, or enzyme (E) FAD. As shown in the lower portion of Figure 4, the rate of β-oxidation can be accelerated by increased respiration as a result of increased mechanical work in cardiac muscle (28). This increase in β-oxidation was associated with a decrease in the acetyl-CoA:FACoA ratio, a decrease in mitochondrial NADH:NAD ratio (8, 25, 27), and presumably a decrease in the $FADH_2$:FAD ratio also. In ischemic hearts, levels of acetyl-CoA decreased and FACoA increased (15), indicating that β-oxidation was inhibited in association with a large increase in the NADH:NAD ratio. These observations indicate that the rate of β-oxidation depends on the rates of oxidation of the reduced nucleotides by electron transport and acetyl-CoA by the citric acid cycle.

ACETYL TRANSFER AND TRANSPORT

In heart muscle, acetyl-CoA produced by β-oxidation can be used at appreciable rates only for oxidation by the citric acid cycle. The only alternative route for the disposal of mitochondrial acetyl-CoA is to transfer the acetyl unit across the mitochondrial membrane to cytosolic carnitine (Fig. 5), where it is stored as acetylcarnitine. This transfer of acetyl units across the mitochondrial membrane is accomplished by a system of transferases and an acylcarnitine translocase similar to the one described for the long-chain acyl derivatives. At present there is no evidence that the translocase for the acetyl units is different from the one for long-chain acylcarnitine. The acetyltransferase system has a very high activity in cardiac muscle (4, 9), but does not seem to have an obvious function. It is virtually a dead-end pathway since there are no apparent uses for either acetyl-CoA or acetylcarnitine in the cytosol. One function assigned to this system is storage of acetyl units in the cytosol as acetylcarnitine (28). There is about 10 times as much carnitine as CoA in cardiac muscle. Storage of excess acetyl units as cytosolic acetylcarnitine would provide a buffer against large changes in mitochondrial acetyl-CoA.

We have attempted to ascribe to this system a second function as a feedback control of long-chain fatty acid activation and transfer to carnitine in the cytosol. This system would be expected to function in the following manner: when the supply of fatty acids exceeds the rate of oxidation, excess acetyl-CoA is formed in the mitochondrial matrix. To make more CoA available, the excess acetyl units are transferred across the mitochondrial membrane and converted to acetyl-CoA and acetylcarnitine in the cytosol. Accumulation of acetyl-CoA and acetylcarnitine in the cytosol would lower the levels of both free carnitine and CoA, thus limiting the availability of CoA for long-chain fatty acid activation and of carnitine for the transferase reaction. Since CoA is normally present in the cytosol at concentrations near the K_m for fatty acid activation, a lower cytosolic CoA concentration

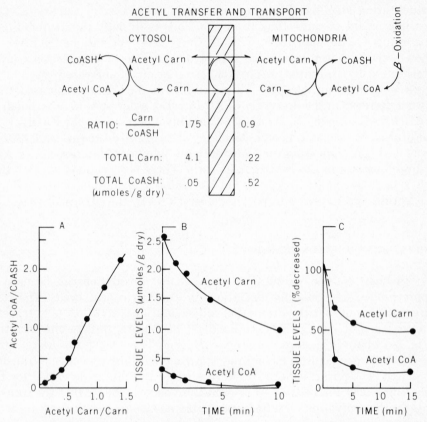

FIG. 5. Acetyl transfer and transport. Effect of fatty acid concentration (0–1.2 mM bound to 3% albumin) on mass-action ratio of carnitine acetyltransferase in hearts developing 60 mmHg ventricular pressure (*A*). Decrease in tissue levels of acetylcarnitine and acetyl-CoA when ventricular pressure development was increased to 120 mmHg in hearts perfused with 1.2 mM fatty acid is shown in *B*. *C* illustrates the decrease in tissue levels of acetylcarnitine and acetyl-CoA after induction of ischemia in hearts perfused with 1.2 mM fatty acid. Ratio of carnitine:CoA in cytosolic and mitochondrial compartments was calculated for hearts performing low levels of mechanical work. Levels of total carnitine and CoA in these compartments are expressed as micromoles per gram of dry tissue.

would have a very pronounced effect on activation. Evidence that this scheme might function in the intact heart is indicated by the ability of these reactions to remain at or near equilibrium. As shown in Figure 5*A*, when hearts were perfused with buffer containing several concentrations of palmitate the ratios of acetyl-CoA:CoA and acetylcarnitine:carnitine increased in a linear manner (28). At low concentrations of palmitate and relatively low acetyl-CoA levels, acetylcarnitine accumulated faster than acetyl-CoA. This would keep mitochondrial levels of CoA high and β-oxidation would not be limited by availability of this substrate. As more acetyl-CoA was produced by β-oxidation, its level increased linearly with respect to acetylcarnitine. With increased cardiac work and increased oxidation of acetyl-CoA, the system would reverse and transfer acetyl units from the cytosol back into the mitochondria. The result would be an increase in the CoA and carnitine concentrations in the cytosol that could accelerate fatty acid activation to meet the new energy demands of the tissue. As illustrated in Figure 5B, tissue levels of both acetyl-CoA and acetylcarnitine were high in hearts performing low levels of cardiac work (0-time values) and the levels of both compounds decreased after an increase in work. This transport system therefore may function to couple the rate of acetyl-CoA oxidation in mitochondria with fatty acid activation in the cytosol, thus providing a negative-feedback loop in the pathway.

In well-oxygenated hearts, only low levels of long-chain acyl-CoA and carnitine derivatives accumulate; in the presence of high levels of exogenous fatty acid, most of the CoA and carnitine present is used to store excess acetyl units. However, under conditions where oxygen becomes limiting, i.e., ischemia and/or hypoxia, the inhibition of β-oxidation results in low levels of acetyl-CoA and acetylcarnitine. The decrease in levels of these compounds after induction of ischemia is shown in Figure 5C. The free CoA and carnitine formed as the levels of their acetyl derivatives decreased were used to form the corresponding long-chain derivatives as illustrated previously.

To summarize how the coupling of mitochondrial oxidation of acetyl-CoA to cytosolic fatty acid activation and uptake may function in the intact cell, the entire pathway of fatty acid oxidation is illustrated in Figures 6 and 7. Flux through the citric acid cycle has been shown to be geared to the rate of oxidative phosphorylation (17) through feedback control of the cycle by changes in the levels of high-energy phosphates and NADH. When hearts were perfused with high levels of fatty acids (1.2 mM) at low levels of cardiac work (Fig. 6), flux through the citric acid cycle was fairly constant (28). Under these conditions, the rate of FFA oxidation was limited by the rate of acetyl-CoA oxidation through the citric acid cycle and acetyl-CoA accumulated. Excess acetyl units produced from β-oxidation were transferred to the cytosol and stored there as acetyl derivatives of CoA and carnitine. Long-chain acyl derivatives of both CoA and carnitine also accumulated but to a lesser extent than the acetyl derivatives (28). As a result of the increased levels of acetyl and long-chain derivatives of CoA and carnitine, the levels of free CoA and carnitine decreased to below their respective K_m values for activation and acyl transfer. This limited the rate of activation and resulted in higher tissue levels of FFA. Thus the gradient for diffusion of FFA into the cells was reduced and the rate of FFA uptake was limited by the rate of intracellular removal.

In contrast to the above situation where the supply of FFA greatly exceeded the rate of FFA oxidation, Figure 7 illustrates the changes that occurred when the rate of oxidation was accelerated. The intermediates that became elevated when the level of cardiac work was increased are shown in boldface. The rates of oxidative phosphorylation and flux through the citric acid cycle were increased, as indicated by faster rates of O_2 consumption and

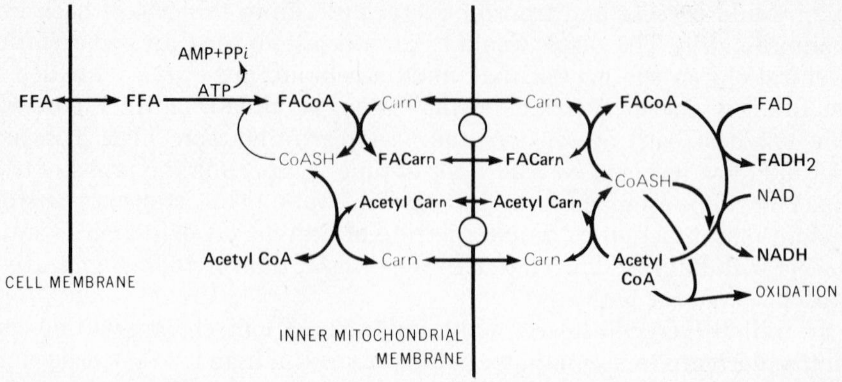

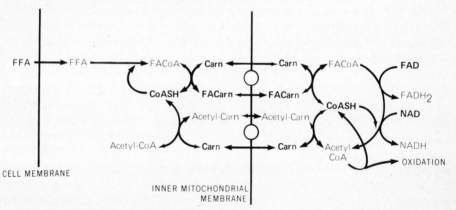

FIG. 6. Pathway for fatty acid oxidation in heart muscle. Metabolic intermediates that are elevated when hearts were perfused with 1.2 mM fatty acid at 60 mmHg ventricular pressure development are shown in boldface. This figure illustrates the 2 transferase systems for acyl units, each located on the inner and outer surfaces of the inner mitochondrial membrane (IMM). It includes the compartmentalization of CoA in 2 noninterchangeable pools (cytosolic and mitochondrial matrix). Carnitine translocase is shown on the IMM between the 2 transferase systems. At low rates of energy utilization and excess fatty acid supply, most of the CoA and carnitine are converted to their acetyl derivatives.

FIG. 7. Pathway for fatty acid oxidation in which metabolic intermediates that were elevated when hearts were perfused with 1.2 mM fatty acid at 120 mmHg ventricular pressure are shown in heavier print. Levels of FACarn increased but it is uncertain if the increase occurred in both cellular compartments. Most, if not all, of the increase was restricted to the cytosolic compartment.

CO_2 production, and levels of acetyl-CoA and acetylcarnitine were rapidly diminished (28). β-Oxidation was stimulated and the levels of long-chain acyl-CoA decreased. Since most of the CoA is located in the mitochondria, this decrease in whole-tissue FACoA probably reflected changes that occurred primarily in the matrix space. Most likely the cytosolic level of FACoA increased as more CoA was made available. This increase is not indicated in Figure 7 because only changes in whole-tissue levels of FACoA were measured. The rise in cytosolic CoA, carnitine, and FACarn as indicated in Figure 7 with no increase in FACoA should not imply that the transferase reaction is displaced from equilibrium but simply indicates lack of data on changes in cytosolic and mitochondrial levels of these compounds. Simultaneously, the levels of free CoA and free carnitine increased, the rate of FFA activation was accelerated, and the decrease in tissue FFA accelerated uptake. Under these conditions, the slowest step for fatty acid utilization appeared to be the capacity of the cells to transport acyl units across the inner mitochondrial membrane and levels of acylcarnitine increased.

The rise in FACarn most likely occurred in the cytosol, but because of the lack of data Figure 7 indicates increased levels in both compartments. With an increase in matrix CoA, FACarn levels in this compartment would be expected to decrease. The rise in FACarn in the cytosol probably accounted for faster rates of transport into the mitochondria because of a higher cytosolic-to-matrix concentration gradient.

Under oxygen-deficient conditions, i.e., ischemia and anoxia, the amount of oxygen available to support oxidation by the citric acid cycle is reduced. The levels of $FADH_2$ and NADH increase, and β-oxidation becomes inhibited. Long-chain acyl derivatives of CoA and carnitine increase to very high levels (Fig. 8) and the activation and uptake of FFA are reduced. Activation may be inhibited due to higher levels of both FACoA and AMP (26) and reduced uptake probably resulted from higher levels of tissue FFA. High levels of fatty acyl-CoA have been shown to inhibit some enzymes [long-chain acyl-CoA synthetase (29, 31) and adenine nucleotide translocase (5, 6, 32)] in a specific manner and many other enzymes in a nonspecific manner (24). Free fatty acids (16) and long-chain acylcarnitine (41), in addition to having a detergent effect at high concentrations, have recently been shown to inhibit Na^+-K^+-ATPase (16, 41). Myocardial ischemia, therefore, in addition to resulting in a reduced capacity for ATP synthesis, also results in the accumulation of compounds that potentially are very detrimental to myocardial function and metabolism.

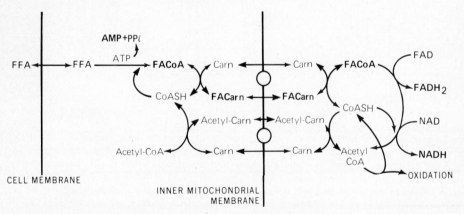

FIG. 8. Pathway for fatty acid oxidation illustrating metabolic intermediates that were elevated during ischemia in hearts perfused with 1.2 mM fatty acid.

Because of the 1:1 exchange transport system through the inner mito-chondrial membrane for carnitine and its acyl derivatives, the normal heart should maintain constant levels of carnitine in the cytosolic and matrix spaces. When long-chain acylcarnitine accumulates in ischemic hearts, however, there is a net transfer of carnitine from the cytosol to the mitochondrial matrix (15). The concentration of total carnitine decreased by only a small amount in the cytosol, but because of the relatively small volume of the matrix space, the concentration in the mitochondria increased some sixfold (Fig. 9). This shift in total carnitine represented an increase in both long-chain acylcarnitine and acid-soluble components (free carnitine plus acetylcarnitine). The same redistribution of carnitine occurs in isolated mitochondria that are incubated with high levels of the long-chain derivative. At the present time, neither the significance nor the mechanism of this observation is known. It may be due to a detergent effect of high levels of acylcarnitine on the mitochondrial membrane, which allows it to become leaky, or it could represent an inward transport of acylcarnitine that is independent of the exchange transporter but only functions at high concen-

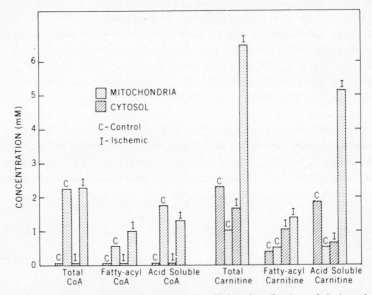

FIG. 9. Effects of myocardial ischemia on cellular distribution of CoA and carnitine derivatives. Hearts were perfused with 1.2 mM fatty acid for 15 min at a coronary flow of 5 ml/min, then switched to a washout buffer containing a respiratory inhibitor (2 hearts/determination). Mitochondria were prepared and resuspended in the presence of respiratory inhibitor. Levels of total CoA and carnitine and of acid-soluble (acetyl + free) and long-chain acyl derivatives of CoA and carnitine were determined on tissue homogenates, postmitochondrial supernatant, and resuspended mitochondria. Levels of mitochondrial metabolites were extrapolated to whole-tissue levels with a value of 58 mg mitochondrial protein/g wet wt of heart muscle. This value was obtained with mitochondrial marker enzymes (cytochrome c oxidase and citrate synthase). Metabolites were expressed as concentrations with 1 μl H_2O/mg mitochondrial protein for the mitochondrial matrix levels and 2 ml H_2O/g dry tissue for cytosolic concentrations.

trations. The cellular distribution of CoA and its acyl derivatives appeared to be maintained in ischemic tissue (Fig. 9). The calculated changes in the levels of FACoA indicated an increase in both the cytosol and matrix spaces as shown in Figure 8, but the rise in the cytosol was very small compared to that in the matrix (Fig. 9).

REFERENCES

1. BEINERT, H., AND W. LEE. Electron-transferring flavoproteins from pig liver and beef liver. *Methods Enzymol.* 5: 424–430, 1963.
2. BORENSZTJN, J., AND D. S. ROBINSON. The effects of fasting on the utilization of chylomicron triglyceride fatty acids in relation to clearing factor lipase (lipoprotein lipase) releasable by heparin in the perfused rat heart. *J. Lipid Res.* 11: 111–117, 1970.
3. BRADSHAW, R. A., AND B. E. NOYES. L-3-Hydroxyacyl-CoA dehydrogenase from pig heart muscle. *Methods Enzymol.* 35: 122–128, 1975.
4. BRESSLER, R. Physiological-chemical aspects of fatty acid oxidation. In: *Lipid Metabolism,* edited by S. J. Wakil. New York: Academic, 1970, p. 49–75.
5. CHONG, H. H., AND S. V. PANDE. On the specificity of the inhibition of adenine nucleotide translocase by long-chain acyl-coenzyme A esters. *Biochim. Biophys. Acta* 369: 86–94, 1974.
6. CHUA, B., AND E. SHRAGO. Reversible inhibition of adenine nucleotide translocase by long-chain acyl-CoA ester in bovine heart mitochondria and submitochondrial particles: comparison with atractylate and bongkrekic acid. *J. Biol. Chem.* 252: 6711–6714, 1977.
7. DE HAAN, E. J., G. S. P. GROOT, H. R. SCHOLTE, J. M. TAGER, AND E. M. WIT-PEETERS. Biochemistry of muscle mitochondria. In: *The Structure and Function of Muscle,* edited by G. H. Bourne. New York: Academic, 1973, p. 417–469.
8. ILLINGWORTH, J. A., W. C. L. FORD, K. KOBAYASHI, AND J. R. WILLIAMSON. Regulation of myocardial energy metabolism. *Recent Advan. Stud. Cardiac Struct. Metab.* 8: 271–289, 1975.
9. FRITZ, I. B. The metabolic consequences of the effects of carnitine on long-chain fatty acid oxidation. In: *Cellular Compartmentalization and Control of Fatty Acid Metabolism.* Oslo: Universitetsforlaget, 1968, p. 39–63.
10. FRITZ, I. B., AND K. T. N. YUE. Long-chain carnitine acyltransferase and the role of acylcarnitine derivatives in the catalytic increase of fatty acid oxidation induced by carnitine. *J. Lipid Res.* 4: 279–288, 1963.
11. GEHRING, U., AND F. LYNEN. Thiolase. In: *The Enzymes,* edited by P. D. Boyer. New York: Academic, 1972, vol. 7, p. 391–405.
12. GLOSTER, J., AND P. HARRIS. Fatty acid binding to cytoplasmic proteins of myocardium and red and white skeletal muscle in the rat. A possible new role for myoglobin. *Biochem. Biophys. Res. Commun.* 74: 506–513, 1977.
13. HALL, C. L., L. HEIJKENSKJÖLD, T. BARTFAI, L. ERNSTER, AND H. KAMIN. Acyl-coenzyme A dehydrogenases and an electron-transferring flavoprotein from beef heart mitochondria. *Arch. Biochem. Biophys.* 177: 402–414, 1976.
14. HEIMBERG, M., H. C. WILCOX, G. D. DUNN, W. F. WOODSIDE, K. T. BREEN, AND C. SOLER-ARGILAGA. Studies on the regulation of secretion of the very low density lipoprotein and on ketogenesis by the liver. In: *Regulation of Hepatic Metabolism,* edited by F. Lund-

quist and N. Tygstrup. Copenhagen: Munksgaard, 1974, p. 119–141.
15. IDELL-WENGER, J. A., AND J. R. NEELY. Effects of ischemia on myocardial fatty acid oxidation. In: *Pathophysiology and Therapeutics of Myocardial Ischemia,* edited by A. M. Lefer, G. J. Kelliher, and M. J. Rovetto. New York: Spectrum Publ., 1977, p. 227–238.
16. LAMERS, J. M. J., AND W. C. HÜLSMANN. Inhibition of $(Na^+ + K^+)$-stimulated ATPase of heart by fatty acids. *J. Mol. Cellular Cardiol.* 9: 343–346, 1977.
17. LANOUE, K. F., W. J. NICKLAS, AND J. R. WILLIAMSON. Control of citric acid cycle activity in rat heart mitochondria. *J. Biol. Chem.* 245: 102–111, 1970.
18. MALLOV, S., AND A. A. ALOUSI. In vitro effect of epinephrine on lipase activity of heart. *Am. J. Physiol.* 216: 794–799, 1969.
19. McGARRY, J. D., AND D. W. FOSTER. The metabolism of (−)-octanoylcarnitine in perfused livers from fed and fasted rats. *J. Biol. Chem.* 249: 7984–7990, 1974.
20. McGARRY, J. D., C. ROBLES-VALDES, AND D. W. FOSTER. Role of carnitine in hepatic ketogenesis. *Proc. Natl. Acad. Sci. US* 72: 4385–4388, 1975.
21. McGARRY, J. D., P. H. WRIGHT, AND D. W. FOSTER. Hormonal control of ketogenesis. Rapid activation of hepatic ketogenic capacity in fed rats by anti-insulin serum and glucagon. *J. Clin. Invest.* 55: 1202–1209, 1975.
22. MEIJER, A. J., AND K. VAN DAM. The metabolic significance of anion transport in mitochondria. *Biochim. Biophys. Acta* 346: 213–244, 1974.
23. MOLE, P. A., L. B. OSCAI, AND J. O. HOLLOSZY. Adaptations of muscle to exercise: increase in levels of palmityl-CoA synthetase, carnitine palmityl-transferase and palmityl-CoA dehydrogenase and in the capacity to oxidize fatty acids. *J. Clin. Invest.* 50: 2323–2330, 1971.
24. MOREL, F., G. LAUQUIN, J. LUNARDI, J. DUSZYNSKI, AND P. V. VIGNAIS. An appraisal of the functional significance of the inhibitory effect of long chain acyl-CoA's on mitochondrial transports. *Fed. European Biochem. Soc. Letters* 39: 133–138, 1974.
25. NEELY, J. R., AND H. E. MORGAN. Relationship between carbohydrate and lipid metabolism and the energy balance of heart muscle. *Ann. Rev. Physiol.* 36: 413–459, 1974.
26. NEELY, J. R., M. J. ROVETTO, J. T. WHITMER, AND H. E. MORGAN. Effects of ischemia on function and metabolism of the isolated working rat heart. *Am. J. Physiol.* 225: 651–658, 1973.
27. NEELY, J. R., K. M. WHITMER, AND S. MOCHIZUKI. Effects of mechanical activity and hormones on myocardial glucose and fatty acid utilization. *Circulation Res.* 38: I-22-I-30, 1976.
28. ORAM, J. F., S. L. BENNETCH, AND J. R. NEELY. Regulation of fatty acid utilization in isolated perfused rat hearts. *J. Biol. Chem.* 248: 5299–5309, 1973.
29. ORAM, J. F., J. I. WENGER, AND J. R. NEELY. Regulation of long-chain fatty acid activation in heart muscle. *J. Biol. Chem.* 250: 73–78, 1975.
30. PANDE, S. V. A mitochondrial carnitine acylcarnitine

translocase system. *Proc. Natl. Acad. Sci. US* 72: 883–887, 1975.

31. PANDE, S. V. Reversal by CoA of palmityl-CoA inhibition of long-chain acyl-CoA synthetase activity. *Biochim. Biophys. Acta* 306: 15–20, 1973.

32. PANDE, S. V., AND M. C. BLANCHAER. Reversible inhibition of mitochondrial adenosine diphosphate phosphorylation by long-chain acyl coenzyme A thioesters. *J. Biol. Chem.* 246: 402–411, 1971.

33. PANDE, S. V., AND R. PARVIN. Characterization of carnitine acylcarnitine translocase system of heart mitochondria. *J. Biol. Chem.* 251: 6683–6691, 1976.

34. RAMSAY, R. R., AND P. K. TUBBS. Exchange of the endogenous carnitine of ox heart mitochondria with external carnitine and its possible relevance to fatty acyl transport into mitochondria. *Biochem. Soc. Trans.* 2: 1285–1286, 1974.

35. ROBINSON, D. S., AND D. R. WING. Regulation of adipose tissue clearing factor lipase activity. In: *Adipose Tissue,* edited by R. Levine and E. F. Pfeiffer. New York: Academic, 1970, p. 41–45.

36. SPECTOR, A. A. Fatty acid binding to plasma albumin. *J. Lipid Res.* 16: 165–179, 1975.

37. SPECTOR, A. A. Metabolism of free fatty acids. *Progr. Biochem. Pharmacol.* 6: 130–176, 1971.

38. SPECTOR, A. A., D. STEINBERG, AND A. TANAKA. Uptake of free fatty acids by Erhlich ascites tumor cells. *J. Biol. Chem.* 240: 1032–1041, 1965.

39. STANLEY, K. K., AND P. K. TUBBS. The role of intermediates in fatty acid oxidation. *Biochem. J.* 150: 77–88, 1975.

40. WIT-PEETERS, E. M., H. R. SCHOLTE, F. VAN DEN AKKER, AND I. DE NIE. Intramitochondrial localization of palmityl-CoA dehydrogenase, β-hydroxyacyl-CoA dehydrogenase and enoyl-CoA hydratase in guinea-pig heart. *Biochim. Biophys. Acta* 231: 23–31, 1971.

41. WOOD, J. M., B. BUSH, B. J. R. PITTS, AND A. SCHWARTZ. Inhibition of bovine heart Na^+, K^+-ATPase by palmitylcarnitine and palmityl-CoA. *Biochem. Biophys. Res. Commun.* 74: 677–684, 1977.

ABBREVIATIONS

ABL	abetalipoproteinemia	HMG-CoA reductase	3-hydroxymethyl-3-glu-taryl coenzyme A reductase
ACAT	acyl-CoA:cholesterol acyl-transferase		
ANS	8-anilinonaphthalene-1-sulfonic acid	IDL	intermediate-density lipo-protein(s)
ARP	arginine-rich protein	IR	infrared
BAM	bile acid micelle	LCAT	lecithin:cholesterol acyl-transferase
CCK-PZ	cholecystokinin-pancreo-zymin	LDL	low-density lipoprotein(s)
CD	circular dichroism	LPL	lipoprotein lipase
CE	cholesteryl ester	MBcGMP	monobutyryl cyclic GMP
CHL	combined hyperlipidemia	NMR	nuclear magnetic reso-nance
CNBr	cyanogen bromide		
ConA	concanavalin A	ORD	optical rotary dispersion
CPIB	chlorophenoxyisobutyrate	PAGE	polyacrylamide gel electro-phoresis
DBcAMP	dibutyryl cyclic AMP		
DES	diethylstilbestrol	PC	phosphatidylcholine
DFDNB	1,5-difluoro-2,4-dinitroben-zene	PE	phosphatidylethanolamine
		PG	prostaglandin
DG	diglyceride	PHLA	postheparin lipolytic activ-ity
DHAP	dihydroxyacetone-PO_4		
DMPC	dimyristoyl phosphatidyl-choline	PIA	N^6-(phenylisopropyl)-adenosine
DSC	differential scanning calo-rimetry	PL	phospholipid
		RER	rough endoplasmic reticu-lum
EDTA	ethylenediaminetetraacetic acid	SDS	sodium dodecyl sulfate
EPR	electron-spin paramagnetic resonance	SER	smooth endoplasmic reticu-lum
ER	endoplasmic reticulum	T_3	3,5,3'-triiodothyronine
FA	fatty acid (*also* fatty acyl)	TCA	trichloroacetic acid
FABP	fatty acid-binding protein	TEMPO	2,2,6,6-tetramethylpiperi-dine-1-oxyl
FACoA	fatty acyl-CoA		
FFA	free fatty acid	TG	triglyceride
FH	familial hypercholestere-mia	UV	ultraviolet
		UWL	unstirred water layer
GSL	glycosphingolipids	VLDL	very-low-density lipopro-tein(s)
HDL	high-density lipoprotein(s)		

INDEX